Forensic Neuropsychiatric Ethics

Balancing Competing Duties In and Out of Court

Forensic Neuropsychiatric Ethics

Balancing Competing Duties In and Out of Court

Edited by

William Connor Darby, M.D.
Robert Weinstock, M.D.

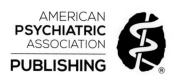

AMERICAN
PSYCHIATRIC
ASSOCIATION
PUBLISHING

If you wish to buy 50 or more copies of the same title, please go to www.appi.org/specialdiscounts for more information.

Copyright © 2025 American Psychiatric Association Publishing
ALL RIGHTS RESERVED

First Edition

Manufactured in the United States of America on acid-free paper

29 28 27 26 25   5 4 3 2 1

American Psychiatric Association Publishing
800 Maine Avenue SW, Suite 900
Washington, DC 20024–2812

www.appi.org

Library of Congress Cataloging-in-Publication Data
Names: Darby, William Connor, editor. | Weinstock, Robert, editor.
Title: Forensic neuropsychiatric ethics : balancing competing duties   in and out of court / edited by William Connor Darby, Robert Weinstock.
Description: First edition. | Washington, DC : American Psychiatric Association Publishing, [2025] | Includes bibliographical references and index.
Identifiers: LCCN 2024050915 (print) | LCCN 2024050916 (ebook) | ISBN 9781615374076 (paperback ; alk. paper) | ISBN 9781615374083 (ebook)
Subjects: MESH: Neuropsychiatry--ethics | Forensic Psychiatry--ethics | Mental Competency--legislation & jurisprudence | Informed Consent--ethics | Informed Consent--legislation & jurisprudence
Classification: LCC RC455.2.E8 (print) | LCC RC455.2.E8 (ebook) | NLM WM 102 | DDC 174.2/9689--dc23/eng/20241205
LC record available at https://lccn.loc.gov/2024050915
LC ebook record available at https://lccn.loc.gov/2024050916

British Library Cataloguing in Publication Data

A CIP record is available from the British Library.

Contents

Contributors ix

Foreword xv

1 The Modern History and Evolution of Forensic Psychiatric Ethics Leading Up to Dialectical Principlism 1
William Connor Darby, M.D., Robert Weinstock, M.D.

2 Dialectical Principlism 15
William Connor Darby, M.D., Robert Weinstock, M.D.

3 Narrative and Ethics in Forensic Psychiatry 33
Ezra E. H. Griffith, M.D.

4 Robust Professionalism: Forensic Psychiatry's Identity and Purpose 51
Richard Martinez, M.D., M.H., Philip Candilis, M.D.

5 Ethical Report Writing 67
Michael A. Norko, M.D., M.A.R., Alec Buchanan, M.D., Ph.D., Paul Bryant, M.D.

6 Ethical Challenges While Testifying 81
Gregory B. Leong, M.D., Mendel Feldsher, M.D.

7 Ethical Implications for the Use of Neuroscience, Neuroimaging, and Artificial Intelligence in the Courtroom 89

Michael R. MacIntyre, M.D., Richard G. Cockerill, M.D., R. Ryan Darby, M.D.

8 Ethical Issues in the Forensic Psychiatric Use of Psychological and Neuropsychological Testing 105

Daniel A. Martell, Ph.D.

9 How to Interpret the Role of the Forensic Psychiatrist to Promote Ethical Work 119

Jennifer Piel, M.D., J.D., Drew Calhoun, M.D.

10 Is Impartiality Attainable in Forensic Work? Managing Bias and Subjectivity in Psychiatric Expert Testimony................143

Aryeh Goldberg, M.D., M.A.

11 Death Penalty: Ethics Considerations for Participating in Capital Cases 155

Gregory B. Leong, M.D., Michael Kanell, M.D., Dustin B. Stephens, M.D., Ph.D.

12 The Tarasoff Duty to Protect: Unintended Consequences and New Liability Concerns..............................165

Alexander C. Sones, M.D., William C. Darby, M.D., Robert Weinstock, M.D.

13 Balancing Ethical Considerations for Assisted Outpatient Treatment 183

Michael R. MacIntyre, M.D., Jeffrey W. Swanson, Ph.D., Jon E. Sherin, M.D., Ph.D., Marvin Swartz, M.D.

14 Ethical Issues in Forensic Psychiatry: Mental Health Firearm Prohibitions 201
Joseph R. Simpson, M.D., Ph.D.

15 Ethical Challenges When Interacting With Professional Organizations, Governmental Agencies, and Community Mental Health Programs 217
Matthew W. Grover, M.D., Bridget McCoy, M.D., Debra A. Pinals, M.D.

16 Ethical Challenges Regarding Informed Consent, Reporting Laws, and Confidentiality Violations.................... 233
Katrina Hui, M.D., M.S., Steven K. Hoge, M.D., Carl Erik Fisher, M.D.

17 Termination of Pregnancy, Ethics, and Decisional Capacity 249
Susan Hatters Friedman, M.D., Jacqueline Landess, M.D., J.D., Nina Ross, M.D., Aimee Kaempf, M.D.

18 Clinical Requests for Hastened Death in Individuals With Mental Illness: An Examination of Advance Directives and Physician Assistance in Dying 269
Michael F. Zito, M.D.

19 Structural and Implicit Bias in Violence Risk Assessments...................................... 287
Shoba Sreenivasan, Ph.D., Melinda DiCiro, Psy.D., ABPP, James Rokop, Ph.D., Linda E. Weinberger, Ph.D.

20 Structural Racism and Ethics.................... 303
Cheryl D. Wills, M.D.

21 Priority-Setting in the COVID
Pandemic: Perspectives From Sweden....313
*Lars Sandman, Ph.D., Manne Sjöstrand, M.D.,
Ph.D., Svante Nyberg, M.D., Ph.D., Christoffer
Rahm, M.D., Ph.D., Niklas Juth, Ph.D.*

Index...329

Contributors

Paul A. Bryant, M.D.
Assistant Professor of Psychiatry, Yale University School of Medicine, Law & Psychiatry Division

Alec Buchanan, M.D., Ph.D.
Professor Emeritus of Psychiatry, Yale University School of Medicine

Drew Calhoun, M.D.
Chief Medical Officer, Civil Center for Excellence, Western State Hospital, Washington State Department of Social and Health Services

Philip J. Candilis, M.D., DFAPA
Professor of Psychiatry, George Washington University School of Medicine; Director of Medical Affairs, Saint Elizabeths Hospital, Washington, District of Columbia

Richard G. Cockerill, M.D.
Assistant Professor of Psychiatry, Northwestern University Department of Psychiatry and Behavioral Sciences, Chicago, Illinois

R. Ryan Darby, M.D.
Assistant Professor of Neurology and Director, Frontotemporal Dementia Clinic, Vanderbilt University, Nashville, Tennessee

William Connor Darby, M.D.
Health Sciences Assistant Clinical Professor, Department of Psychiatry and Biobehavioral Sciences, David Geffen School of Medicine, University of California, Los Angeles

Melinda DiCiro, Psy.D., ABPP
Deputy Director, Forensic Services, Department of State Hospitals, Roseville, California

Mendel Feldsher, M.D.
Assistant Clinical Professor, Department of Psychiatry, School of Medicine, Loma Linda University, Loma Linda, California

Carl Erik Fisher, M.D.
Assistant Professor of Clinical Psychiatry, Department of Psychiatry, Columbia University and New York State Psychiatric Institute, New York

Aryeh Goldberg, M.D., M.A.
Medical Director, General Adult and Forensic Psychiatrist, Goldberg Psychiatry, Los Angeles, California

Ezra E. H. Griffith, M.D.
Professor Emeritus of Psychiatry and African American Studies, Yale University, New Haven, Connecticut

Matthew W. Grover, M.D.
Assistant Clinical Professor, Program in Psychiatry, Law, and Ethics, Department of Psychiatry, University of Michigan, Ann Arbor, Michigan

Susan Hatters Friedman, M.D., M.St.
The Phillip Resnick Professor of Forensic Psychiatry, Professor of Psychiatry, Pediatrics, Reproductive Biology, and Law, Case Western Reserve University, Cleveland, Ohio

Steven K. Hoge, M.D.
Clinical Professor, Director, Columbia-Cornell Forensic Psychiatry Fellowship Program, Department of Psychiatry, Columbia University and New York State Psychiatric Institute, New York

Katrina Hui, M.D., M.S.
Fellow, Department of Psychiatry, University of Toronto, Toronto, Ontario, Canada

Niklas Juth, Ph.D.
Full Professor of Clinical Medical Ethics, Department of Public Health and Caring Sciences, Centre for Research Ethics and Bioethics, Uppsala University, Uppsala, Sweden

Aimee Kaempf, M.D.
Clinical Associate Professor, Department of Psychiatry, University of Arizona College of Medicine, Tucson, Arizona

Michael Kanell, M.D.
Staff Psychiatrist, Los Angeles County Office of Diversion and Reentry, Los Angeles, California

Jacqueline Landess, M.D., J.D.
Training Director, Forensic Psychiatry Fellowship, Medical College of Wisconsin, Milwaukee, Wisconsin

Gregory B. Leong, M.D.
Adjunct Clinical Professor (Voluntary), Department of Psychiatry and Behavioral Sciences, Keck School of Medicine, University of Southern California, Los Angeles, California

Michael R. MacIntyre, M.D.
Health Sciences Assistant Clinical Professor, Department of Psychiatry and Biobehavioral Sciences at the David Geffen School of Medicine, University of California, Los Angeles, Los Angeles, California

Daniel A. Martell, Ph.D.
Forensic Neuropsychologist, Park Dietz & Associates, Inc., Newport Beach, California

Richard Martinez, M.D., M.H.
Robert D. Miller Professor of Forensic Psychiatry; Director, Forensic Psychiatry Services and Training, University of Colorado at Anschutz Medical School, Denver, Colorado

Bridget McCoy, M.D.
Assistant Professor, Department of Psychiatry and Behavioral Neuroscience, Saint Louis University School of Medicine, Saint Louis, Missouri

Michael A. Norko, M.D., M.A.R.
Professor of Psychiatry, Yale University School of Medicine, Law & Psychiatry Division

Svante Nyberg, M.D., Ph.D.
Chief Medical Officer, Stockholm Health Care Services, Region Stockholm, Sweden

Jennifer Piel, M.D., J.D.
Associate Professor, Director, Center for Mental Health, Policy & the Law, Department of Psychiatry and Behavioral Sciences, University of Washington, Seattle, Washington

Debra A. Pinals, M.D.
Clinical Professor of Psychiatry, Director, Program in Psychiatry, Law, and Ethics, Department of Psychiatry, University of Michigan, Ann Arbor, Michigan

Christoffer Rahm, M.D., Ph.D.
Associate Professor of Psychiatry, Centre for Psychiatry Research, Department of Clinical Neuroscience, Karolinska Institutet & Stockholm Health Care Services, Region Stockholm, Sweden

James Rokop, Ph.D.
Chief Psychologist, Forensic Services, Department of State Hospitals, Sacramento, California

Nina Ross, M.D.
Assistant Professor of Psychiatry, Case Western Reserve University, Cleveland, Ohio

Lars Sandman, Ph.D.
Professor of Health Care Ethics, Director, National Centre for Priorities in Health, Department of Health, Medicine and Caring Sciences, Linköping University, Linköping, Sweden

Charles L. Scott, M.D.
Clinical Professor, Department of Psychiatry and Behavioral Sciences; Chief, Division of Psychiatry and the Law; Director, Forensic Psychiatry Fellowship Program, UC Davis School of Medicine, San Francisco, California

Jon E. Sherin, M.D., Ph.D.
Former Director, Los Angeles County Department of Mental Health, Los Angeles, California

Joseph R. Simpson, M.D., Ph.D.
Adjunct Clinical Associate Professor (Voluntary), Department of Psychiatry and Behavioral Sciences, Keck School of Medicine, University of Southern California, Los Angeles, California; Clinical Adjunct Faculty, University of Nevada, Reno, Reno, Nevada

Manne Sjöstrand, M.D., Ph.D.
Docent of Medical Ethics, Centre for Psychiatry Research, Department of Clinical Neuroscience, Karolinska Institutet & Stockholm Health Care Services, Region Stockholm, Sweden

Alexander C. Sones, M.D.
Clinical Instructor (Voluntary), Department of Psychiatry and Biobehavioral Sciences at the David Geffen School of Medicine, University of California, Los Angeles, Los Angeles, California

Shoba Sreenivasan, Ph.D.
Forensic Psychologist, California Department of State Hospitals; Adjunct Clinical Professor, Keck School of Medicine of the University of Southern California, Los Angeles, California

Dustin B. Stephens, M.D., Ph.D.
Assistant Professor of Psychiatry, Semel Neuropsychiatric Institute at the David Geffen School of Medicine, University of California, Los Angeles, Los Angeles, California

Jeffrey W. Swanson, Ph.D.
Professor of Psychiatry and Behavioral Sciences at Duke University School of Medicine, Durham, North Carolina

Marvin Swartz, M.D.
Professor of Psychiatry and Behavioral Sciences at Duke University School of Medicine, Durham, North Carolina

Linda E. Weinberger, Ph.D.
Professor of Clinical Psychiatry and Behavioral Sciences, Keck School of Medicine, University of Southern California; Chief Psychologist, USC Institute of Psychiatry, Law, and Behavioral Science, Los Angeles, California

Robert Weinstock, M.D.
Health Sciences Clinical Professor, Department of Psychiatry and Biobehavioral Sciences, David Geffen School of Medicine, University of California, Los Angeles, California

Cheryl D. Wills, M.D.
Associate Professor of Psychiatry, Case Western Reserve University, Cleveland, Ohio

Michael F. Zito, M.D.
Assistant Clinical Professor, Department of Psychiatry and Biobehavioral Sciences, David Geffen School of Medicine at UCLA; Staff Psychiatrist, VA Greater Los Angeles Health Care System, Los Angeles, CA

Disclosures

The following contributor has indicated a financial interest in or other affiliation with a commercial supporter, manufacturer of a commercial product, and/or provider of a commercial service as listed below:

Philip J. Candilis, M.D., DFAPA
Stock ownership: Pfizer, Merck; expert testimony: U.S. Drug Enforcement Administration

The following contributors stated that they had no competing interests during the year preceding manuscript submission:

P.A. Bryant, M.D.; A. Buchanan, M.D., Ph.D.; D. Calhoun, M.D.; R.R. Darby, M.D.; W.C. Darby, M.D.; M. DiCiro, Psy.D., ABPP; M. Feldsher, M.D.; C.E. Fisher, M.D.; A. Goldberg, M.D., M.A.; E.E.H. Griffith, M.D.; M.W. Grover, M.D.; S. Hatters Friedman, M.D., M.St.; S.K. Hoge, M.D.; K. Hui, M.D., M.S.; N. Juth, Ph.D.; A. Kaempf, M.D.; M. Kanell, M.D.; J. Landess, M.D., J.D.; G.B. Leong, M.D.; M.R. MacIntyre, M.D.; D.A. Martell, Ph.D.; R. Martinez, M.D., M.H.; B. McCoy, M.D.; M.A. Norko, M.D., M.A.R.; S. Nyberg, M.D., Ph.D.; C. Rahm, M.D., Ph.D.; J. Rokop, Ph.D.; N. Ross, M.D.; L. Sandman, Ph.D.; J.R. Simpson, M.D., Ph.D.; A.C. Sones, M.D.; D.B. Stephens, M.D., Ph.D.; J.W. Swanson, Ph.D.; M. Swartz, M.D.; L.E. Weinberger, Ph.D.; R. Weinstock, M.D.; C.D. Wills, M.D.; M.F. Zito, M.D.

The following contributors did not supply information regarding disclosures:

R.G. Cockerill, M.D.; J. Piel, M.D., J.D.; D.A. Pinals, M.D.; C.L. Scott, M.D.; J.E. Sherin, M.D., Ph.D.; M. Sjöstrand, M.D., Ph.D.; S. Sreenivasan, Ph.D.

Foreword

Charles L. Scott, M.D.

The word "forensics" derives from the Latin word *forensis*, which means "of the forum." In Ancient Rome, the forum was a general meeting place or market where people gathered to discuss business and public affairs. *Forensics* is practiced in courts of law where scientific principles are applied to legal matters. The word "ethics" originates from the Greek word *ethos*, referencing one's character or morality. Thus, in quite simplistic terms, forensic ethics can be defined as a combination of these two ancient principles, resulting in the application of scientific principles in a moral manner and with good character. On a practical level, however, this definition falls quite short.

Mental health clinicians and evaluators of a person's mental health for legal purposes must address highly nuanced and possibly conflicting goals that arise in their work. Is there a resource that provides practical principles to serve as an ethical foundation for forensic evaluations and the provision of patient care? The textbook *Forensic Neuropsychiatric Ethics: Balancing Competing Duties In and Out of Court* is the definitive answer to this critical question.

Forensic Neuropsychiatric Ethics consists of 21 chapters that review real-life dilemmas facing practitioners who work in the field of mental health. The first two chapters ground the reader in the modern history and evolution of forensic ethics. Chapter 2, "Dialectical Principlism," highlights an approach that was developed to assist forensic psychiatrists and other health professionals to analyze the complex situations that occur when ethical duties and principles conflict with each other. Through dialectical principlism, the authors provide an ethical path forward in gray areas of practice when one needs to rank, balance, and integrate ethics guidelines from key thought leaders in the field and medical and forensic organizations. Subsequent chapters provide practical direction on a range of important topics, including maintaining robust professionalism, writing an ethical report, testifying ethically, applying ethics principles when in different professional roles, participating in capital cases, managing bias and subjectivity, incorporating testing into one's opinion, and working in leadership roles.

This book also excels through the application of ethics principles in real-life situations commonly faced by clinicians and evaluators. Specific chapters address how to incorporate ethics when providing informed consent, violating confidentiality, considering advance directives and physician assistance in dying, and fulfilling the Tarasoff duty to protect. Of note, this book wisely includes emerging and timely issues with chapters that focus on ethics considerations related to assisted outpatient treatment, the assessment and potential removal of firearms, the termination of pregnancy and decisional capacity, and implications for the use of neuroscience and artificial intelligence in the courtroom. An important highlight of this book is the discussion of how ethnic and minority groups must be considered in the context of clinical and forensic work. Chapters on ethics guidelines for the use of cultural formulation, the presence of structural racism in evaluations, and the recognition of structural and implicit bias in violence risk assessments serve as important reminders of inequities between dominant and nondominant group members in our society.

Forensic Neuropsychiatric Ethics: Balancing Competing Duties In and Out of Court represents a must-have resource for all clinicians, forensic evaluators, educators, administrators, lawyers, and judges. Through the consistent use of practical vignettes and the clear application of ethics guidelines, this remarkable book provides a guiding light through murky moral dilemmas in complex situations. The editors have brilliantly created the modern forum for discussing how to create a better tomorrow through the application of ethics in the valuable work that we do.

The Modern History and Evolution of Forensic Psychiatric Ethics Leading Up to Dialectical Principlism

William Connor Darby, M.D.

Robert Weinstock, M.D.

The modern era of forensic psychiatry is marked by major developmental milestones such as the founding of the American Academy of Psychiatry and Law (AAPL) in 1969, the creation of the American Board of Forensic Psychiatry in 1976, the subsequent advent of formal forensic psychiatry fellowship training programs, and the recognition of forensic psychiatry as a subspecialty by the American Board of Medical Specialties on September 17, 1992 (Prentice 1995). Before the founding of AAPL in 1969, forensic psychiatry was developed by individual practitioners incorporating an apprenticeship model for training and educating other psychiatrists in how to ethically operate as forensic experts. Two of the most prominent and highly respected forensic psychiatrists during this dawn of the modern era, Bernard Diamond,

M.D., and Seymour Pollack, M.D., helped shape and define an ethics-based role for psychiatrists operating in legal contexts as being distinct from their role as "general" psychiatrists (i.e., in a treatment role). This was critical, because most of the forensic opinions offered to the courts during this time period came from general psychiatrists regarding their patients rather than forensic psychiatrists serving a third party (Rappeport 1982). The confusion over a psychiatrist's role and agency and the conflicts for those venturing into the courtroom created a dire need for clarification in distinguishing the forensic role from the treatment role.

Diamond and Pollack agreed that the forensic role entailed the application of their psychiatric skills, techniques, knowledge, theories, and science to assist the legal system in its resolution of disputes (Weinstock et al. 2017). They both asserted that psychiatrists entering the forensic role had a duty to be honest and to mitigate the effects of bias in their opinions that could unfairly mislead the trier of fact (Weinstock et al. 2017). They differed, however, in their views on whether forensic psychiatrists must completely divorce themselves from the medical value systems from which their skill and expertise derived when performing this forensic function (Weinstock et al. 2017). Diamond (1959) favored an approach to forensic work in which he carefully selected cases in which his honest opinion would align with the values of a physician; thus, he chose to be an expert only on the defense side in criminal cases, under the stipulation that the defense attorney would cooperate with him to present the whole psychiatric truth. Additionally, he approached ambiguities in psycholegal questions from a medical and psychiatric perspective, which allowed him to fully articulate and expand on his reasoning regarding relevant psychiatric issues without believing he was restricted in doing so by more narrow legal interpretations of statutes and case law (Diamond 1959). Pollack (1974), in contrast, believed that forensic psychiatrists should ground themselves in the legal value system and orientation to maximize objectivity and avoid problems of "therapeutic misconception." He argued that forensic psychiatrists should attempt to determine the legal intent of case law and statutes, much as an attorney would opine on what the law alone, not the field of psychiatry, believed was relevant (Pollack 1974).

As described by Ciccone (2013), in the late 1970s, AAPL created a Committee on Ethics to help define the forensic role and guide experts on ethics dilemmas inherent in the field. Jonas Rappeport, M.D., one of the founding members of AAPL, was the first chair of the Committee on Ethics and presided over the initial draft of the AAPL Ethics

Guidelines that was presented to members for feedback. Following Rappeport as chair in the early 1980s, Henry Weinstein, M.D., further developed the AAPL Ethics Guidelines with the committee, which included Robert Weinstock, M.D. The Ethics Guidelines were adopted by AAPL in May 1987. The following year, Weinstock became chair and led efforts to change the language in the guidelines that created an impossible requirement that forensic psychiatrists be completely impartial and objective to a more attainable standard: "honesty and striving for objectivity."

Before the approval of AAPL's first ethics guidelines in May 1987, Alan Stone, M.D., delivered the keynote luncheon address at the 1982 AAPL Annual Meeting, "The Ethics of Forensic Psychiatry: A View From the Ivory Tower," which had profound effects in shaping today's landscape of forensic psychiatric ethics.

Stone's Critique of Forensic Psychiatric Ethics

During the luncheon address that was later a published chapter, Stone (1985) provided four ethical boundary problems plaguing forensic psychiatry. Stone elucidated these primary challenges for forensic psychiatrists and credited them for why he personally would never again take the stand to act as an expert witness. Although Stone acknowledged his inability to reconcile these problems, his questions challenged and motivated others to develop ethics theories to guide forensic work.

In his address, Stone was very concerned about the role he played as a forensic expert on a case involving a Black U.S. Army sergeant who was being court-martialed for stealing government property. As discussed further by Appelbaum (1990), Stone narrowly focused on the psycholegal question of whether the sergeant had kleptomania or any other psychiatric disorder that would excuse him from criminal responsibility. Although Stone was sympathetic to the racism the army sergeant suffered in the military at the time and believed it was the major contributor to his stealing federal property, he elected not to include this consideration, as he determined it was beyond the scope of the forensic question he was being asked to assess. Stone testified as a U.S. Army psychiatrist in the military trial, and the sergeant was sentenced to 5 years of hard labor. Stone elaborated on his regrets for not describing the motives of the sergeant (i.e., addressing the racial facets that led to the sergeant's sense of moral justification to take the property that he believed was his in return for enduring harsh societal discrimination). Although this social origin context did not meet criteria for any psychiatric disorder at the time and was not legally exculpatory, Stone nonetheless believed that the information could have served as an important mitigating factor, reducing the severity of the sergeant's punishment.

Stone reacted to this experience by vowing to stay out of the courtroom because he believed honest forensic testimony like his could paradoxically facilitate unjust outcomes. Reflecting on the experience, Stone critiqued the implications of forensic psychiatric work in his 1982 AAPL keynote address. Stone (1985) asserted that the first boundary issue is the basic legitimacy question of forensic psychiatry: "Does psychiatry have anything true to say that the courts should listen to?" That is, in opining on a particular psychiatric-legal issue, do forensic psychiatrists "have true answers to the legal and moral questions posed by the law?" (Stone 1985). Stone described Immanuel Kant, Sigmund Freud, and Heinz Hartmann as proponents of the "purist position" that our psychiatric science is inadequate to address moral questions of criminal responsibility. For example, in the case of the Black army sergeant, Stone could argue that attempts to explain the sergeant's motives in the narrow psychopathological model of the time (i.e., whether the sergeant met the strict DSM criteria at the time for kleptomania) were insufficient and gave the false impression of the lack of significant mitigating factors (e.g., the profound effects of societal discrimination). Stone described five intellectual problem areas that support this purist position: the problem of the fact-value distinction, determinism versus free will, deconstruction of the self, the mind-brain problem, and the chasm between "normal science" and morality.

Stone's first question raised serious issues for forensic psychiatrists to grapple with at the time, even though it addressed only a narrow area of the wide range of psycholegal cases in which forensic psychiatrists participate. It would be easy to dismiss Stone's question of the legitimacy of forensic psychiatric testimony in civil areas of medical malpractice, such as whether a treatment psychiatrist properly provided informed consent for antipsychotic medications, erred in discharging a Tarasoff duty when one was triggered, or failed to meet adequate standards of psychiatric practice in the management of a suicidal patient. It is clear and obvious that forensic psychiatrists are fully capable of providing relevant and truthful information that is probative for these malpractice issues. Additionally, many types of forensic assessments deal with issues of capacity or competency: for example, testamentary capacity, competence to make health care decisions, competence to manage financial affairs, competence to enter into a contract, guardianship assessments, competence to stand trial, and competence to waive Miranda rights. Again, it is easy to reject Stone's challenge—whether psychiatry has "anything true to say that the courts should listen to"—in these types of competence evaluations that have significant parallels to the capacity evaluations performed by psychosomatic psychiatrists in treatment settings.

The moral questions of criminal responsibility represent only a small fraction of the work forensic psychiatrists do, such as evaluations of criminal insanity defense, diminished actuality, diminished capacity, and imperfect self-defense. Additionally, Stone's critique in this area may be more of a reflection of his era, when psychodynamic testimony was more prominently used in expert testimony as the primary rationale for experts' opinions (although Stone was adamant that these conceptual problems apply even to the "hard science part of psychiatry"). Although we acknowledge that criminal-responsibility forensic assessments (in which opinions are formulated with a reasonable degree of medical certainty) can be some of the most difficult and complex areas for forensic psychiatrists, we believe it is a fairly settled and uncontroversial position today that forensic psychiatrists provide significant probative value to the courts on these issues. That is, we reject the purist notion that psychiatrists lack the skills and tools to opine on moral issues such as criminal responsibility; the entire field of forensic psychiatry is built on addressing these types of problems and is fully capable of doing so.

Consider insanity defense cases in jurisdictions with a morality test. Are forensic psychiatrists capable of assessing whether a person's mental state was such that they truly could not appreciate the moral wrongfulness of their criminal action? We would answer unequivocally in the affirmative: forensic psychiatrist experts have much truth-telling to offer the trier of fact in these cases. For example, situations in which the defendant suffers from a psychotic disorder and has persecutory delusions that lead to defensive actions against a perceived threat of serious harm. These cases follow a straightforward logic: the defendant suffers from a psychotic illness, and symptoms from that illness alter the defendant's mental state such that they believe they are acting morally to protect themselves against imminent, serious harm from another person or evil entities.

Forensic psychiatrists play an important role in these cases to differentiate defendants who feign such persecutory delusions (malingering) from those who truly meet the legal criteria for not guilty by reason of insanity. People who feign psychosis, even the most sophisticated and intelligent actors, are detected by skilled forensic psychiatrists because malingerers report atypical hallucination and delusional symptoms (i.e., rare and unusual symptoms), overact and call attention to their psychotic symptoms, are inconsistent in their report of symptoms, do not provide the classic time course and onset of symptoms (e.g., they rarely report the prodromal symptoms that typically precede psychotic symptoms), show a discrepancy between what they are reporting and how they behave, behave differently when they know they are being observed, and fail to describe coping strategies for how they mitigate distress from the psychotic symptoms. Moreover, people who feign psychosis are generally incapable of faking grossly disorganized speech and thus do not exhibit this symptom. Malingerers are also unlikely to be aware of and successfully imitate negative symptoms of psychotic disorders, which would require sophisticated acting skills that would be rare to encounter. Additionally, it is unlikely that people who feign psychosis would have evidence of psychotic symptoms and odd behaviors in medical, psychiatric, or other records as well as corroborated observations of psychotic behaviors from collateral sources. For example, it would be highly unlikely that someone feigning psychosis would have a documented history of significant mental illness and have observable psychotic symptoms in multiple settings long before the offense for which they are charged.

As far as the concerns related to narrow questions of criminal responsibility, as in Stone's case involving the Black army sergeant, one work-around to the critique of being unable to provide a sufficient explanation would be to address this question more broadly. That is, Stone could have opted to include cultural context regarding the sergeant's belief that he was morally justified to take the government property as payback for all the social injustices and racial discrimination he had endured. Although at the time this social motive would not have met a strict biological psychiatric definition for a disorder or even the criteria for a psychiatric diagnosis, it could be seen as falling within the broader scope of psychiatric expertise within the current biopsychosocial model understanding of psychiatric illness. It also could have been part of a psychodynamic assessment that was prevalent at the time. Ezra Griffith has championed a narrative approach, highlighting how cultural facets are important parts of forensic work (Griffith 1998, 2005). Griffith (1998, 2005) observed that a "culture-free" model of forensic psychiatric ethics would fall short in maximizing objective truth-telling and respect for persons, and he proposed his cultural formulation and narrative approaches as solutions to such an oversight (see later section, "Responses to Stone's Critique").

Thus, in addressing Stone's first basic legitimacy question to forensic psychiatrists—whether they have anything of truthful value to provide to the courts—these examples demonstrate that forensic psychiatrists can and do satisfy this requirement to enter the courtroom. Stone's thought-provoking questions in this area can now best be used by psychiatrists who stay within their scope of expertise and carefully qualify the limitations of their opinions so as to not fall victim to determinism versus free will, mind-brain, or other potential pitfalls. Philosophers have been unable to resolve those sorts of problems, and there is no persuasive reason to hold psychiatrists in the courtroom to such an impossibly high standard. The legal system itself cannot meet this standard.

Stone's next ethical boundary question for forensic psychiatrists asks, "Is one twisting justice to help the evaluee?" Psychiatrists acting in the forensic role may be confused or tempted to promote beneficence and nonmaleficence above all else, as they would in the treatment role with their patients. For example, in the case involving the army sergeant, Stone may have been tempted (because he sympathized with the racial injustices the sergeant suffered and wanted to help him avoid what he believed would be cruel punishment that was disproportionate to the crime) to opine that the sergeant suffered from kleptomania or another psychiatric disorder that would excuse him from criminal responsibility. However, Stone avoided doing so because it would be dishonest and a distortion of the truth. Thus Stone ponders how forensic psychiatrists can facilitate good in such situations in which honest testimony can be used by the legal system to produce seemingly unjust outcomes and unfair punishment for evaluees. Moreover, even if the punishment were to fit the crime, Stone wonders how psychiatrists— who are trained to use their expertise for healing purposes—reconcile the consequences of their honest forensic testimony, which can cause significant harm in those they are evaluating.

With his third ethics boundary question, Stone turned to the flip side of the risk of distorting truth to help the evaluee: "Is one deceiving the evaluee to serve justice?" That is, forensic psychiatrists could go too far in the other direction, like a police detective misleading the evaluee to obtain information, believing that it is warranted to maximally serve justice. One problem is that evaluees are more likely to erroneously believe that a forensic psychiatrist (unlike a police detective) is trying to help them or assist them on their case, even when the expert clearly states at the onset of an evaluation that they have been retained by the opposing side or prosecution. Given the societal expectations of medical doctors as healers working to advance the welfare of others consistent with the traditional treatment role, evaluees may be confused about the expert's role and divulge inculpating information that they would not otherwise share. There is a risk that forensic psychiatrists would use their therapeutic skills to coax the evaluee into revealing information that is damaging to their criminal or civil case. A forensic psychiatrist aspiring to be as ethical as possible in their work may rightfully question where to draw the line between a skillful evaluation that elicits necessary information and an unethical evaluation that misleads the evaluee into divulging crucial evidence.

Defendants who have not previously been involved with the legal system might be the most vulnerable to misunderstanding the forensic psychiatrist's role and overly trusting doctors. Such a defendant might even misinterpret the forensic psychiatrist's explanation of their role as further evidence of the expert's helpfulness. In contrast, defendants with antisocial personality disorder, psychopathic traits, and long criminal histories will be less likely to falsely trust an expert.

These dangers are present in forensic work, but in our opinion, they are not reasons to stay out of the courtroom. Instead, they are reasons to be vigilant when performing forensic work.

Finally, Stone's fourth ethics question asked, "Is one prostituting the profession by becoming an advocate?" Stone discussed the temptation that forensic psychiatrists could submit to being a "hired gun," distorting their opinions to please the attorney or side that retained them. That is, forensic psychiatrists could mistake their role for that of the attorney trying to win the case. Different variations and motives of the hired gun exist. The most commonly discussed motivation for "prostituting" the profession in such a way is avarice, as experts are financially incentivized to distort the truth to help the side that hired them.

Another possibility is that the forensic expert exaggerates their findings in the pursuit of some ideological agenda—for example, a forensic expert who is morally opposed to the death penalty and feels justified in distorting their opinion to prevent someone from being sentenced to death. Conversely, a forensic expert may be seduced by the criminal justice system and believe that they are helping carry out justice or protecting society by overstating how dangerous a defendant is, leading to a harsher punishment.

These cases represent some of the most egregious ethics violations in the field of forensic psychiatry. Rather than seeing them as a reason to stay out of the courtroom, as Stone did, we view this as an area of opportunity to develop ethical guidance for experts to avoid these traps and provide the field of forensic psychiatry with checks and balances to discourage and deter bad actors. For example, a forensic psychiatrist can be a consultant to an attorney to help cross-examine an expert who is thought to be a hired gun.

Responses to Stone's Critique

Although many forensic psychiatrists reacted to Stone's critique with shock and anger, Appelbaum (1997, 2008), who like Weinstock was a student of Stone, responded to these four ethical boundary questions by formulating "A Theory of Ethics for Forensic Psychiatry," his 1996 AAPL Presidential Address. Although he ignored Stone's primary philosophical question, whether psychiatry has any truth to offer the law (most likely as a result of psychiatry having more and more scientifically sound data to present in court and a shift away from opinions based on psychoanalytic interpretations), Appelbaum with his principlism approach addressed the other three of Stone's problem areas for forensic psychiatrists: 1) the potential for psychiatrists to overidentify as a treating psychiatrist and distort the psychiatric truth to benefit the evaluee; 2) the potential for psychiatrists to deceive a patient to maximize truth-telling to promote the interests of justice; and 3) the potential for psychiatrists to prostitute the profession by becoming an advocate (a hired gun). Appelbaum (1997, 2008) asserted that the primary societal value of forensic work is to advance the interests of justice, and he distilled two primary principles to guide forensic psychiatrists: truth-telling (both subjective and objective) and respect for persons (to respect the humanity of the person being evaluated and not to engage in deception, exploitation, or needless invasion of privacy). According to Appelbaum, the potential for overidentifying as treating psychiatrists advocating for the evaluee would be rectified by establishing a distinct set of ethics for forensic psychiatry, separate from the treatment psychiatry role. Citing how it was already widely accepted that research psychiatrists have a unique set of ethics principles governing their work, Appelbaum drew a parallel that in both research and forensic roles, psychiatrists did not have a traditional physician-patient relationship and thus were exempt from the traditional medical ethics principles of beneficence and nonmaleficence. Instead, forensic psychiatrists had the duty to use their psychiatric expertise to tell the truth and facilitate justice rather than to try to help and mitigate harm to the person being evaluated. But, as we describe in the next chapter on dialectical principlism, psychiatrists in these other roles maintain (or should maintain) some of their traditional medical ethics values and obligations.

Appelbaum's second principle of respect for persons answered Stone's question about the possibility of deceiving the person being evaluated as an arm of justice. This principle entails that forensic psychiatrists should not coerce or deceive the evaluee as a means to an end of obtaining information, even if doing so would maximize truth-telling to foster justice. Additionally, this respect for persons encompasses the disclosure of information obtained through forensic evaluations. Although physician-patient confidentiality does not apply in forensic settings, psychiatrists should still limit the information disclosed in written and oral reports to only that which is probative to answering the legal question honestly. Irrelevant and prejudicial information should not be disclosed, and the disclosure of information should be limited as much as possible to the legal participants involved in the cases. Appelbaum was of the view that forensic psychiatrists owe the same sorts of duties to evaluees that they have to any person. In our opinion, although we agree there is no traditional physician-patient relationship or duty as in treatment, there may be some special obligations as physicians to not undertake certain types of forensic roles.

Appelbaum further elaborated that truth-telling is composed of both subjective and objective components, which can be applied to Stone's concern of the hired-gun problem and the more insidious seduction of the legal system to unconsciously demean the profession. That is, it is clear that a hired gun violates Appelbaum's truth-telling principle by being dishonest and distorting data to help the side that hired them. Stone alluded to a related pitfall to which forensic psychiatrists may fall victim, where the power of the adversarial legal system influences a forensic psychiatrist to unconsciously identify their role as being similar to the attorney's role to advocate for one side. This characterizes a potential unconscious bias that leads forensic psychiatrists to favor the side that hires them. That is, the forensic psychiatrist may unintentionally approach the case in a way that is likely to yield an opinion aligned with that bias, and in so doing, fail to reach an appropriate level of objective truth-telling.

AAPL Ethics Guidelines elaborate on practical methods for forensic psychiatrists to strive for objective truth-telling that could be interpreted as ways to avoid potential pitfalls related to unconscious biases (American Academy of Psychiatry and the Law 2005):

> Psychiatrists practicing in a forensic role enhance the honesty and objectivity of their work by basing their forensic opinions, forensic reports, and forensic testimony on all available data. They communicate the honesty of their work, efforts to attain objectivity, and the soundness of their clinical opinion, by distinguishing, to the extent possible, between verified and unverified information as well as among clinical "facts," "inferences," and "impressions."

Confirmation bias—the tendency to search for, interpret, and favor information that affirms a particular hypothesis—is a serious land mine that threatens the objectivity of a forensic practitioner's work and the credibility of the entire profession. AAPL guidelines recognize this problem and suggest the partial remedy of obtaining all the relevant information and performing due diligence to demarcate whether the information is verified. That is, forensic psychiatrists should not stop prematurely, for whatever reason, in collecting additional evidence that may conflict with their initial hypothesis.

A year after Appelbaum's Presidential Address, Ezra Griffith delivered the 1997 AAPL Presidential Address, "Ethics in Forensic Psychiatry: A Cultural Response to Stone and Appelbaum" (Griffith 1998). Griffith (1998, 2005) observed that a "culture-free" model of forensic psychiatric ethics would fall short in maximizing objective truth-telling and respect for persons, and he proposed his cultural formulation and narrative approaches as solutions to this oversight. Griffith said that forensic work that ignores cultural context—and specifically the dynamics of dominant versus nondominant groups of people in society—will inherently be biased against nondominant individuals. To Griffith, ethical forensic work calls for efforts to discover, understand, and convey an individual's narrative within a cultural context, recognizing the power dynamics at play in society. Griffith's approach can be understood as one method for combating certain types of implicit bias that are incompatible with one's conscious values but nevertheless lead to prejudiced forensic opinions (see Dr. Griffith's contribution to this volume, Chapter 3, "Narrative and Ethics in Forensic Psychiatry").

Michael Norko (2018) described the importance of presence, empathy, compassion, and centering to elevate the search for truth from a mechanical to a spiritual exercise, which he outlined in his 2017 AAPL Presidential Address. Norko emphasized how compassion should be integrated into forensic work (Norko 2005, 2018; see also Chapter 6,

"Ethical Challenges While Testifying"). Candilis and Martinez developed their aspirational robust professionalism model to highlight integrity in forensic work, with experts integrating personal morality with their professional role (Candilis et al. 2001; Martinez and Candilis 2005; see their contribution to this volume, Chapter 4, "Robust Professionalism: Forensic Psychiatry's Identity and Purpose").

Conclusion

The field of forensic psychiatry has been advanced by the development of ethics guidelines, principles, and considerations that accelerated with the founding of AAPL in 1969, the academic dialogue between Pollack and Diamond, Stone's critique, and subsequent responses by Appelbaum, Griffith, Norko, Martinez, Candilis, and others. These important contributions have better clarified the roles and responsibilities for forensic psychiatrists, as distinct from psychiatrists in the traditional treatment role.

In the next chapter, we discuss dialectical principlism, first introduced in Weinstock's 2014 AAPL Presidential Address. The model prioritizes duties according to role, integrating Norko's compassion, Griffith's narrative, Appelbaum's principlism, Candilis and Martinez's robust professionalism, and other approaches to help psychiatrists identify, weigh, and balance the competing considerations that guide ethical decision-making for a given situation (Darby 2021; Darby and Weinstock 2017, 2018a, 2018b; Darby et al. 2022; Weinstock 2015).

References

American Academy of Psychiatry and the Law: Ethics Guidelines for the Practice of Forensic Psychiatry. Adopted May 2005. Bloomfield, CT, American Academy of Psychiatry and the Law, 2005. Available at: https://www.aapl.org/ethics-guidelines. Accessed October 1, 2020.

Appelbaum PS: The parable of the forensic psychiatrist: ethics and the problem of doing harm. Int J Law Psychiatry 13(4):249–259, 1990 2286491

Appelbaum PS: A theory of ethics for forensic psychiatry. J Am Acad Psychiatry Law 25(3):233–247, 1997 9323651

Appelbaum PS: Ethics and forensic psychiatry: translating principles into practice. J Am Acad Psychiatry Law 36(2):195–200, 2008 18583695

Candilis PJ, Martinez R, Dording C: Principles and narrative in forensic psychiatry: toward a robust view of professional role. J Am Acad Psychiatry Law 29(2):167–173, 2001 11471782

Ciccone JR: Commentary: forensic education and the quest for truth. J Am Acad Psychiatry Law 41(1):33–37, 2013 23503173

Diamond BL: The fallacy of the impartial expert. Arch Crim Psychodyn 3(2):221–236, 1959

Darby WC: Ethics challenges for presenting genetic data in forensic settings. J Am Acad Psychiatry Law 49(2):179–186, 2021 33972350

Darby WC, Weinstock R: Prescribing stimulants in college populations: clinical and ethical challenges. Adolesc Psychiatry (Hilversum) 7(3):179–189, 2017

Darby WC, Weinstock R: The limits of confidentiality: informed consent and psychotherapy. Focus Am Psychiatr Publ 16(4):395–401, 2018a 31975932

Darby WC, Weinstock R: Resolving ethics dilemmas in forensic practice, in Ethics Dilemmas in Forensic Psychiatry and Psychology Practice. Edited by Griffith E. New York, Columbia University Press, 2018b, pp 7–22

Darby WC, MacIntyre M, Weinstock R: Pragmatic approaches to COVID-19 related ethics dilemmas for psychiatrists. J Am Acad Psychiatry Law 50(4):566–576, 2022 36220157

Griffith EEH: Ethics in forensic psychiatry: a cultural response to Stone and Appelbaum. J Am Acad Psychiatry Law 26(2):171–184, 1998 9664254

Griffith EEH: Personal narrative and an African-American perspective on medical ethics. J Am Acad Psychiatry Law 33(3):371–381, 2005 16186203

Martinez R, Candilis PJ: Commentary: toward a unified theory of personal and professional ethics. J Am Acad Psychiatry Law 33(3):382–385, 2005 16186204

Norko MA: Commentary: compassion at the core of forensic ethics. J Am Acad Psychiatry Law 33(3):386–389, 2005 16186205

Norko MA: What is truth? The spiritual quest of forensic psychiatry. J Am Acad Psychiatry Law 46(1):10–22, 2018 29618531

Pollack S: Forensic Psychiatry in Criminal Law. Los Angeles, CA, University of Southern California Press, 1974

Prentice SE: A history of subspecialization in forensic psychiatry. Bull Am Acad Psychiatry Law 23(2):195–203, 1995 8605403

Rappeport JR: Differences between forensic and general psychiatry. Am J Psychiatry 139(3):331–334, 1982 7058947

Stone AA: The ethics of forensic psychiatry: a view from the ivory tower, in Law, Psychiatry, and Morality. Edited by Stone AA. Washington, DC, American Psychiatric Press, 1985, pp 57–75

Weinstock R: Dialectical principlism: an approach to finding the most ethical action. J Am Acad Psychiatry Law 43(1):10–20, 2015 25770274

Weinstock R, Leong GB, Piel JL, et al: Defining forensic psychiatry: roles and responsibilities, in Principles and Practice of Forensic Psychiatry. Edited by Rosner R, Scott CL. Boca Raton, FL, CRC Press, 2017, pp 7–15

2

Dialectical Principlism

William Connor Darby, M.D.
Robert Weinstock, M.D.

W e believe that most people enter psychiatry with a desire to act
ethically, and that most are interested in doing the right (or most
ethical) action when faced with challenges. This aspiration does not
disappear when we enter the forensic realm, but it does become more
complex, operating at the intersection of law and psychiatry. To aid
forensic psychiatrists, we present a method of resolving ethical dilemmas, named *dialectical principlism*.

Dialectical principlism was developed to assist forensic psychiatrists and other health professionals in analyzing the complex dilemmas that occur when ethics duties and principles conflict with one
another. Dialectical principlism is most helpful in and best reserved
for special situations in which ethics guidelines are not sufficiently
applicable or compete with one another. In these gray areas, there is
likely no risk of professional or organizational sanctions regardless of
the action chosen. And thus, dialectical principlism is an aspirational
model for psychiatrists who are motivated to "do the right thing" in
situations where there is no clear consensus on what the right thing
is. That is, dialectical principlism was developed for those practitioners striving to determine the most ethical action in difficult situations,
going beyond merely staying out of trouble and avoiding sanctions. For
being an ethical citizen, "not breaking the law" is a low bar; similarly,

15

not committing ethics violations is only the bare minimum of being an ethical forensic psychiatrist.

Dialectical principlism operates by identifying the relevant ethics duties and principles, prioritizing them (i.e., ranking their relative importance), and balancing them (i.e., weighing all the ethics considerations favoring the proposed action against all the considerations opposing the action). Opposing duties and principles are ranked based on the particular role of the practitioner and the specific contextual factors. The dialectical principlism method integrates ethics guidelines such as those from medical and forensic organizations (e.g., American Medical Association [AMA] [2001]; American Psychiatric Association [2013, 2014]; American Psychological Association [2010]; American Academy of Psychiatry and the Law [AAPL] [2005, 2013]; and American Academy of Forensic Sciences [AAFS]); ethics theories such as principlism, casuistry, narrative, ethics of caring, and normative ethics; and ethics models specific to forensic professionals such as the principlism approach of Appelbaum (1997), the narrative approach of Griffith (1998), the robust professionalism of Candilis and Martinez (Candilis et al. 2001), and the compassion model of Norko (2005, 2018).

In this chapter, we demonstrate the special features of dialectical principlism, including how it affords the balance of conflicting ethics criteria in determining the most ethical action. The framework strives to achieve this goal by prioritizing ethics considerations according to a practitioner's specific professional role. We distinguish between *proximal* and *distal* duties (previously referred to as "primary" and "secondary" but changed for clarity) to highlight how the model weighs principles in a manner dependent on the role of the practitioner.

For example, a treating psychiatrist has a set of proximal duties based on the primary societal value for the treatment role that differs from that of the forensic role; thus, a different calculus occurs in these two settings. In the treatment role, the primary societal value is to advance patient welfare, with the greatest relative weight given to principles most related to promoting that value (beneficence, nonmaleficence, autonomy) when balanced with other competing considerations and principles. We call these *proximal duties* to differentiate them from *distal duties* that are less related to promoting patient welfare (but are important considerations that sometimes can outweigh proximal duties in the balancing process). An example of a distal duty outweighing proximal duties occurs with reporting child or elder abuse: the duty to protect the most vulnerable in our society outweighs beneficence, nonmaleficence, and autonomy considerations to patients. This is rare;

most of the time, ethics-based clinical treatment decision-making will be guided by what is best to promote patient welfare via considerations of autonomy, nonmaleficence, and beneficence and not what is in the best interest of third parties who are not our patients.

In forensic psychiatry, the primary societal value is to advance justice. Thus, the proximal duties in the forensic role change to truth-telling and respect for persons, because those are more relevant to the aims of promoting justice than the treatment role's aims of promoting patient welfare. As in the treatment role, in extreme cases, proximal duties can be outweighed by distal considerations in terms of guiding our most ethical behavior. For example, determining whether to accept certain forensic cases may be driven more by distal duties such as considering the evaluee's welfare, societal expectations for physicians, and personal values. The proximal duties of truth-telling and respect for persons would guide the forensic psychiatrist in how to perform the evaluation but offer little guidance on the ethical selection of cases or how to choose and control the use of our expertise in forensic settings.

The context of the situation and the unique set of personal, cultural, and societal values created from a practitioner's narrative are used to assign weights to proximal and distal duty principles. Finally, these principles are balanced by using the reflective equilibrium method of Rawls (1971) to decide what is the most ethical action for that specific individual, in that specific role, given that specific situation.

Special Ethics Considerations at the Intersection of Law and Psychiatry

Ethics in forensic work for psychiatrists, as well as other mental health and medical experts, presents special challenges. Forensic work operates at the intersection of two disparate fields. Psychiatry is a branch of medicine, with patient welfare as its primary concern. Treating psychologists and other physicians such as neurologists also prioritize their patients' welfare. In the legal system, though, the major focus is to settle disputes and achieve legal justice. When engaged in forensic practice, forensic professionals bring to the legal system their own methods, goals, rules, ethics, and values, which are distinct from those of the legal system. Ethical dilemmas may arise when the ethics principles and rules that govern forensic practice are in conflict with those that govern attorneys. Ethical dilemmas also occur when the ethics principles relevant to forensic practice are themselves in conflict, thereby creating questions about which principles to prioritize.

Organizational Guidelines

To help forensic experts facing these conflicting obligations to the law and their practice, many organizations have ethics guidelines for forensic work that frame the boundaries of what is or is not ethical practice. These organizations include the AMA, American Psychiatric Association, American Psychological Association, AAPL, and AAFS. AAPL requires that practitioners be honest and strive for objectivity in their forensic work and that they give notice to evaluees regarding the nature and purpose of the evaluation and limits of its confidentiality (American Academy of Psychiatry and the Law 2005).

Ethical dilemmas occur when practitioners encounter competing guidelines. If one guideline is completely neglected for another, then the risk of unethical action increases. That is, following any guideline rigidly while neglecting all others is potentially problematic; such actions may cause conflict with other duties, responsibilities, and guidelines.

For example, consider a situation in which a forensic expert initially informs an evaluee of the nature and purpose of the forensic evaluation, but it becomes evident later in the evaluation that the evaluee did not understand the advisement. The forensic expert would not technically violate AAPL's ethics guidelines by not reminding the evaluee of their role, having given the initial notice. Moreover, the expert may believe that to maximize AAPL's other guideline of striving for objectivity, a reminder of their role and purpose later in the evaluation could prevent them from obtaining critical information probative to the legal question. But this would entail being dishonest with the evaluee and violating a respect-for-persons principle. This example, which we have discussed previously to illustrate the dialectical principlism model (Darby and Weinstock 2018b), demonstrates how attempting to adhere to only one guideline to the exclusion of all others risks violating fundamental ethics values. Familiarity with the guidelines is important so that practitioners can adhere to them and identify when conflicts exist. Such situations require them to determine which guidelines to prioritize. This process of prioritizing may subsequently lead to different conclusions on how to act most ethically.

To deal with conflicting ethics guidelines, forensic experts may implement relevant ethics theories and models to help lay out and emphasize what criteria should be considered.

Ethics Theories Pertinent to Forensic Psychiatry

Some of the major ethics theories relevant to forensic work are normative ethics (including virtue, deontology, and consequentialism), ethics of caring, principlism, narrative, and casuistry (closely related to and possibly including narrative).

Virtue ethics originated in the virtues delineated by Plato and Aristotle. In recent years, it has had a resurgence, emphasizing the need to have moral character to behave ethically and to be reflected in the usual practice of virtuous professionals (Candilis et al. 2007). That is, it is insufficient to have been educated on ethics theories or to be aware of the important considerations; it is also necessary to have moral character and the intent or desire to carry out the right action.

Other types of *normative ethics* include duty (deontological ethics) and consequentialism (utilitarian ethics). *Consequentialism* contends broadly that the morality of an action be judged based on its consequences: the right action is the one that produces the best outcome or the most good (Hope 2004). *Deontological ethics*, conversely, judges the morality of an action based on rules such as "always tell the truth." For example, a deontologist might argue that it is never moral to lie or not to tell the whole truth, and also that it is never ethical to kill a person (Hope 2004).

There are limits to how far either of these methods alone can determine our most ethical action. For example, most would disagree with killing one person to harvest their organs so that a number of other people could live; nevertheless, doing so could be argued as an extension of consequentialism, producing the most good by saving the most lives. In this situation, the strong deontological principle of not killing others would be determinative. In a parallel manner, strictly adhering to deontological ethics values alone might lead to serious consequences, such as the Gestapo in Nazi Germany asking citizens where to find hidden Jewish people; not lying would lead to the capture and torture of innocent individuals.

Gilligan's (1982) *ethics of caring*, which is in part an outgrowth of feminist ethics, is an alternative to Kohlberg's *developmental principlist* model of moral development. Kohlberg (1984) considered thinking in terms of principles to explain that the morality of an action is the highest stage of moral development, and that most people never achieve it. It has been argued that developmental principlism can lead to a "cold" kind of morality. For example, should we as individuals (in contrast to society as a whole) really aspire to treat all people the same? Should we give our family, our friends, and ourselves no more consideration than anybody else?

The two major conceptions of the practice of bioethics include principlism and casuistry (Cudney 2014). Modern *principlism* such as that proposed by Beauchamp and Childress (2013) involves balancing context-dependent conflicting principles. Beauchamp and Childress (2013) developed four principles of *biomedical ethics*: autonomy, beneficence, nonmaleficence, and distributive justice. *Distributive justice* is not legal justice. It refers specifically to the fair allocation of limited medical resources. Various editions of their book have contained incremental revisions of their views. In the 2013 edition, they clearly asserted that common morality is relevant. When the four principles of medical ethics conflict with one another or with common morality, they need to be balanced using Rawls's *reflective equilibrium* to determine the most ethical action.

Principlism is often contrasted with *casuistry* (or a version of it called *narrative*). Casuistry in the past was used pejoratively and equated with ethical relativism, devoid of higher principles and theory. Modern casuistry and principlism have been moving closer to each other in recent years (Cudney 2014). Contemporary advocates of casuistry such as Jonsen and Toulmin argued for a more "bottom-up" approach of drawing from paradigm cases to formulate the relevant principles, rights, and rules to apply to new cases (Paulo 2015).

When one is faced with a new situation, a paradigm case is selected that has a similar ethical dilemma, implying a similar solution. It is not unusual, however, for disagreements to arise regarding how much weight to apply to one facet of the case over another and which paradigm to use. This requires identifying the relevant facets to consider. These facets can then be weighed using the reflective equilibrium method of Rawls as described by Beauchamp and Childress (2013); the method then becomes similar to that of principlists, who apply and balance mid-level principles.

Models of Forensic Professional Ethics

In forensic professional ethics, principlism has best been applied by Appelbaum. As discussed in Chapter 1 ("The Modern History and Evolution of Forensic Psychiatric Ethics Leading Up to Dialectical Principlism"), in response to Stone's (1985) challenge to provide an ethics framework for the field, Appelbaum (1997, 2008) developed principles for forensic psychiatry to distinguish it from treatment psychiatry. Appelbaum claimed that ethics requirements are determined by the role of the profession. In forensic psychiatry, the goal is to promote legal justice. That goal is fostered ethically by subjective and objective truth-telling, as well as by demonstrating respect for persons.

Although Appelbaum's model accurately defines the principles to help practitioners act ethically in most forensic contexts, there are some limitations to how it can guide ethical behavior. When principles in his model conflict with one another, which should take precedence? That is, what do we do when fostering justice comes into conflict with showing respect for persons? Should we intervene when the legal system is not showing respect for the evaluee? Should we reject a case if we think the goal of an attorney is inappropriate or unethical, even if allowed by the law? That is, does answering the legal question honestly trump respecting persons when the two conflict, or vice versa? Additionally, other principles, outside of truth-telling and showing respect for persons, are important to consider and can be determinative in unique situations.

Weinstock initially developed a forensic ethics approach that involved answering legal questions but also considered that psychiatrists had traditional medical ethics responsibilities, as physicians trained in medicine and applying their medical expertise to legal matters, to consider the welfare of those they evaluate and the societal consequences of their work (Weinstock et al. 1990). Weinstock, who was mentored by Bernard Diamond, agreed with Diamond (1959) that forensic psychiatrists should retain some of their medical values when applying their skills and expertise in the forensic role. Appelbaum appropriately cautioned that forensic psychiatrists risk misleading the evaluee when they simultaneously adhere to the duties of a forensic role while also taking the ethical position of a treating psychiatrist, what he calls a "mixed model" (Appelbaum 1997). Appelbaum shared similar concerns that Pollack (1974) articulated earlier related to "therapeutic bias." Appelbaum's rationale was that an evaluee can mistake the forensic psychiatrist as trying to help them even when hired by the opposing side. Appelbaum contended that the risk is greatest if psychiatrists are confused about their role as a result of considering principles of traditional medical ethics.

Weinstock was persuaded by the arguments of Appelbaum and worked on modifying his position to take these concerns into account while still asserting a role for traditional medical ethics in forensic work. This critique was the impetus for efforts that culminated in the dialectical principlism that Weinstock developed in conjunction with Darby.

Another model of forensic ethics, *robust professionalism*, maintains a role for traditional medical ethics in the field (Candilis 2011; Candilis and Martinez 2012; Candilis et al. 2001; Martinez and Candilis 2005). In this model, the forensic professional acts most ethically by going beyond just answering the legal question to include efforts to resolve underlying conflicts and problems that benefit the individual being assessed. For example, this model could be used to achieve the most ethical outcome when the forensic expert is consulted to make end-of-life decisions involving initial conflict between patient and family (Candilis et al. 2007). Theorists have argued that going beyond the narrowly defined forensic role is a central tenet of the forensic practitioner's robust professional duty and not merely an afterthought.

Robust professionalism has elements related to narrative, in that they both assert that as more information about the situation is obtained, the most ethical action becomes apparent. However, like Appelbaum's principlism model, robust professionalism does not clearly address how a forensic expert should resolve conflicting ethics considerations. It also is not evident whether Candilis and Martinez developed paradigm cases or principles to compare and apply to new cases as in modern casuistry and whether their model implements Rawls's reflective equilibrium in the balancing process seen in modern principlism.

Griffith (1998, 2003, 2005) developed a narrative model to help guide ethical behavior in forensic work. His model is a way to determine what is ethical in a case by fleshing out details, motivation, and background. It includes an emphasis on cultural considerations and the special problems faced by nondominant groups. Norko (2005, 2018) advocated for compassion to be part of the narrative of an ethical forensic assessment, even if the evaluation leads to an opinion that does not help the person evaluated.

Narrative clearly plays an important role in ethics analysis when no conflicting obligations exist. But when faced with conflicting duty considerations in forensic work (e.g., answering the legal question, showing respect for persons, consideration of cultural factors, societal discrimination, biomedical ethics principles related to the evaluee), narrative alone does not necessarily guide decision-making because it is not clear what considerations take primacy in the forensic context.

Dialectical Principlism

Dialectical principlism is our method of laying out, prioritizing, and balancing conflicting ethics considerations to help practitioners act most ethically (Darby 2021; Darby and Weinstock 2017, 2018a, 2018b; Darby et al. 2022; Weinstock 2015). Dialectical principlism developed as a way to address the challenge faced by forensic psychiatrists to ethically assist the legal system using our medical expertise, while not entirely divorcing ourselves from the traditional medical ethics associated with that expertise. We assert that forensic psychiatrists should not solely answer psycholegal questions without regard to the implications. This is consistent with early theories of Weinstock (Weinstock et al. 1991), who argued that traditional Hippocratic ethics play a role in forensic practice, because our expertise is borne from our training in traditional ethics settings, and psychiatrists are not completely divorced from those ethics—even in nontreatment roles. This loyalty to traditional medical ethics is supported by surveys of AAPL forensic psychiatrists in 1991 and 2018: respondents validated strong agreement that "medical and psychiatric ethics remain a consideration when performing a forensic evaluation" (Darby et al. 2021; Weinstock et al. 1991).

This model builds from and encompasses all the ethics models, theories, and guidelines mentioned earlier. For example, narrative is an essential component of this ethics analysis. It is the starting point from which to ascertain the relevant role and is used to assign weights to the principles based on contextual factors and the practitioner's unique personal ethics and values. Appelbaum's principlism is paramount to defining the proximal duty principles for the forensic expert role. Robust professionalism highlights the importance of ethics considerations outside a narrowly defined forensic role, what dialectical principlism refers to as *distal duty principles*. The balancing process of our model is essentially Rawls's reflective equilibrium and has similarities to Dworkin's (1986) model of legal interpretivism.

Dialectical principlism, as a method to analyze complex ethical dilemmas, incorporates the other ethics theories and approaches (rather than competing with them) when ethics guidelines do not

suffice. Dialectical principlism establishes a hierarchy of ethics considerations prioritized according to the role of the practitioner. Proximal
duties are distinguished from distal duties based on professional role,
and then the relevant principles are weighed accordingly in the reflective equilibrium-like balancing process. The conflicting considerations
could be conflicting ethics guidelines, theories, or models.

Principlism Under the Dialectical Principlism Model

Under the dialectical principlism model, *principlism* refers to the
emphasis on principles in the broadest sense of the term. Principles
include meeting duties as prioritized for a specific role and context;
professional ethics, which may be influenced by organizational guidelines; personal ethics and values, which may be shaped by various ethics theories; societal expectations for the specific professional role; and
culturally based principles distinctive to individual practitioners and
set by their unique personal and professional narrative.

Dialectical principlism assigns weighted values to principles based
on the practitioner's professional role, the specific context of the situation, and the unique set of personal, cultural, and societal values created from an individual's unique narrative. Although it incorporates
rather than competes with other models, dialectical principlism distinguishes itself by establishing a hierarchy of ethics considerations
ranked according to the role of the physician or other professional
forensic practitioner. We define *proximal* and *distal* duties based on how
integral they are in promoting the primary societal value for that specific role type. Forensic psychiatry experts and other practitioners may
disagree on the formulation of proximal and distal duties. We present
our theoretical conception to assist in analyzing complex ethical dilemmas (Table 2.1).

Dialectical principlism demarcates proximal versus distal duties
depending on the practitioner's role. In the treatment setting, proximal-duty principles differ from those of other roles such as forensic, research, or administrative. Practitioners in treatment, forensic,
research, and administrative roles face competing obligations and
ethics considerations that are weighed differently based on the role.
For example, the proximal duties in the treatment role include the
Beauchamp and Childress bioethical principles related to advancing individual patient welfare (i.e., beneficence, nonmaleficence, and

Table 2.1 Duties of a health professional working in various roles as described by dialectical principlism

	Forensic role	Treatment role	Research role	Administrative role
Primary societal value	Advancing justice	Advancing patient welfare	Advancing scientific knowledge	Advancing distributive justice
Proximal duties	1. Truth-telling 2. Respect for persons	1. Respect for autonomy 2. Beneficence 3. Nonmaleficence	Fostering the internal and external validity of experiments	Allocation of resources for maximal good in the system
Distal duties	1. Consideration of evaluee's welfare 2. Consideration of retaining attorney's case 3. Consideration of societal expectations for physicians 4. Consideration of personal values	1. Protecting vulnerable third parties 2. Distributive justice and other societal considerations 3. Consideration of employer or organization 4. Consideration of personal well-being or safety	Consideration of research subject's welfare via 1. Fair subject selection 2. Favorable risk-benefit ratio 3. Safety	Consideration of welfare of the individual patient receiving care via 1. Autonomy 2. Beneficence 3. Nonmaleficence 4. Informed consent 5. Respect for persons

autonomy). We consider their distributive justice principle to be a distal duty, however, because it is less central to how physicians and other mental health professionals help their patients and more relevant to how care is delivered fairly on a macro level. Although proximal duties will most often outweigh distal duties, in special contexts a distal duty may be so strong as to trump competing proximal-duty considerations.

As discussed earlier, reporting suspected elder or child abuse is a distal duty. Another example is a Tarasoff-type duty to protect others in situations triggered by the patient's credible threat of imminent violence. In both examples, the context of extreme harm to vulnerable third parties adds significant weight to the distal duty, giving it priority over breaching confidentiality to prevent or mitigate violence.

In the forensic role, we designate Appelbaum's truth-telling and respect for persons as proximal duties because they are central to advancing the interests of justice. Distal duties include considerations to the evaluee and retaining attorney, personal ethics, and societal expectations for physicians and other mental health professionals.

In the research role, as Appelbaum (1997) noted, psychiatrists and other researchers have conflicting duties in advancing scientific understanding. We define research proximal duties as principles that maximize the internal and external validity of experiments and distal duties as principles related to fairness, respect, safety, and beneficence for research participants. An example of a distal duty trumping a proximal one is when research projects are stopped prematurely to protect subjects' interests when unexpected harm occurs or when it is clear that subjects in one arm of the study are forgoing important benefits (whether or not an institutional review board requires it).

Conflation of research and treatment roles may lead clinical trial participants to underestimate risks and overestimate potential benefits of experimental interventions because they believe the professional leading the study is considering their individual well-being as primary, when it realistically may be secondary to the study. This risk is highest when the researcher is also the treating doctor. Hospital administrators and managed care reviewers can be seen to have proximal duties to maximize resource allocation, with significant distal duties to patient welfare. A similar phenomenon may occur in forensic settings: evaluees may falsely perceive that forensic psychiatrists and other professionals are there to help them even if properly informed of forensic roles and who retained them.

Dialectics in Dialectical Principlism

Dialectics refers to the balancing of competing principles to arrive at a synthesis of considerations that direct action. This is akin to the reflective equilibrium model of Rawls (1971).

Examples of Dialectical Principlism

The analysis framed by dialectical principlism is best reserved for situations in which there is a conflict between ethics principles, especially when a distal duty is uniquely relevant. In the treatment setting, organizational ethics guidelines will usually suffice, and otherwise, practitioners will be guided by principles of beneficence, nonmaleficence, and autonomy to maximally advance patient welfare. We discussed earlier how dialectal principlism can be used in special circumstances, such as breaching confidentiality to report elder and child abuse or fulfilling a Tarasoff duty, illustrating that the distal duty to vulnerable third parties can outweigh proximal duties to the patient. Additionally, we have previously written about the application of dialectical principlism in treatment role situations to address dilemmas related to stimulant prescriptions in college-age populations (Darby and Weinstock 2017), as well as pandemic-related dangerousness assessments and distinguishing psychosis from delusion-like beliefs (Darby et al. 2022).

In the forensic role, the primary societal value is to advance justice, with proximal duties being Appelbaum's truth-telling and respect for persons and distal duties being the evaluee's welfare, societal expectations for physicians, and personal values. Again, for most forensic scenarios, following AAPL's ethics guidelines and Appelbaum's principlism model will be sufficient to inform ethical forensic work as experts opine on legal questions honestly, striving to be as objective as possible and showing adequate respect for persons. However, a number of potential conflicts and situations involving distal duty considerations are uniquely salient; applying dialectical principlism can help experts analyze competing considerations to resolve dilemmas. We have previously described examples in which dialectical principlism could help practitioners strive to be as ethical as possible, including determining whether to accept cases for the prosecution solely to present aggravating factors at the penalty phase of capital cases (i.e., as distinguished from rebutting mitigating factors); whether to accept referrals from sources believed to be unethical (Weinstock 2015); slippage of initial forensic advisements (Darby and Weinstock 2018b); issues related to implicit bias in capital cases (Darby et al. 2018, 2020); considerations for presenting psychiatric genetic data, neuroimaging, and artificial intelligence in forensic settings (Darby 2021); and questions regarding breaching attorney-client work privilege to protect against imminent violence or danger (Darby et al. 2022).

Some experts may not consider conflicts that arise commonly in forensic work, such as not disclosing privileged information when forming an opinion that does not help the side that hired you. If we were to blindly follow the principle of truth-telling to the extreme without consideration of other principles, it could be rationalized that disclosing the opinion to the opposing side would best foster justice. However, doing so would be such an egregious example of violating the distal duty to the retaining attorney (in addition to potentially creating legal liability for the expert) that few, if any, forensic psychiatrists would consider it.

Other conflicts involve a distal duty to the person being evaluated. One example would be, after conducting a sanity assessment, notifying jail physicians that a defendant is suicidal. This act would be going beyond just answering the narrow psycholegal question of sanity as well as the respect-for-persons principle. Another example would be choosing not to evaluate the competency to be executed of a person who clearly has no mental illness and no real chance of being found incompetent; this pertains to choosing carefully how our forensic psychiatric expertise is used and not being an instrument of unethical ends (i.e., by being used to greenlight an execution), even if it is legal and does not violate official ethics guidelines.

There are also examples of the distal duty to a psychiatrist's personal ethics and values (including societal expectations of physicians) trumping proximal duty considerations. Forensic psychiatrists may reject being retained by organizations that they deem extremely unethical (e.g., racist groups, violent cults). Experts may choose not to participate in certain capital punishment roles out of a belief that the death sentence is immoral at a societal level or antithetical to societal expectations of physicians given their medical training.

Conclusion

Dialectical principlism can help experts select cases in an ethical manner. On a macro level, this ethical decision-making process can lead to improved resource allocation of forensic psychiatric expertise to promote greater social good. Many experts fail to consider or use an ethics-based approach to decision-making when faced with situations in which ethics considerations conflict. Psychiatrists may instead resort to other options, such as seeking advice from colleagues, referring to organizational ethics guidelines, or consulting with their malpractice insurance carrier or legal professionals regarding liability concerns. Use of one method may be insufficient on its own, however, when one aspires to reach the most ethical decision. For instance, although it may be useful to consult with colleagues with more experience or more knowledge about ethics questions, those colleagues may not be able to provide guidance on how to weigh and balance competing considerations. Ethics guidelines from medical and psychiatric organizations cannot apply to every nuanced situation; further, they can conflict with one another without any indication as to which should take priority, so they cannot always help determine what is most ethical for the multitude of unique situations that arise in practice. The goal of malpractice carriers and risk management professionals is to instruct practitioners on how best to prevent or reduce liability, and not necessarily about what is most ethical or most protective to third parties. Moreover, depending on their agency, they may guide practitioners on what is best to limit an employer's liability rather than the individual practitioner's.

Practitioners striving to act most ethically and do what is best for their patients and society may sometimes be more willing to assume a slightly increased liability risk. Ethical decisions related to the practice of forensic psychiatry should not be outsourced to attorneys or risk management professionals, because their roles and ethics responsibilities differ from those of psychiatrists in the forensic role. Instead, risk management professionals and attorneys should be advisors, not deciders, in these contexts to help experts minimize liability when doing what is right.

Dialectical principlism illustrates how psychiatrists can make ethics-based decisions when faced with dilemmas. Most situations do not require the complex analysis of dialectical principlism, but when they do, dialectical principlism provides a framework to inform ethics-based decision-making via identifying, prioritizing, and balancing competing considerations based on role and context. Dialectical principlism can help psychiatrists determine which action is ethically best for an individual across various roles and situational contexts. The model provides a structure both to understand what factors led to a particular ethics-based action and to articulate the rationale for the action to others.

References

American Academy of Psychiatry and the Law: Ethics Guidelines for the Practice of Forensic Psychiatry. Adopted May 2005. Bloomfield, CT, American Academy of Psychiatry and the Law, 2005. Available at: https://www.aapl.org/ethics-guidelines. Accessed October 1, 2020.

American Academy of Psychiatry and the Law: Ethics Questions and Answers: Opinions of the AAPL Committee on Ethics. Adopted May 2013. Bloomfield, CT, American Academy of Psychiatry and the Law, 2013. Available at: https://aapl.org/docs/pdf/Ethics%20Questions%20and%20Answers.pdf. Accessed October 1, 2020.

American Medical Association: Principles of Medical Ethics. Chicago, IL, American Medical Association, 2001

American Psychiatric Association: The Principles of Medical Ethics with Annotations Especially Applicable to Psychiatry. Arlington, VA, American Psychiatric Association, 2013

American Psychiatric Association: Opinions of the Ethics Committee on the Principles of Medical Ethics with Annotations Especially Applicable to Psychiatry. Arlington, VA, American Psychiatric Association, 2014

American Psychological Association: Ethical Principles of Psychologists and Code of Conduct. Washington, DC, American Psychological Association, 2010

Appelbaum PS: A theory of ethics for forensic psychiatry. J Am Acad Psychiatry Law 25(3):233–247, 1997 9323651

Appelbaum PS: Ethics and forensic psychiatry: translating principles into practice. J Am Acad Psychiatry Law 36(2):195–200, 2008 18583695

Beauchamp TL, Childress JF: Principles of Biomedical Ethics, 7th Edition. New York, Oxford University Press, 2013

Candilis PJ: Commentary: a new chapter for forensic ethics. J Am Acad Psychiatry Law 39(3):342–344, 2011 21908750

Candilis PJ, Martinez R: Reflections and narratives: new to the journal and to professional ethics. J Am Acad Psychiatry Law 40(1):12–13, 2012 22396337

Candilis PJ, Martinez R, Dording C: Principles and narrative in forensic psychiatry: toward a robust view of professional role. J Am Acad Psychiatry Law 29(2):167–173, 2001 11471782

Candilis PJ, Weinstock R, Martinez R: Forensic Ethics and the Expert Witness. New York, Springer Science, 2007

Cudney P: What really separates casuistry from principlism in biomedical ethics. Theor Med Bioeth 35(3):205–229, 2014 24846659

Darby WC: Ethics challenges for presenting genetic data in forensic settings. J Am Acad Psychiatry Law 49(2):179–186, 2021 33972350

Darby WC, Weinstock R: Prescribing stimulants in college populations: clinical and ethical challenges. Adolesc Psychiatry (Hilversum) 7(3):179–189, 2017

Darby WC, Weinstock R: The limits of confidentiality: informed consent and psychotherapy. Focus Am Psychiatr Publ 16(4):395–401, 2018a 31975932

Darby WC, Weinstock R: Resolving ethics dilemmas in forensic practice, in Ethics Dilemmas in Forensic Psychiatry and Psychology Practice. Edited by Griffith E. New York, Columbia University Press, 2018b, pp 7–22

Darby WC, Appelbaum PS, Martinez RP, et al: Applying Differing Forensic Ethics Approaches in a Death Penalty Case. Presented at the American Academy of Psychiatry and the Law Annual Meeting, Austin, Texas, October 2018

Darby WC, Weinstock R, Griffith E, et al: Can We Overcome Our Biases to Reach an Objective Opinion? Presented at the American Academy of Psychiatry and the Law Annual Meeting, virtual, October 2020

Darby WC, Stephens DB, Weinstock R: Evolving forensic ethics: revisiting an AAPL survey 27 years later. Paper presented at the annual meeting of the American Academy of Psychiatry and the Law, virtual, October 2021

Darby WC, MacIntyre M, Weinstock R: Pragmatic approaches to COVID-19 related ethics dilemmas for psychiatrists. J Am Acad Psychiatry Law 50(4):566–576, 2022 36220157

Diamond BL: The fallacy of the impartial expert. Archives of Criminal Psychodynamics 3(2):221–236, 1959

Dworkin R: A Matter of Principle. Cambridge, MA, Harvard University Press, 1986

Gilligan C: In a Different Voice: Psychological Theory and Women's Development. Cambridge, MA, Harvard University Press, 1982

Griffith EEH: Ethics in forensic psychiatry: a cultural response to Stone and Appelbaum. J Am Acad Psychiatry Law 26(2):171–184, 1998 9664254

Griffith EEH: Truth in forensic psychiatry: a cultural response to Gutheil and colleagues. J Am Acad Psychiatry Law 31(4):428–431, 2003 14974797

Griffith EEH: Personal narrative and an African-American perspective on medical ethics. J Am Acad Psychiatry Law 33(3):371–381, 2005 16186203

Hope T: Medical Ethics: A Very Short Introduction. New York, Oxford University Press, 2004

Kohlberg L: Essays on Moral Development, Vol 2: The Psychology of Moral Development: The Nature and Validity of Moral Stages. San Francisco, CA, Harper and Row, 1984

Martinez R, Candilis PJ: Commentary: toward a unified theory of personal and professional ethics. J Am Acad Psychiatry Law 33(3):382–385, 2005 16186204

Norko MA: Commentary: compassion at the core of forensic ethics. J Am
    Acad Psychiatry Law 33(3):386–389, 2005 16186205
Norko MA: What is truth? The spiritual quest of forensic psychiatry. J Am
    Acad Psychiatry Law 46(1):10–22, 2018 29618531
Paulo N: Casuistry as common law morality. Theor Med Bioeth 36(6):373–389,
    2015 26576963
Pollack S: The role of psychiatry in the rule of law. Psychiatr Ann 4:16–31,
    1974
Rawls J: A Theory of Justice. Cambridge, MA, Belknap Press of Harvard
    University Press, 1971
Stone AA: The ethics of forensic psychiatry: a view from the ivory tower, in
    Law, Psychiatry, and Morality. Edited by Stone AA. Washington, DC,
    American Psychiatric Press, 1985, pp 57–75
Weinstock R: Dialectical principlism: an approach to finding the most ethical
    action. J Am Acad Psychiatry Law 43(1):10–20, 2015 25770274
Weinstock R, Leong GB, Silva JA: The role of traditional medical ethics in
    forensic psychiatry, in Ethical Practice in Psychiatry and the Law. Edited
    by Rosner R, Weinstock R. New York, Plenum Press, 1990
Weinstock R, Leong GB, Silva JA: Opinions by AAPL forensic psychiatrists on
    controversial ethical guidelines: a survey. Bull Am Acad Psychiatry Law
    19(3):237–248, 1991 1777687

3

Narrative and Ethics in Forensic Psychiatry

Ezra E. H. Griffith, M.D.

Narrative has earned a place in the ethical praxis of forensic psychiatry. Lewis Mehl-Madrona (2010) noted that "stories unlock the mysteries of psychophysical suffering that declarative facts cannot reveal" and that stories can "confirm our intuitive grasp of the relationships between our life events and our bodies" (pp. 4–5). They define our identities, clarify the meanings and intentions of our actions, and describe our theories about the world. He argued that narratives establish relationships among us and are helpful in improving our connections to each other. They may be useful in medicine and general psychiatry and may also influence personal growth and healing (Mehl-Madrona 2010).

In recent years, the ubiquity of storytelling has been reinforced. There are "narratives about minority groups, children, many different professional and vocational groups, conflict, politeness, the acquisition of identity, the loss of identity, groups with particular illnesses, resilience and adversity, life change, immigration, atrocities, incest, death, and so on" (Griffith 2017, p. 128). There is also the political dimension of narrative. This is to say that storytellers often, but not always, present their accounts with the intent to influence the audience's efforts to reach a conclusion about the story's meaning. Consequently, storytelling is not always an act of gratuitous amusement.

Peter Brooks (2006) has reminded us that narrative has the potential and the power to mislead. Brooks emphasized a simultaneous struggle: on the one hand, the inevitability and irreplaceability of narrative as a vehicle of emotion; and on the other hand, its possible use to reinforce logic and reasoning. As we explore narrative in this chapter, we must continually keep in mind the imperative of framing it in the context of forensic ethics. I argue that narrative is an important tool in the work of forensic psychiatrists. Nevertheless, I will underline Brooks's point that narrative is not a simplistic ornament. Its use requires care and reflection.

I turn to Janet Malcolm's story titled "Iphigenia in Forest Hills" (Malcolm 2010). She described the trial of a female physician who was convicted of hiring a man to kill her husband. Malcolm's account provoked the following reaction from a reader: "Malcolm's mesmerizing account of the ... trial portrays it as a contest of competing narratives, where evidence is subject to opposing interpretations, and she points out the shaky details of the prosecution's case" (Miller 2010). The reader hypothesized that the guilty verdict resulted from the prosecution's ability to offer a clearer explanation than what was provided by the defense to explain the motive for the killing. The prosecution's proposed story was that the defendant's anger and desire for revenge were due to her losing custody of her daughter to the estranged husband. In Malcolm's tale, we have an analysis that includes reference to court performance by actors in the trial, opposing narratives presented in court, the problem of bias, and the jury's task of contending with contradictory stories flowing from the same facts. I make use of Malcolm's narrative to emphasize that employing narrativity in our forensic work has its risks. The search for truth may at times be elusive and uncertain.

In this chapter, I make clear that the recounting of stories is important. There is room for narrativity in our work. I discuss how narratives have entered medicine and forensic psychiatry. I touch on some of what we have learned about their construction and analysis from other disciplines. I review how forensic psychiatrists have recently sought to improve their use of narrative by exploring elements such as empathy, dignity, performance, and cultural context. Throughout my discussion I am mindful of the important task, articulated by Adshead (2014), of combining a narrative approach in forensic psychiatry with a narrative approach to ethics. Then I contemplate the practical problems inherent in applying narrative to forensic work.

In concluding this introduction, I present these words from Brooks (2006, p. 13):

> Narratives do not simply recount happenings; they give them shape, give them a point, argue their import, proclaim their results. And to do so, they necessarily espouse some sort of "point of view" or perspective, however hidden it may be, even from narrators themselves.

Narrative in Medicine

Rita Charon called it "narrative medicine" and pointed out that the health care professions began to take note sometime after World War II that the "most fertile and clinically salient information we derive about patients comes from listening to them talking about their illnesses" (Charon 2006, p. 192). Clinicians gradually began to understand more clearly the significance of listening to the patient's experience of living with illness. Both patients and caregivers need these stories to make sense of the patient's illness.

Charon (2006) emphasized that these conversations between patients and clinicians were an essential early step in a process of self-examination that led to mutual recognition and respect, reflection on the relationship, and eventual change in their interactions. This transformation was aided by broader social movements such as feminism and consumerism. In the 1970s, the academic discipline of literature and medicine began to flower, with doctors entering the patient's narrative world with greater ease and seeing themselves and the stories as broader therapeutic agents. Charon cited the example of the physician's developing anew the skill of staying the course, "accompanying patients with presence instead of abandoning them to fear" (Charon 2006, p. 197).

Annemarie Mol (2002) deepened understanding of "talking bodies," of penetrating these conversations that should go on among health professionals but also between clinician and patient. Mol dissolved the old distinction between disease and illness, between pathology and the psychosocial. She wanted the narrative to include an understanding of the practicalities of living daily with a diseased body. Part of the clinical task is being aware of what clinicians do to "make things visible, audible, tangible, knowable" (Mol 2002, p. 33). Thus, there is an ethnographic dimension to narrative medicine that is fundamental to conceptualizing narrative in forensic psychiatry. Mol agreed that the pathologist and internist may discuss differently the blockage of an artery. However, she pointed out that the enactments of pathologist, internist, and other specialists will be used interactively to make sense of the therapeutic plan. That plan should be developed with attention to the storied complaints of the patient and consideration of how the patient lives with the disease of atherosclerosis.

There are two powerful recent examples of narrative medicine that I would recommend to readers. The first exemplifies the effort of a physician to talk about a patient's disease. The author is Arthur Kleinman (2019). The story is about his wife, Joan, who is suffering from Alzheimer's disease. A physician and medical anthropologist, Kleinman recognized that his role as caregiver changed and took on new meaning when he assumed his wife's care at home. Her doctors wanted to talk biomedicine while he wanted to chat about the impact of the disease on his wife and on himself. It was challenging, too, as she progressively lost the capacity to contribute to her own story.

The second text that I call to readers' attention is by Véronique Griffith (Griffith et al. 2020). It is an ethnographic illustration of Mol's theorizing, focused this time on endometriosis. In the text, patients with endometriosis talk about their diseased bodies and what it means to live with the pain and stigma of the disease. In addition, Griffith observes the enactments practiced by physicians and nurses in endometriosis clinics. We have reports of what patients say about their own bodies, their interactions with caregivers, and their complaints about being ignored and left to suffer. Griffith demonstrates the power of narrative, even including patients' visual art accounts of their suffering, reinforcing the intended meanings of the patients' verbal accounts. Griffith's use of the patients' art amplifies their voices and enhances the dialogue between patient and caregiver, while contextualizing the patients' suffering.

Narrative and Ethics in Forensic Psychiatry

The use of verbal and visual storytelling recalls the efforts by Gergen and Gergen (2006) to illustrate different methodological uses of narrative in general psychiatry. They illustrated examples of what they called *narratives in action*: in psychotherapy, organizational transformation, and conflict resolution. This is a reminder that narratives have had a place in psychiatry for a long time, which is no doubt why Mehl-Madrona (2010) talked of the promise of narrative psychiatry. Here I consider the reemergence of narrative in forensic psychiatry during the last few decades. In doing so, however, I point out that the alienist Dr. Walter Channing was pleased to use narrative in discussing expert forensic testimony delivered in a New Hampshire murder trial more than a century ago (Channing 1898).

I suggest that the renewal of narrative in forensic psychiatry coincided with developments in forensic psychiatry ethics. Observers often say that a major conversation about forensic psychiatry ethics started in 1982 when Alan Stone delivered a lecture at the annual meeting of the American Academy of Psychiatry and the Law (Stone 1984). In his presentation, Stone rejected all the ethics principles that forensic psychiatrists could use as a moral anchor for their forensic work and characterized forensic psychiatry as "a quintessentially lawless activity" (Appelbaum 1997, p. 234). Appelbaum emphasized Stone's point that the "bedrock principles of beneficence and nonmaleficence, to which medicine had looked historically, were outside the clinical realm" (Appelbaum 1997, p. 234). In reaction to this bleak view of the ethics basis for forensic psychiatry practice, forensic psychiatrists began to comment on possible ways of responding by suggesting elements that might constitute a theory of forensic psychiatry ethics.

The American Academy of Psychiatry and the Law also began to focus more attention on contemplating ethics principles that might govern the practice activities of its members. The next milestone came when Appelbaum (1997) published his theory of ethics for forensic psychiatry practice. In it, he articulated the concepts of "truth-telling" and of "respect for persons" that he wished to be applied to forensic psychiatry. Appelbaum noted that the primary value in such a theory was to advance the interests of justice. This was different from the values of clinical psychiatrists that were embedded in the traditional physician-patient relationship. Because the evaluees in forensic psychiatry are not considered patients, the bedrock physician-patient relationship of clinical work could not be of use in conceptualizing ethics for forensic psychiatry.

In 1998, I critiqued these ideas offered by Stone and Appelbaum and offered suggestions (Griffith 1998). There is no way of getting past my objections to Stone's claims. He wanted forensic experts out of the courtroom, and I was disheartened by his desire (Griffith 1998). It saddened me because, as a Black forensic psychiatrist, I could not see how any minority-group defendants could benefit from a lack of access to the help of forensic specialists. At the time, I had in mind the image of a thoughtful, well-prepared forensic psychiatrist carrying out a thorough forensic evaluation and then explaining in court how the findings could shed light on biomedical and psychosocial factors related to the index event that had brought the defendant to court. One might say that I felt there was, in Stone's thesis, a modicum of inattention to the needs of minorities.

What about the theory of ethics that Appelbaum advanced for the discipline of forensic psychiatry? While agreeing that he made an important and useful contribution to the field, I believed that his position needed to be fleshed out and made more directly relevant to the special needs of minority groups (Griffith 1998). I did not disagree with him about the general utility of truth-telling and respect for the defendant's person. While those values represented reasonable guidelines, they did not reflect recognition of the status of nondominant professionals and group members in the broad cultural scheme of the United States. In other words, the pursuit of truth-telling and respect for persons did not consider the inequities between dominant and nondominant group members that so permeate our society. I was concerned that, for example, some psychiatrists might carry out their forensic evaluations with greater thoroughness and attention to truth-telling and respect for persons when evaluating dominant group members as opposed to others. After all, these inequities in care were well known.

I searched for a method that would enhance thoroughness in our work and sharpen focus on the usual problem of disparities in medical practice. I recommended use of the cultural formulation in forensic psychiatry. In practice, this meant that "the evaluating forensic specialist understand the subject's personal perspective on the incident under review; the cultural identity of the individual such as behavioral or ideological ethnicity; cultural factors relevant to the individual's illness; cultural factors relating to the individual's social environment and functioning; and any relevant intercultural elements of the relationship between the evaluator and his subject. ... The cultural formulation should serve to construct a fuller story of how the forensic event occurred" (Griffith 1998, p. 181). One could agree that Appelbaum's emphasis on the ethics elements should improve forensic praxis. However, I felt a need for a more robust effort to integrate those cultural elements into our work. Hence the reliance on a mechanism, such as the cultural formulation, that is integrated into the narrative we create to communicate our findings. It should therefore be clear that I was not advocating the use of narrative in forensic psychiatry devoid of ethics elements such as truth-telling and respect for persons. The integration of the cultural formulation into narrative tends to enhance the fullness of the story, which in turn augments truth-telling and respects the humanity of our evaluees.

I have found this renewed discussion of narrative in forensic psychiatry to be an important arena of progress in the profession. The interest in narrative has catalyzed a special body of work by a cadre of forensic psychiatrists who have examined what constitutes, in Mol's terminology (Mol 2002), the enactments carried out by forensic specialists. This work has focused in large part on ways to improve forensic narrative while keeping an eye on the ethics principles that serve as a guardrail to maintain the boundaries of ethics-based praxis. I believe that a useful summary of this basic work is captured in essays by Candilis and colleagues (2001), Griffith (2005), Martinez and Candilis (2005), and Norko (2005).

Norko (2005) pointed out that "thoroughness" in our work cannot be relied on to transform our work. He preferred to focus on "compassion" and argued that its use extends the boundaries of the forensic psychiatrist's task and illustrates how narrative might effectively protect disadvantaged evaluees. The expert who uses compassion in evaluations extends the work in a context of human endeavor and places the work on a bedrock of authentic struggle. This leads us to "engage the humanity of all the subjects of our evaluations" (Norko 2005, p. 389).

Martinez and Candilis (2005) approached their argument from a different vantage point. They argued that narratives of our personal and professional lives serve as sources of our moral compass. It is through our personal narratives that we create the values so important in our lives. They stated that ethics lacked power if built merely on principles, without narrative. To them, narrative enriched ethics principles. Furthermore, they saw value in having the principles tested against the stories of our vulnerable defendants. I was drawn also to another point by Martinez and Candilis, that the professionalism of our discipline should involve principles as well as evolving moral aspirations. Personal and cultural stories should help us think about what the profession stands for and how we can remain self-critical. This is advocacy for their views of robust professionalism (Candilis et al. 2001).

Other scholars have been looking at different enactments involved in creation of the forensic narrative. For example, Brodsky and Wilson (2013) examined the role of empathy in forensic evaluations, arguing that it may be a useful assessment tool. Others have written extensively about the different narratives that emerge from the different terrains that characterize the geographic and social context of a crime. Examples are stories from prisons, refugee camps, sex offender clinics, and juvenile detention facilities. Darby and Weinstock (2018), while making use of narrative and other approaches to forensic psychiatry praxis, have emphasized the ethics dimension of the work. Their dialectical-principlism model integrates narrative, principlism, and other approaches to help forensic specialists identify, weigh, and balance the competing considerations that guide ethics decision-making.

Narrative Construction and Analysis

Forensic psychiatrists should be aware that in the last several decades, relevant discourse about narrative has been flowering. Candilis et al. (2007) approached their discussion of narrative from an ethics framework. Buchanan and Norko (2011) focused squarely on conceptualization of the forensic report. Griffith and colleagues (2017) thought of narrative in the context of overall changes in the evolution and modernization of forensic psychiatry. I note, too, that scholars have examined narrative in the operation of United States asylum hearings (Feldman 2012), a venue that has been of increasing interest to the forensic expert.

Gwen Adshead (2011, 2014) asserted that the criminal court is a place for the examination of tragedy, akin to the early ideas of the Greek tragedians. She pointed out that the forensic report acts as a tragic narrative that humanizes defendants and makes them into actors in a drama. In the context of Greek tragedy, however, the defendant-protagonist is often caught up in something violent, unreasonable, and irreparable. Adshead theorized that the tragic narrative in our forensic work may represent an attempt to make meaning out of meaningless suffering. She noted the presence of the defendant's voice in the report and commented insightfully that the process of weighting the defendant's voice often presented an important ethics dilemma.

Adshead (2011) described the forensic narrator's task of creating a story about the evaluee, enunciating choices along the way based on a point of view, a personalized construction of the world, and personal values. The narrator reveals the evaluee's voice but then adds layers of nuance and meaning. This is where language and metaphor come into play in the written report, and diction and other stylistic uses of the narrator's body enter the court presentation. Adshead (2014) has drawn attention to the expert's interest in refashioning the evaluee's identity in the story. She has particularly emphasized the narrator's penchant for telling monster stories that tend to frighten the community.

She underlined the common reality that under our adversarial legal system, even stories of monsters may be readjusted by sympathetic listeners to be narratives of individuals who have been temporarily lost in life's thickets of bad luck. In this context, then, she insisted that forensic experts should appreciate that they engage in the construction of competing narratives. This opens the door to potential ethics dilemmas. She concluded that forensic experts must strive to be aware of what they are doing in their work and why they are doing it. They should also work at understanding the relation between their enactments and their beliefs and values, both conscious and unconscious (Adshead 2011, 2014).

Adshead (2011) highlighted another point that deserves our attention and that, to my knowledge, has not been explored thoroughly in the forensic literature. She explained that in the usual criminal court system, the adversarial context serves as a constraint to keep limits on the breadth of the stories we create. The cross-examination tests the narrator and imposes certain cultural limits on the stories so that they are not inherently outlandish and beyond the understanding of the audience. However, she suggested that in other courts, such as family court, where the adversarial struggle is not so pronounced and part of the established court ritual, these constraints may not be as evident. She went so far as to argue that in family court, dramatic narratives may detract from the task of finding solutions that contribute to the flourishing of the child and family. In another example, the immigration court, Adshead (2011) and Feldman (2012) suggested that the focus on the credibility of the immigrant-refugee may ultimately raise questions about the stories recounted in these courts, as the foundational basis of the narrative is often hard to verify.

Comments by Brooks (2006) on the construction and analysis of narrative also deserve discussion. He focused on narratology in the law, but I think his line of argument is instructive and relevant to our purposes. At the outset, I note that Brooks appreciated the power of narrative to contribute to the understanding of human action and human beings. As I stated in the chapter introduction, however, he understood the potential of narrative to mislead and to misconvict. Still, he recommended that "the law needs to become more conscious of its storytelling functions and procedures" (Brooks 2006, p. 28). I would make the same recommendation to the discipline of forensic psychiatry. Brooks's emphatic point was that "narrative is not reducible to other kinds of speech and argument, and since it is not, it demands analytic consideration in its own right" (Brooks 2006, p. 5).

Brooks was not timid in his critique of narrative related to the law. He scoffed at lawyers' narratives that took on a tone of decisiveness when they were full of contradictions. He talked of narrative as "an act of ventriloquism" when the narrator pretends that the account is the direct words of a witness, but it is in fact indirect language or "narrated monologue" (Brooks 2006, p. 8). He pointed out that narrators may slip readily into errors of authenticity and integrity in their stories. He thought of these kinds of mistakes as a way of avoiding responsibility in the telling of the story. Thus, little imagination is necessary to understand why we tell our trainees to work hard at verifying aspects of stories by seeking different witnesses who can report on an event. Brooks also mentioned the problem of "perspectival narrative," which can result in our having "four different retellings of what we know is the 'same' story—the story of what happened between a man and a woman one night" (Brooks 2006, p. 10).

He suggested that one might explain this difference in meaning by noting how the "narrative glue" used by each narrator to combine the incidents and events in the story is different (Brooks 2006, p. 10). The glue derives from the narrator's perspective and may consequently lead to the situation where, in a single case, some observers reach a narrative conclusion of consensual sex and others reach a conclusion of rape. These results may have been influenced by narrators' values, beliefs, and conscious and unconscious conceptual notions linked to culture. A telling point from Brooks is that even judges at the appeals-court level don't always seem to grasp how they recast stories from the trial court to arrive at their desired legal judgments. Thus, the connections among facts and events may be established, by expediency, to create a single coherent narrative from a collection of possibilities. It is the urge to make sense of the evidence in disarray before us that drives us to put things into narrative order.

Brooks (2006) briefly contemplated how these difficulties appear when we engage in creating reports that describe the future dangerousness of an evaluee, such as victim impact statements and death penalty reports. Adshead (2011, 2014) cautioned us about reports that center on the monstrous dimensions of our evaluees. Most forensic experts quickly appreciate the pitfalls in describing how a civil event has affected the day-to-day functioning of an evaluee. These narratives are obviously subject to conscious and unconscious use of prejudice, exaggeration, distortion, and descriptive richness. The trouble is that while we are committing all these sins in the narrative, we may be insisting that what we say is neutral. We enjoy thinking that we are merely describing events as they unfolded in the forensic happening.

There is good reason for lawyers to study narrative, but Brooks recommended caution. We should not let stories manipulate us to the point where we begin to think that storytelling is the same as real life. I think it commonplace for experts to jump to a conclusory storyline based on skimpy facts, instead of working to see what witnesses have to say about what transpired during the actual incident. For example, one may learn that a man invited a young woman to his apartment. The expert never asked what happened in the apartment, but assumed he knew what transpired because it is common knowledge how men behave once they have invited a woman to private quarters. The basis of the assumption is unclear. The expert's conclusion may appear, in Brooks's language, "sufficiently plausible." However, the lack of a verified factual basis suggests that the expert may well be unaware of the problem of "irresponsible authorship" of narrative (Brooks 2006, p. 27).

There are some other elements that I wish to reemphasize in this section of the chapter. Forensic narratives are rarely meant simply to transmit information to an audience. Generally, we intend to persuade the audience to accept the narrative that we are presenting. Thus, there is political intent in our work (Griffith and Baranoski 2011) and the espousing of a point of view (Brooks 2006). There is also coloring of the narrative because our personal identities flow into what we write and influence our perspectives. Sometimes we are invited to represent our evaluees, to compensate for their weakness or absence of voice (Cavallo 2000). These elements are significant in understanding the complexity of narrative as applied to the praxis of forensic psychiatry. This supports the need for a narratology in forensic psychiatry training, at least because the narrative is intertwined with forensic ethics.

Truth, Empathy, Compassion, and Dignity

Michael Norko declared boldly at the beginning of his disquisition that "the search for truth is a foundational aim and value of forensic psychiatry" (Norko 2018, p. 10). He elevated truth-telling in our work to the place of a spiritual exercise, seemingly substantially higher than the position to which Appelbaum (1997) originally allocated it. In fact, Norko (2018, p.10) claimed that there are certain attitudes and activities that "occupy the groundwork of forensic practice and form pathways to truth." In his view, several constitutive values were presence, empathy, compassion, and centering. Searching for truth and truth-telling in our work is not a simplistic, palpably objective pursuit. The forensic expert does not turn on a searchlight and go looking for truth in secret corners. The expert must be thoughtful about purpose and meaning in the work. This is where a willingness to be present, compassionate, and empathic comes into play.

By this point in the chapter, I hope that it is clearer how and why Norko (2018, p. 15) felt justified in asserting that "empathy and compassion are the tools of presence." By pulling together contributions from many scholars, he integrated these elements into a tool that can be used in the creation of narrative, oral or written. I have often imagined the forensic expert sitting quietly, preparing for the start of an evaluation. This is a time to recall the elements that help establish contact and initiate an inquiry into the event that led to the individual being an evaluee in a forensic context.

Scholars have considered other elements in discussing these foundational aims and values of forensic psychiatry. Buchanan (2015) and Griffith and Greenidge (2020) contributed to conversations about human dignity and its relation to forensic psychiatry ethics. Briefly, their thesis rests on the notion that our interactive evaluation of an individual may be influenced by our thoughts about the individual's humanity. Seeing the individual as having human dignity will get us closer to balanced stories and away from Adshead's tales of tragic monsters that may essentially represent one-sided pictures of complex human beings.

Other work of this genre has focused on the problem of bias. One good example is a contribution by Sidhu and Candilis (2018) on biased attitudes against women that may permeate our work; another is an editorial by Martinez and Candilis (2020) that reminds forensic specialists about the necessity of being attuned to the stories of individuals caught in systems and institutions that perpetuate racism and injustice. The authors highlighted distinctive attitudes, commonly found in the general community, that can have deleterious effects via the distortion of narrative. Related psychoanalytic scholarship has shed light on attitudes derived from "experiences of hating and being hated" (White 2002). For example, some minority groups may be objects of destructive racist attributions—of being hated. Some may internalize insults that result in their hating themselves. Others may respond with their own racialized hatred, characterized by externalized violence and destruction. This work may well deepen the possibility of more explanatory mechanisms being used in narrative. It may also minimize the presence of bias in what we do.

Gherovici and Christian (2019) edited a text focused on the use of psychoanalysis in Latinx barrios. The text criticized the notion that poor people are underdeveloped and reachable only as objects of charitable activities. The objective was to make clear that working psychoanalytically with poor people is no longer some sort of suspicious activity. Poor people have an unconscious. This position reinforces the notion that seeing the humanity in others may affect how we offer ourselves as helpers and caregivers to others who are disadvantaged. This expansion of forensic narrative explication is a welcome dimension of our work. It should enhance forensic professionalism and the connection between narrative and ethics through truth-telling and respect for persons.

Application to Forensic Praxis

I have provided considerable theorizing to this point in discussing narrative and ethics in forensic psychiatry. I have reviewed my own dissatisfaction with Stone's position, that we have little to offer. I have stated how I arrived at the conclusion that narrative offers a useful framework for reconceptualizing what we do in our profession. I have been mindful of several pitfalls to avoid in developing a forensic narrative. I look finally to the task of integrating these principles and ideas into the art of creating the narrative. This is a brief review, as Buchanan and Norko (2011) and Griffith et al. (2010) have set out in detail fundamental concepts concerning forensic narrative. It should now be clear that the forensic narrative is not a simplistic recitation of information from the evaluation. It is the refashioning of the information into the narrative that makes the work performative (Griffith et al. 2010).

Initiating a forensic narrative assumes that the narrator has carried out the requisite evaluation, interviewed relevant witnesses, reviewed pertinent documents, and studied other data that bear directly or indirectly on the matter at hand. The forensic expert should also think about whether consultation with other experts may contribute value to the narrative. Thoroughness in these activities must be understood as a fundamental mark of respect for the evaluee. It also sharpens and deepens precision in the narrative.

The narrative is usually structured into three major parts. The introduction describes the purpose of the report, identifies who has hired the expert and who has been examined and interviewed, and reviews documents (including video and audio recordings and other forms of information such as medical reports, wills, or statutes). The introduction is usually the shortest of the report's three sections.

Nevertheless, scrutiny of it can reveal bias or simple dereliction of duty. Cross-examiners critique this all the time—for example, why did the doctor see the defendant only once for 2 hours in a murder case? Or why is there no listing of an examination done by a psychologist in a case of claimed psychological deficits?

The second part of the report is informative, with an emphasis on describing the information collected from the sources enumerated in the introduction. Performative techniques come into play here, although not as boldly as in the third section of the report. Here the narrator claims to report authentically what the defendant said, but then emphasizes or deemphasizes the defendant's words. This is where we see the problems of perspectival narrative mentioned earlier. In this section, it is easy to take the medical report from a treating physician and heighten or diminish its relevance depending on the desired outcome in the conclusion of the report.

The third part of the report is the discussion and the conclusion. The narrator describes the form of narrative adopted in the specific case. Emphasis may be put on how much the plaintiff has suffered in a discrimination case or an instance of personal injury. The narrator supports the adopted storyline and cites from the professional literature to buttress a particular claim. This section may be replete with the sufficiently plausible arguments cited before and lack serious support from the major event or the collateral witnesses. It is, too, the natural terrain for practical use of compassion, empathy, and dignity in tasks of representation and identity within the narrative.

Conclusion

Darby and Weinstock (2018) stated:

> [W]hen faced with conflicting duty considerations in forensic work (e.g., answering the legal question, showing respect for persons, consideration of cultural factors, societal discrimination, biomedical ethics principles related to the evaluee), narrative alone does not necessarily guide decision making, because it is not clear what considerations take primacy in the forensic context." (pp. 12–13)

They then noted that in a 2016 lecture, I acknowledged this problem and endorsed an integrative approach of applying the technique of ethics principlism to the narrative model to resolve this difficulty in practice. They were right.

Darby and Weinstock usefully reemphasized their point, which affords me the opportunity to underline an important issue at this juncture. No rigid application of any ethics approach will serve forensic psychiatrists well in their work. This comes up as pointedly in the application of principlism, when one is trying to balance proximal and distal commitments, as in the enactment of narrative. Darby and Weinstock noted that the weighing of ethics principles derived from "the unique set of personal, cultural, and societal values created from an individual's unique narrative" (Darby and Weinstock 2018, p. 14). I agree and argued this point when I discussed the connection between personal narrative and ethics (Griffith 2005). It is clear to me now that melding narrative (with the emphasis on psychocultural elements) and ethics butts against the question of whether there are universal norms that apply to all cultures. Prograis and Pellegrino (2007) discussed this matter in reviewing the place of an African American perspective in bioethics. Their conclusion was that it is currently difficult to resolve this debate, especially in the face of increasing emphasis on diversity in Western culture. Flexible integration of narrative and ethics principles seems necessary, as we continue the discussion.

References

Adshead G: Commentary: thereby hangs a tale—the creation of tragic narratives in forensic psychiatry. J Am Acad Psychiatry Law 39(3):364–369, 2011 21908753

Adshead GMJ: Commentary: stories and histories in forensic psychiatry. J Am Acad Psychiatry Law 42(4):437–442, 2014 25492069

Appelbaum PS: A theory of ethics for forensic psychiatry. J Am Acad Psychiatry Law 25(3):233–247, 1997 9323651

Brodsky SL, Wilson JK: Empathy in forensic evaluations: a systematic reconsideration. Behav Sci Law 31(2):192–202, 2013 23188692

Brooks P: Narrative transactions: does the law need a narratology? Yale J Law Humanities 18:1–28, 2006

Buchanan A: Respect for dignity and forensic psychiatry. Int J Law Psychiatry 41:12–17, 2015 25888501

Buchanan A, Norko MA (eds): The Psychiatric Report: Principles and Practice of Forensic Writing. New York, Cambridge University Press, 2011

Candilis PJ, Martinez R, Dording C: Principles and narrative in forensic psychiatry: toward a robust view of professional role. J Am Acad Psychiatry Law 29(2):167–173, 2001 11471782

Candilis PJ, Weinstock R, Martinez R: Forensic Ethics and the Expert Witness. New York, Springer, 2007

Cavallo S: Witness: the real, the unspeakable, and the construction of narrative. J Midwest Mod Lang Assoc 33:1–2, 2000

Channing W: Medical expert testimony in the Kelley murder trial. Am J Insanity 54:385–417, 1898

Charon R: The self-telling body. Narrative Inq 16:191–200, 2006

Darby WC, Weinstock R: Resolving ethics dilemmas in forensic practice, in Ethics Challenges in Forensic Psychiatry and Psychology Practice. Edited by Griffith EEH. New York, Columbia University Press, 2018, pp. 7–22

Feldman C: A Truthful Accounting of Events: The Roles of Linguistic Strategy, Narrative, and Performance in United States Hearings, 2012. Senior Projects, Spring, 2012. Paper 1. Available at: http://digitalcommons.bard.edu/senproj_s2012/1. Accessed January 2, 2021.

Gergen MM, Gergen KJ: Narratives in action. Narrative Inq 16:112–121, 2006

Gherovici P, Christian C (eds): Psychoanalysis in the Barrios: Race, Class and the Unconscious. London, Routledge, 2019

Griffith EEH: Ethics in forensic psychiatry: a cultural response to Stone and Appelbaum. J Am Acad Psychiatry Law 26(2):171–184, 1998 9664254

Griffith EEH: Personal narrative and an African-American perspective on medical ethics. J Am Acad Psychiatry Law 33(3):371–381, 2005 16186203

Griffith EEH: Narrative and performance in forensic psychiatry and psychology practice, in Bearing Witness to Change: Forensic Psychiatry and Psychology Practice. Edited by Griffith EEH, Norko MA, Buchanan A, et al. Boca Raton, FL, CRC Press, 2017, pp 117–134

Griffith EEH, Baranoski M: Oral performance, identity, and representation in forensic psychiatry. J Am Acad Psychiatry Law 39(3):352–363, 2011 21908752

Griffith EEH, Greenidge NE: Dignity and transcultural forensic consultation. J Am Acad Psychiatry Law JAAPL.200021–20, 2020 32675331

Griffith EEH, Stankovic A, Baranoski M: Conceptualizing the forensic psychiatry report as performative narrative. J Am Acad Psychiatry Law 38(1):32–42, 2010 20305072

Griffith EEH, Norko MA, Buchanan A, et al (eds): Bearing Witness to Change: Forensic Psychiatry and Psychology Practice. Boca Raton, FL, CRC Press, 2017

Griffith VAS: Healers and Patients Talk: Narratives of a Chronic Gynecological Disease. Lanham, MD, Lexington Books, 2020

Kleinman A: The Soul of Care: The Moral Education of a Husband and a Doctor. New York, Viking, 2019

Malcolm J: Iphigenia in Forest Hills. The New Yorker, May 3, 2010, pp. 34–63

Martinez R, Candilis PJ: Commentary: toward a unified theory of personal and professional ethics. J Am Acad Psychiatry Law 33(3):382–385, 2005 16186204

Martinez R, Candilis P: Ethics in the time of injustice. J Am Acad Psychiatry Law 48(4):428–430, 2020 32900819

Mehl-Madrona L: Healing the Mind Through the Power of Story. Rochester, VT, Bear & Co., 2010

Miller C: On trial. The New Yorker, May 24, 2010

Mol A: The Body Multiple: Ontology in Medical Practice. Durham, NC, Duke University Press, 2002

Norko MA: Commentary: compassion at the core of forensic ethics. J Am Acad Psychiatry Law 33(3):386–389, 2005 16186205

Norko MA: What is truth? The spiritual quest of forensic psychiatry. J Am Acad Psychiatry Law 46(1):10–22, 2018 29618531

Prograis L, Pellegrino ED (eds): African American Bioethics: Culture, Race, and Identity. Washington, DC, Georgetown University Press, 2007

Sidhu N, Candilis P: Feminism and forensic ethics, in Ethics Challenges in Forensic Psychiatry and Psychology Practice. Edited by Griffith EEH. New York, Columbia University Press, 2018, pp 23–39

Stone AA: The ethical boundaries of forensic psychiatry: a view from the ivory tower. Bull Am Acad Psychiatry Law 12(3):209–219, 1984 6478062

White KP: Surviving hating and being hated. Contemp Psychoanal 38:401–422, 2002

4

Robust Professionalism

Forensic Psychiatry's Identity and Purpose

Richard Martinez, M.D., M.H.

Philip Candilis, M.D.

As a relatively young subspecialty, forensic psychiatry has slowly recognized the unique dilemmas peculiar to its practice. Torn between its historical roots in the traditions of medicine and its practice within the institutions and rituals of law, forensic psychiatry has struggled to define its identity and purpose. The law provides social order; the ethical value of adversarial advocacy is foundational to its identity and purpose. Psychiatry's foundational values derive from the values of medicine—avoiding harm, providing benefit, and caring for and healing patients. They define psychiatry's identity and purpose. Before the American Academy of Psychiatry and the Law (AAPL) came to be more than 50 years ago and formal fellowship training began more than 30 years ago, most forensic psychiatrists were clinical psychiatrists (Rappeport 1982). Subsequently, forensic psychology followed developments in forensic psychiatry, becoming its own subspecialty within the social sciences.

Early forensic thinkers identified unique ethical dilemmas in forensic practice, including potential conflicts with informed consent and confidentiality, the problem of *dual roles* (Strasburger et al. 1997). Others underscored the dilemma of applying traditional medical ethics principles to evaluations responding to legal questions (Candilis and Martinez 2017). Some focused on standards in reports (Simon 2007); others applied clinical ethics and case studies to ethical problems (Ciccone and Clements 1984a, 1984b, 2001). Robert Weinstock (1986, 1988, 1989) assessed the profession's perceptions about ethical problems, and Thomas Gutheil and colleagues explored the unique challenges experts face in the courtroom (Gutheil et al. 2003).

Although forensic psychiatry emerged from general psychiatry as a specialized practice within the legal system, a clear consensus on its purpose or goals has yet to develop. The long-standing debate about whether forensic psychiatry is a specialized practice within the ethical framework of medicine or a practice beholden to legal goals has hampered the development of such a consensus. Our own work over the last 20 years has encouraged an integrated model for professionalism in forensic psychiatry that we label *robust professionalism*—an approach to this tension between medicine and law (Candilis et al. 2001; Martinez and Candilis 2005).

Ethical Approaches

In general, the issue of what is ethical can best be appreciated by an examination of ethical dilemmas, positing obligations for and against an action or inaction and considering the consequences. What ethical conflicts exist when a psychiatrist is in a clinical role and has a duty to inform third parties about a potentially dangerous patient? How does a psychiatrist weigh the duty to maintain confidentiality against breaching it because of dangers to a third party, the so-called Tarasoff duty? What ethical conflict exists when a psychiatrist decides to place an involuntary hold on a patient in an emergency setting, depriving the patient of liberty but acting to provide a beneficial intervention that avoids greater harm? These are not uncommon situations for treating psychiatrists.

Performing a competency assessment on a psychotic patient sentenced to death (a rare event in forensic practice) provides a dramatic example of ethical dilemmas peculiar to forensic psychiatrists. In a less dramatic setting, the expert must assess insanity knowing that the opinion is fraught with uncertainty and limited by the jurisdiction's statutory definition. How does one offer an opinion to a jury that is faced with the ultimate legal-moral challenge? This ethical dilemma pits the forensic psychiatrist's duty to respond to the legal question against the professional obligation to be transparent, honest, and within the scope of practice.

Before determining professional principles, rules, virtues, actions, or consequences, we advocate for better understanding of the professional basis for forensic psychiatry and, equally, an understanding of the foundational goals and purposes of the profession. What are the social goods that, to be achieved, require certain professional values and standing?

Historically, scholars in forensic psychiatry have addressed professional ethics by examining the subspecialty from three perspectives. Some have focused on the specific question of how to analyze specific ethical quandaries by applying ethical theory and decision-making; they weigh specific tensions between professions and values (Ciccone and Clements 1984a, 1984b, 2001; Gutheil et al. 1991). Others have offered a theory of ethical principles that guide professional behavior (Appelbaum 1997). Still others have addressed the specific qualities or attributes of the ethical forensic practitioner (Norko 2005).

A different approach, pursued in our work, is to ask what it means to be a professional person. How do the common goals and purposes of the subspecialty—the social goods—guide our understanding of how to be and what to do?

Goals and Purposes of Forensic Psychiatry

First, we advocate for common overarching goals and purposes of forensic psychiatry that guide all practitioners. Our subspecialists are no longer the group of individuals who first identified and formed organizations such as AAPL—forensic practice has grown to include a variety of dedicated professionals, working in diverse and varied settings, including many individuals from nondominant groups whose personal stories have shaped their perspectives.

Early scholarship on the ethical basis of forensic psychiatry was narrowly focused on the role of "forensic experts" engaged in activities of evaluation and testimony. With the expansion of professional activities to clinical services, consultative roles, administrative leadership, forensic testing, and assessment, forensic psychiatry must continue to consider its evolving professional identity and purpose. These factors affect the professional decisions and ultimate consequences for individuals and the systems in which they practice.

We begin with the presumption that forensic practice is a privilege with unique moral requirements. Forensic practice contains a diverse group of professional practitioners whose identities (e.g., ethnic, racial, gender) energize and define the profession. Forensic practitioners are in the unique position to bear witness to what they see and hear and must consider often complicated narratives in making judgments and forming opinions that result in profound consequences for other human beings.

Facing an ethical crisis of economics and organization in the 1980s, medicine defined the goals of health care that guide professional activity (Hanson and Callahan 1999); forensic mental health has yet to establish a set of goals or purposes that anchor its common social goods in those shared by medicine and law. With increased recognition of the injustices and inequities within societal systems (Martinez and Candilis 2020), we have come to appreciate that forensic mental health must move toward a consensus on goals and purposes that are unique to its practice. Here we define social goods that are obtained by an approach to professionalism that we consider *robust*.

The AAPL Ethics Guidelines begin with a definition of forensic psychiatry, but the 2005 revision does not provide a consensus statement on the social goods of forensic psychiatry (American Academy of Psychiatry and the Law 2005). Similarly, the American Psychological Association's "Specialty Guidelines for Forensic Psychologists" from 1991 (revised in 2013) describes its history but not its social goods. We consequently support efforts to prioritize a practical and theoretical professionalism that identifies the concepts, behaviors, products, or outcomes that are essential to the ethics of forensic experts, scholarship that considers attributes and virtues of the forensic professional, and strategic approaches to decision-making that provide guidance for practitioners encountering specific dilemmas. However, in the absence of a consensus about our goals and purposes—the social goods we provide—these approaches will have limitations. Just as medicine identified its core social goals and purposes, we believe it is important that forensic practice formulate a set of common goals, overarching social goods that protect both vulnerable values of justice and fairness and individuals caught in the justice system.

We have consequently identified the following goals and purposes for forensic practice (Martinez 2018; Martinez and Candilis 2020):

- To provide knowledge and understanding of people diagnosed with mental illness within legal, regulatory, administrative, governmental, public, and clinical settings.
- To provide competent and respectful care to people with mental illness in correctional and other clinical settings.
- To contribute to the nondiscriminatory truth-seeking and fairness goals of the legal system.
- To witness and narrate from forensic psychiatry's and forensic psychology's unique perspectives the suffering and inequities that accompany mental illness.
- To advocate for the destigmatization and decriminalization of people with mental illness.
- To advocate for alternatives to the narratives of polarization common in the adversarial legal system.
- To remain mindful of and address the suffering of those with mental illness.
- To advocate for research and public policy that increase understanding of mental illness, address inequities in the behavioral health system, and move toward the development of forensic and treatment interventions that decrease suffering.

Background on Ethical Approaches to Forensic Psychiatry

In the modern period, Bernard Diamond and Seymour Pollack, two prominent clinicians and scholars, contributed perspectives that continue to define the debate on the goals of the forensic expert in the courtroom. Pollack promoted the view that forensic psychiatrists must be guided by the values of the legal system. Because forensic psychiatrists are guests in the house of law and its adversarial rituals, the forensic psychiatrist must act in support of its social goods (Pollack 1971, 1974a). Pollack, a founding member of AAPL, believed that forensic psychiatry has a "specific instrumental function, the use of psychiatry for legal purposes" (Pollack 1974b, p. 18). He argued that the first principle for forensic psychiatry must be the "principle of legal dominance," and that therapeutic goals and values of psychiatry are subservient to it (Pollack 1971). Although Pollack supported advocacy through traditional activities outside the forensic role, he believed that neutrality, detachment, and objectivity were the values of the forensic psychiatrist in the role of expert evaluator.

Diamond was a prominent California forensic psychiatrist (Choper et al. 1990), an advocate for the "diminished capacity" defense, and an influence on California legislative decisions involving the interplay of psychiatry and the law (Diamond 1959). He proposed that the forensic psychiatrist should resist—even refuse to participate in—situations where one's findings would be used to distort justice. He understood that the role of the forensic psychiatrist is different from the fiduciary one of the traditional physician-patient relationship, but he did not interpret that difference to mean that the forensic psychiatrist should adapt, abandoning traditional physicianly values and becoming no more than a tool of the legal system. He wrote, "The psychiatrist is no mere technician to be used by the law as the law sees fit, nor is the science, art, and definitions of psychiatry and psychology to be redefined and manipulated by the law as it wishes" (Diamond 1992, p. 123). In contrast to Pollack's belief in objectivity and detachment, Diamond understood that "there is no such thing as a neutral, impartial witness" (Diamond 1959, p. 229). He believed that the forensic evaluator should care about how their opinion might be used in the adversarial system.

Although he did not use the same language later developed by Ezra Griffith, Diamond appreciated that the adversarial legal system involved a contest of narratives, each side attempting to promote a version of truth. Of course, the risks of distortion by diminishing complexity and obfuscating nuance work against the law's claim of seeking justice and uncovering truth. Diamond was aware of this problem and made it clear that when the expert's work would lead to "use and consequences [that] would be contrary to the professional and/or ethical judgment of the expert," the forensic psychiatrist should refuse to participate. Diamond was aware of the "hired gun" problem and was an advocate for developing the highest ethical standards to guard against it. Diamond was an early proponent for a forensic expert who was not subservient to the law but was an educator in the courtroom and to the legal profession. The legitimacy of the expert lay in the forensic psychiatrist's medical and psychiatric knowledge and expertise.

Paul Appelbaum attempted to solve this tension with his landmark article in 1997 (Appelbaum 1997). Responding to Alan Stone's (1985) criticism of forensic psychiatry, which raised doubts whether the subspecialty could legitimately operate within the legal system, Appelbaum proposed a theory of ethics that reordered certain classic principles for forensic experts. He made the principles of *truth-telling* and *respect for persons* primary for forensic practice. He did not believe that forensic experts had exclusive access to the ultimate truth, but that reports and testimony should be driven by telling what one honestly believed after a careful and thorough investigation. Integrity, thoroughness, and competency are clearly essential values for the work of forensic psychiatry. Appelbaum limited his theory to those activities that involved evaluations of individuals in administrative and legal settings. Like Pollack, he assumed that the justice system itself is invested in just outcomes and that objectivity could be achieved by honest and truth-seeking experts. He did not acknowledge that the adversarial system itself is based in competing narratives, each striving to persuade juries and judges, sometimes through distortion, bias, oversimplification, and even obfuscation. In addition, he formulated his theory without considering the conscious and unconscious ways experts may be influenced by individual beliefs and incentives; nor did he consider the failings of the systems in which forensic experts practice.

Appelbaum was concerned about the potential misunderstanding that can arise without a firm separation of roles between the roles of clinician and forensic evaluator (Appelbaum 2008). Defendants might assume that the psychiatrist is there to care and treat, an assumption that could be detrimental to their legal predicament. Likewise, by not making clear the difference between expert evaluator and clinician, the psychiatrist evaluator might inadvertently manipulate or even deceive the evaluee. Appelbaum argued, therefore, for a strict divide between the two roles. Appelbaum's framework has been a useful starting point for the last 25 years, but it clearly privileges legal ends above medical or professional ones. His approach allows for purely role-based justifications for harming evaluees. It can have the unintended impact of diminishing the obligations forensic psychiatrists have to refuse certain cases or discouraging advocacy for a more nuanced opinion when a retaining attorney pressures the expert to limit or shape their opinions to their advantage. It does not provide direction in addressing larger systemic deficiencies that result in unfair, unjust outcomes.

The Cultural Formulation and Building an Alternative Ethical Approach

In the 1990s, Ezra Griffith, former editor of *The Journal of the American Academy of Psychiatry and the Law* and a Yale professor, responded to both Appelbaum's theory and Stone's nihilistic view that forensic psychiatry did not belong in the courtroom (Griffith 1998). To understand

Griffith's contribution, one must return to Stone's original paper where he reviews the case of "Dr. Leo" to illustrate his skepticism. Stone used Leo to illustrate the intrinsic biases involved in forensic assessments, biases that discredit the forensic expert in court. Leo was a Jewish physician who in 1801 testified on behalf of a Jewish defendant prosecuted for stealing spoons. Stone portrays Leo as no more than a hired gun, given his history of appearing in other cases involving Jewish defendants, and therefore, prone to subjective and biased testimony.

Griffith used the same Dr. Leo to illustrate a different perspective. He recognized that participation in a system where the dominant culture defines the rules disenfranchises minority groups. Therefore, he argued, Leo must be seen in the context of "history, morality, and human values." Leo is acting morally by jumping into the contest, providing a perspective to counter the dominant culture and its values. Griffith posed a sympathetic view of Leo as he questioned the lost opportunity when "the nondominant group psychiatrist can stay on the outside of a process directed by the dominant group, which cannot be trusted in its dealing with nondominant group members" (Griffith 1998, p. 176).

Additionally, Griffith identified another concern with Appelbaum's approach. He argued that Appelbaum assumed that the justice system is value-neutral, uncontaminated by inequities and deficiencies that lead to unfair or disproportionate outcomes—outcomes that reveal underlying bias and racism. Appelbaum, in elevating legal ends, did not consider the ways the forensic expert may collude with a system containing bias and unfairness. Griffith argued that a mechanism for what he labeled the "cultural formulation" must be incorporated into forensic assessments in the same way that such an approach has improved clinical treatment (Griffith 2003).

In Griffith's writings, there is an approach that supports the conscientious forensic psychiatrist's "capacity to pick one's path through the minefield of forensic work that defines the accomplished expert" (Griffith 1998, p. 182). Although he rejects activism in the courtroom, he articulates why, in an imperfect and flawed justice system, forensic experts should not walk away from this reality. Instead, they should remain mindful of the ways the justice system can use the expert to obfuscate truth and perpetuate unfairness. When professionals in the legal drama distort findings or testimony for purposes of winning, the expert must resist and advocate for a more nuanced narrative (Griffith and Baranoski 2007, 2011; Griffith et al. 2010).

In 2008, Griffith published a series of articles from the 2007 AAPL Annual Meeting that featured a panel including Stone alongside him and Appelbaum. Indeed, Stone focused almost entirely on robust professionalism to moderate his views (Stone and MacCourt 2008). Griffith again argued for the importance of recognizing the inequities of the justice system. Providing a hopeful view of forensic psychiatry's future, he reasserted the reasons that forensic psychiatrists should continue courtroom work. Twenty-five years after Stone's 1982 challenge to forensic psychiatry, it was Griffith's view that the field of forensic psychiatry was evolving and setting new standards of practice. He saw as evidence of improvement the development of core competencies, fellowship training, and increased standardization of forensic evaluations. He wrote, "It is in work such as this that the forensic psychiatrist will evolve a more secure professional identity, one effectively grounded in values and technique and less assailable by the whims and fancy of other disciplines" (Griffith 2008, p. 205).

Building on Griffith's work, Michael Norko, also a Yale professor, provided a convincing argument for the importance of compassion in forensic practice (Norko 2005). Finding support in our call for "compassionate professional involvement" (Candilis et al. 2001, p. 169), Norko stressed that the nature of forensic work—where trauma, violence, and loss are frequent themes—challenges the expert to remain aware and to seek understanding of the humanity of those in the forensic encounter. As president of AAPL, Norko extended his concept of compassion and invited forensic psychiatrists to consider forensic practice a "calling," a true spiritual activity (Norko 2018).

Alec Buchanan, a colleague of Norko's, has advocated forcefully for a related approach that places the inherent dignity or worth of all human beings at the foundation of forensic practice (Buchanan 2014, 2015). Buchanan reminds the profession that even if some evaluations may harm someone, experts should remain contextually aware and avoid objectifying evaluees. Elevating human dignity, even in persons who have committed horrendous crimes, protects both a vulnerable value and vulnerable people, while at the same time reminding the forensic evaluator that a relational encounter lies at the center of all evaluations.

Robust Professionalism

In our writings on professionalism, we embraced Griffith's "cultural formulation." With an appreciation of narrative understanding, skepticism about moral justifications that emerge strictly from role identity, the importance of integrating personal morality with professional roles, and concern about an ethical approach that supports legal goals over traditional medical or professional ones, we began to consider an integrated concept of forensic professionalism (Candilis and Martinez 2006; Martinez and Candilis 2005). During our work toward a theory of professionalism for forensic practice, we coined the term *robust professionalism* (Candilis et al. 2001; Martinez and Candilis 2005). As forensic psychiatrists with backgrounds in professional and health care ethics, we turned to colleagues in the health care ethics literature, with specific attention to the growing literature on professionalism in medical practice (Cruess and Cruess 1997; Cruess et al. 2014; Hafferty and Castellani 2009; Irby and Hamstra 2016).

Cruess and Cruess (1997, 2008), for example, considered professionalism much more than a list of attributes or qualities. They emphasized the importance of the social contract between professions and society, highlighting that professional status is not an inherent right but is negotiated with society based on the trustworthiness of the profession and fulfilling societal expectations. In other words, the status and value of a profession are directly measured by the profession's contribution to the social good.

Managed care reform in the 1980s and 1990s resulted in growing concerns that medicine was losing sight of its core purposes and goals. It required a review and redefinition of its professional identity. The Hastings Center initiated an international effort to redefine the goals and purposes of health care across nations and cultures (Hanson and Callahan 1999). In their publication defining common goals for health care practice, the authors identified four:

1. The prevention of disease and injury and the promotion of and maintenance of health;
2. The relief of pain and suffering caused by maladies;
3. The care and cure of those with a malady and the care of those who cannot be cured;
4. The avoidance of premature death and the pursuit of a peaceful death.

Increasingly, the work of ethicists and others established that professionalism in health care practice can be understood only by linking it to the *social goods* that come from the provision of health care.

The former director of the AMA Institute of Ethics, Matthew Wynia, and colleagues confirmed that professionalism "protects not only vulnerable persons but also vulnerable social values" (Wynia et al. 1999, p. 1612). He defined professionalism as "an activity that involves both the distribution of a commodity and fair allocation of a social good, but that is uniquely defined according to moral relationships" (Wynia et al. 1999, p. 1612). Wynia and colleagues presented an archetypal model of professionalism. Devotion to service, public profession of values, and active participation in negotiating for the values and needs of patients were the main elements of their model. Activism in the public negotiation for the ends of medical practice was included (Wynia et al. 2014). Other frameworks for professionalism considered core virtues in the health care professional and emphasized competencies and milestones (Irby and Hamstra 2016). Cruess and colleagues (2014) likewise promoted a view of professionalism that acknowledges an evolving identity across one's professional life span.

For us, then, forensic practice can be visualized as the patient or evaluee and the forensic practitioner at the center of a spoked wheel (Martinez 2018). Each spoke that radiates to the outer rim represents the moral relational link to all involved in the forensic activity. In a sanity evaluation, for example, although one is primarily assessing the defendant, there are clear relational links to many others involved in the assessment who are affected by the expert's work: the defense attorney, the prosecutor, the judge, the jury, the victim and family, the defendant's family, and the community. The forensic psychiatrist has the responsibility to remain aware of many relationships while weighing the importance of each link.

Whether the encounter involves treatment of a forensic patient, administrative decisions, or forensic expert evaluations and opinions, robust professionalism consequently requires an integrity in forensic practice (here a wholeness or intactness) that makes moral relationships foundational to all forensic activities. It requires mindful awareness of the many connections and consequences inherent to the enterprise.

Robust professionalism recognizes that professional obligations and moral commitments cannot be captured in the language of contracts or the law. We see considerable problems with a concept of the forensic professional captured neatly by a societal role, especially a role defined by another profession. Robust professionalism considers moral dilemmas and obligations, not through strict role justifications, but through the concept of integrity (as an integrated whole), where professional aspirations and duties are joined into a unified professional practice. It is a unity that includes both the historical values of a profession and personal moral perspectives. It is reflected in both the spoken word during testimony and the written report's narrative integrity (Martinez and Candilis 2011). Recent events involving psychologists advising the CIA in torture practices are a glaring example of strict role justifications stripped of personal conscience and leading to disturbing harms (Report of the Senate Select Committee on Intelligence 2014; Rosenberg 2023).

We have similarly described what is necessary to promote aspirational professional qualities (Candilis 2009; Candilis and Martinez 2006; Candilis et al. 2001, 2007). Our traditional review of forensic psychiatry's struggle with divided allegiances rejects the polarizing perspectives of Pollack and Diamond that continue to dominate forensic psychiatry. Instead, we advocate for specific ethical habits and skills for the forensic practitioner. These stress the importance of self-reflection, self-awareness, awareness of role conflicts, and sensitivity to vulnerable individuals.

The formation of professional identity over a lifetime is likewise central to our thinking. As educators in forensic fellowship programs, we are struck by the annual progression of general psychiatry residents into forensic practitioners. As mentors, we work with our fellows as values and professional identity are transformed. Whether performing clinical care in correctional settings, working as an administrator in a forensic hospital, providing expert testimony, or pursuing legislative reform, our trainees can rely on a model that is relevant to all of them.

Conclusion

Our professionalism recognizes that all forensic practitioners are engaged in moral relationships. Robust professionalism requires awareness of the enormous responsibility in making judgments about other human beings, where offering opinions can result in dramatic consequences for those directly and even indirectly involved. Robust professionalism incorporates a kind of aspirational conduct, supporting ethics duties and obligations outside the technical requirements of the job, identifying consensus social goods, limiting moral justifications based on a narrow role identity, and requiring thoughtful consideration of the systemic and personal moral consequences of words and deeds.

The ultimate strength of an approach that functions theoretically to prioritize vulnerable people and values, and to identify habits and skills that overcome inequity, is that it works hand in glove with other approaches. In applying robust professionalism at the practical level for a theory of human rights, for example, practitioners can identify behaviors that operationalize the inherent dignity of an evaluee (Candilis and Griffith 2021). Describing the narrative of an evaluee who has experienced systemic racism, and the associated lack of opportunity, enriches the expert's relationship to the system, the community, and the individual alike. Robust professionalism requires more than an aseptic procedural participation in human dilemmas but asks that one fully engage in the often messy and imperfect moral dimension of the work.

References

American Academy of Psychiatry and the Law: Ethics Guidelines for the Practice of Forensic Psychiatry. Adopted May 2005. Bloomfield, CT, American Academy of Psychiatry and the Law, 2005. Available at: https://www.aapl.org/ethics-guidelines. Accessed October 1, 2020.

American Psychological Association: Specialty guidelines for forensic psychology. Am Psychol 68(1):7–19, 2013 23025747

Appelbaum PS: A theory of ethics for forensic psychiatry. J Am Acad Psychiatry Law 25(3):233–247, 1997 9323651

Appelbaum PS: Ethics and forensic psychiatry: translating principles into practice. J Am Acad Psychiatry Law 36(2):195–200, 2008 18583695

Buchanan A: Respect of dignity as an ethical principle in forensic psychiatry. Leg Criminol Psychol 19:30–32, 2014

Buchanan A: Respect for dignity and forensic psychiatry. Int J Law Psychiatry 41:12–17, 2015 25888501

Candilis PJ: The revolution in forensic ethics: narrative, compassion, and a robust professionalism. Psychiatr Clin North Am 32(2):423–435, 2009 19486823

Candilis PJ, Griffith EEH: Thoughtful forensic practice combats structural racism. J Am Acad Psychiatry Law 49(1):12–15, 2021 33246987

Candilis PJ, Martinez R: Commentary: the higher standards of aspirational ethics. J Am Acad Psychiatry Law 34(2):242–244, 2006 16844806

Candilis PJ, Martinez R: Recent developments in forensic psychiatry ethics, in Bearing Witness to Change: Forensic Psychiatry and Psychology Practice. Edited by Griffith EEH, Norko MA, Buchanan A, et al. Boca Raton, FL, CRC Press, 2017

Candilis PJ, Martinez R, Dording C: Principles and narrative in forensic psychiatry: toward a robust view of professional role. J Am Acad Psychiatry Law 29(2):167–173, 2001 11471782

Candilis PJ, Weinstock R, Martinez R: Forensic Ethics and the Expert Witness. New York, Springer, 2007

Choper JH, Mosk S, Skolnick JH, et al: In memoriam: Dr. Bernard L. Diamond. Calif Law Rev 78(6):1429–1439, 1990

Ciccone JR, Clements CD: The ethical practice of forensic psychiatry: a view from the trenches. Bull Am Acad Psychiatry Law 12(3):263–277, 1984a 6478069

Ciccone JR, Clements C: Forensic psychiatry and applied clinical ethics: theory and practice. Am J Psychiatry 141(3):395–399, 1984b 6703105

Ciccone JR, Clements C: Commentary: forensic psychiatry and ethics—the voyage continues. J Am Acad Psychiatry Law 29(2):174–179, 2001 11471783

Cruess SR, Cruess RL: Professionalism must be taught. BMJ 315(7123):1674–1677, 1997 9448538

Cruess RL, Cruess SR: Expectations and obligations: professionalism and medicine's social contract with society. Perspect Biol Med 51(4):579–598, 2008 18997360

Cruess RL, Cruess SR, Boudreau JD, et al: Reframing medical education to support professional identity formation. Acad Med 89(11):1446–1451, 2014 25054423

Diamond BL: The fallacy of the impartial expert. Arch Crim Psychodyn 3(2):221–236, 1959

Diamond BL: The forensic psychiatrist: consultant versus activist in legal doctrine. Bull Am Acad Psychiatry Law 20(2):119–132, 1992 1633333

Griffith EEH: Ethics in forensic psychiatry: a cultural response to Stone and Appelbaum. J Am Acad Psychiatry Law 26(2):171–184, 1998 9664254

Griffith EEH: Truth in forensic psychiatry: a cultural response to Gutheil and colleagues. J Am Acad Psychiatry Law 31(4):428–431, 2003 14974797

Griffith EEH: Stone's views of 25 years ago have now shifted incrementally. J Am Acad Psychiatry Law 36(2):201–205, 2008 18583696

Griffith EEH, Baranoski MV: Commentary: the place of performative writing in forensic psychiatry. J Am Acad Psychiatry Law 35(1):27–31, 2007 17389341

Griffith EEH, Baranoski M: Oral performance, identity, and representation in forensic psychiatry. J Am Acad Psychiatry Law 39(3):352–363, 2011 21908752

Griffith EEH, Stankovic A, Baranoski M: Conceptualizing the forensic psychiatry report as performative narrative. J Am Acad Psychiatry Law 38(1):32–42, 2010 20305072

Gutheil TG, Bursztajn HJ, Brodsky A, et al: Decision-Making in Psychiatry and the Law. Baltimore, MD, Williams and Wilkins, 1991

Gutheil TG, Hauser M, White MS, et al: "The whole truth" versus "the admissible truth": an ethics dilemma for expert witnesses. J Am Acad Psychiatry Law 31(4):422–427, 2003 14974796

Hafferty FW, Castellani B: A sociological framing of medicine's modern-day professionalism movement. Med Educ 43(9):826–828, 2009 19709007

Hanson MJ, Callahan D (eds): The Goals of Medicine: The Forgotten Issues in Health Care Reform. Washington, DC, Georgetown University Press, 1999

Irby DM, Hamstra SJ: Parting the clouds: three professionalism frameworks in medical education. Acad Med 91(12):1606–1611, 2016 27119331

Martinez R: Professional identity, the goals and purposes of forensic psychiatry, and Dr. Ezra Griffith. J Am Acad Psychiatry Law 46(4):428–437, 2018 30593472

Martinez R, Candilis PJ: Commentary: toward a unified theory of personal and professional ethics. J Am Acad Psychiatry Law 33(3):382–385, 2005 16186204

Martinez R, Candilis PJ: Ethics: Principles of writing, in Psychiatric Report: Principles and Practice of Forensic Writing. Edited by Buchanan A, Norko MA. New York, Cambridge University Press, 2011, pp 56–67

Martinez R, Candilis PJ: Ethics in the time of injustice. J Am Acad Psychiatry Law 48(2):428–430, 2020

Norko MA: Commentary: compassion at the core of forensic ethics. J Am Acad Psychiatry Law 33(3):386–389, 2005 16186205

Norko MA: What is truth? The spiritual quest of forensic psychiatry. J Am Acad Psychiatry Law 46(1):10–22, 2018 29618531

Pollack S: Principles of forensic psychiatry for psychiatric-legal opinion-making, in Legal Medicine Annual 1971. Edited by Wecht CH. New York, Appleton-Century-Crofts, 1971

Pollack S: Forensic Psychiatry in Criminal Law. Los Angeles, CA, University of Southern California Press, 1974a

Pollack S: The role of psychiatry in the rule of law. Psychiatr Ann 4:16–31, 1974b

Rappeport JR: Differences between forensic and general psychiatry. Am J Psychiatry 139(3):331–334, 1982 7058947

Rosenberg, C. (2023, April 13). Ex-C.I.A. Psychologist Re-enacts Interrogation Techniques for Guantánamo Court. The New York Times, April 13, 2023. Available at: https://www.nytimes.com/2023/04/13/us/politics/cia-torture-guantanamo-saudi-detainee-nashiri.html. Accessed January 13, 2025.

Report of the Senate Select Committee on intelligence committee study of the Central Intelligence Agency's detention and interrogation program together with foreword by Chairman Feinstein and additional and minority views. Senate 113th Congress 2d Session S. Report 113-288, 2014

Simon RI: Authorship in forensic psychiatry: a perspective. J Am Acad Psychiatry Law 35(1):18–26, 2007 17389340

Stone AA: The ethics of forensic psychiatry: a view from the ivory tower, in Law, Psychiatry, and Morality. Edited by Stone AA. Washington, DC, American Psychiatric Press, 1985, pp 57–75

Stone AA, MacCourt DC: Ethics in forensic psychiatry: re-imagining the wasteland after 25 years. J Psychiatry Law 36:617–643, 2008

Strasburger LH, Gutheil TG, Brodsky A: On wearing two hats: role conflict in serving as both psychotherapist and expert witness. Am J Psychiatry 154(4):448–456, 1997 9090330

Weinstock R: Ethical concerns expressed by forensic psychiatrists. J Forensic Sci 31(2):596–602, 1986 3711835

Weinstock R: Controversial ethical issues in forensic psychiatry: a survey. J Forensic Sci 33(1):176–186, 1988 3351454

Weinstock R: Perceptions of ethical problems by forensic psychiatrists. Bull Am Acad Psychiatry Law 17(2):189–202, 1989 2758120

Wynia MK, Latham SR, Kao AC, et al: Medical professionalism in society. N Engl J Med 341(21):1612–1616, 1999 10577119

Wynia MK, Papadakis MA, Sullivan WM, et al: More than a list of values and desired behaviors: a foundational understanding of medical professionalism. Acad Med 89(5):712–714, 2014 24667515

5

Ethical Report Writing

Michael A. Norko, M.D., M.A.R.
Alec Buchanan, M.D., Ph.D.
Paul Bryant, M.D.

> There's the story, then there's the real story, then there's the story of
> how the story came to be told. Then there's what you leave out of the
> story. Which is part of the story too.
> —Margaret Atwood (2014, p. 56)

Ethical report writing is a skill requiring training, experience, and continuous self-appraisal. It has many facets, as we explore in this chapter, including the central task of constructing a narrative that tells the story in an honest and objective way, while communicating effectively and defending an expert opinion that seeks to resolve challenging questions about often complex situations of significant importance to the people involved (Buchanan and Norko 2013).

The report is the crafted culmination of all the stages of the forensic evaluation process (Norko and Buchanan 2015). Drafting a report is not merely an effort of sorting and summing data and interactions; it is also how careful experts examine and reexamine data elements, their assumptions and biases, the logic of their conclusions, their fairness to the task, and the professionalism and humanity of their response to the evaluee and others.

An ethical report cannot flow from an evaluation process that is ethically flawed. There is no component of the ethics of forensic psychiatry that is not implicated in the creation of the written report (at least where a report is required). The many contributors to this book thus have also participated in the elucidation of the ethics of report writing; we try not to duplicate their efforts in this chapter.

The multiple deliberations involved in report drafting should identify ethical flaws in the evaluation process and lead to their correction. They should also form a cyclical learning progression that informs future evaluations. We endeavor in this chapter to explore the ethics constituents of this iterative process. An ethical evaluation does not, however, guarantee an ethical report. There are procedural and technical aspects of report writing that are also subject to ethics considerations. We attend to these next. Finally, we address the implications for the ethics of report writing of working within the systems of law and mental health, where substantial inequities exist for the people whose stories we are asked to tell.

Inherent Values

The forensic psychiatric report is where the ethical practice of a forensic psychiatric evaluation is held open for inspection. Some of the ethical values reflected in a forensic psychiatric report are common to other medical and psychiatric specialties. They include respecting human dignity, practicing with compassion, acting honestly, and seeking to advance social justice (American Psychiatric Association 2013). Other values that are relevant to the report relate to the particular circumstances and requirements of forensic psychiatric practice. They include striving for objectivity in answering the legal question (American Academy of Psychiatry and the Law 2005).

Even when the values concerned are shared with other specialties, their application is sometimes different in the circumstances of a forensic evaluation (Buchanan 2015). Honesty seems to require telling the truth, but telling the truth in the forensic context has multiple elements, including a *subjective* component that refers to saying what one believes and an *objective* one that requires something more, including an indication of the limits of the author's knowledge of the subject or the case (Appelbaum 1990, 1997). There is a truth related to context that emerges in the narrative section of a report but is not easily accessed in other ways (Griffith 1998). Compassion should be married to the evaluative task (Norko 2005).

Legally, informed consent is a restriction on data transfer. In forensic psychiatry, however, informed consent is better seen as a dialogue that constrains an evaluator's behavior (Gutheil et al. 1991). Forensic psychiatric evaluations are preceded by giving notice to the person being evaluated of the purpose of the evaluation and of the reasonable anticipated limits to confidentiality. Where collateral information is obtained, equivalent notice is given to the sources of that information. Even when such notice has been given, the person being evaluated may forget or otherwise ignore it in the course of the evaluation. The content of the written report cannot prove that all of these dangers received sufficient attention, but a badly written report can sometimes suggest that they did not.

Consent and Notice to the Person Being Evaluated

Professional ethical guidelines state that consent for the evaluation should be obtained "when necessary and feasible" (American Academy of Psychiatry and the Law 2005). Whether consent is required or not, the introduction to the psychiatric report should describe the notice that was given to the person being evaluated concerning the nature and purpose of the evaluation and the limits of confidentiality. Sometimes—for instance, when criminal charges include sexual abuse—the introduction will also include reference to the evaluator's explanation of the mandatory reporting laws to the evaluee (see Buchanan and Norko 2013, p. 361). When the person being evaluated appears not to understand this, the lack of understanding should be stated in the report.

Obtaining consent is a means of safeguarding respect for the individual being evaluated. When the evaluation is court ordered, the introduction should describe the individual's level of participation. The age at which someone can consent to a psychiatric evaluation varies by jurisdiction; for children and minors, the discussion of consent should involve an appropriately qualified substitute decision-maker. The initial explanation should include reference to the evaluator's sources and the records obtained to complete the evaluation.

In both civil litigation and criminal cases, information is often provided to an evaluator (usually at the outset of an evaluation) without the permission or sometimes even the knowledge of the person being evaluated. When a competency-to-stand-trial evaluation is ordered by a court, for instance, or a state-of-mind evaluation is requested by the prosecution in a criminal trial, the request to conduct an evaluation is typically accompanied by background information that may include medical records, witness statements, and police accounts of what happened.

Sometimes information is included that the person being evaluated would prefer not be used in a report. One question for the person conducting the evaluation will then be, if those wishes are respected, whether the evaluation can still answer the question being asked. A second, broader, question is whether and when information should be used without permission. If no ethically satisfactory solution is found, the evaluation will usually be abandoned without the need for a report. Occasionally, however, it will be possible to provide a conclusion with a qualification regarding the need for review should additional information become available. The ethical questions are usually best addressed with transparency regarding what the evaluator already has access to and in consultation with the person being evaluated and their attorney.

Material that has been obtained cannot be unobtained, and written material that has been read cannot be unread. Sometimes this means that having conducted all or part of an evaluation, the evaluator cannot ethically produce a report. The obvious corollary is that ethical questions should be addressed as soon as they arise rather than when the report is being written.

Collecting Data for the Report

The quality and ethics of the forensic report rely on the quality and ethics of the processes for collecting data in the evaluation. The first consideration occurs when agreeing to conduct an evaluation, when the expert determines whether there are any potential conflicts of interest in accepting the case. Beneath that face-value determination is the need for self-assessment of personal biases and countertransference related to the type of case, the facts of the case, or any of the key figures in the case. Without such awareness, the data the evaluator collects will be subject to unknown biases; as Swinton (2013) observed, our own view of the world shapes what we see or think we see, as well as the way we respond to it. Candilis and Griffith (2021) have noted the value of implicit bias assessment tools in forensic practice to help professionals examine their beliefs.

Other preparation is also necessary before conducting interviews. The forensic expert must be authentically present "to the people and problems at hand," including to the suffering of others. Presence, in turn, requires cognitive, emotional, and even spiritual preparation, as well as mindfulness and an attentive attitude (Norko 2018, pp. 13–14).

Presence in forensic practice involves empathy and compassion. Kohut (2011, p. 207) believed that all psychological observation requires empathy as "vicarious introspection." Multiple authors have described the importance of empathy in forensic work (Norko 2018). Compassion follows empathy, with the added dimension of action, whether that is engaging the humanity of the subject (Norko 2005), the narrative and humanistic quality of the report writing (Candilis et al. 2001), or service to the legal goal of justice (Ciccone and Clements 1984). Effective presence is the ground of the "authentic human understanding of the other" necessary to truth-telling in the forensic report (Norko 2018, p. 14).

Managing Data in the Report

Readers of psychiatric reports and those who make legal decisions based on those reports usually do not use all of the information that a report contains, especially when data and opinions are complex (Norko and Buchanan 2015). They take shortcuts (Goodman-Delahunty and Dhami 2012). When reading insanity reports, for instance, judges and lawyers focus on diagnosis, whether the symptoms meet the applicable legal standard, and the expert's ultimate opinion (Redding et al. 2001). The author of a forensic psychiatric report has to balance the understandable desire to include any significant material against relevance, economy, and the needs of the reader.

The often difficult choice that follows, concerning what kind of information (and how much) to include, should be informed by ethics. If a report is to adequately address inconsistencies in what the person being evaluated has said during the evaluation, or inconsistencies between what they said and what appears in background materials such as medical records, these inconsistencies need to be presented in a way that is honest and also demonstrates proper respect for the person being evaluated. At a minimum, the person being evaluated needs to have been told at the start of the evaluation what question the evaluator is seeking to answer. The ethics approach cannot be inserted at the point the report is written.

Assuming that what is required has been explained and understood, the author of the report still faces the task of presenting and explaining inconsistencies in a way that the reader will understand. Some inconsistency is to be expected, particularly in the details of events that happened a long time ago, but where the inconsistency concerns facts relevant to the conclusion, the report should make that inconsistency explicit.

Less tangible than logical consistency, but a more pervasive challenge to the task of preparing an ethically informed psychiatric report, is the awkward fact that the results of an evaluation frequently do not point uniformly in one direction. Often, some information and aspects of the mental state suggest one conclusion, whereas other information and mental state features suggest another. Ethics considerations are then relevant to what the evaluating psychiatrist writes. First, the need for honesty is best served by ensuring that the body of the report accurately describes the range of information assembled and by seeking to describe in the conclusion not just the answer to the question asked but also the author's confidence in that answer. Second, the search for objectivity will usually be displayed most clearly in a report that is transparent about the process by which that conclusion has been reached (Norko and Buchanan 2011).

Narrative and Voice

The narrative section of the forensic report conveys an essentially linear and chronological account of the relevant events underlying the reason for the evaluation. A traditional approach to report writing is for evaluators to tell the story as they have best understood it, considering all the available data, including collateral interviews. This approach is guided by the ethics principles of honesty and striving for objectivity.

While this method conveys a coherent version of events, it has been criticized on the grounds that it may also obscure potential biases, including those related to cultural and personal characteristics of the author of the report (Candilis and Griffith 2021; see also Buchanan and Norko 2011a). One suggested remedy encourages *giving voice* to the attitudes, perspectives, and experiences of each informant (Griffith and Baranoski 2007; Griffith et al. 2011). This approach endeavors to support the ethics principle of respect for persons. The term *forensic empathy* has been applied to the process of allowing the "true voice" of interviewees to be heard in the forensic report (Appelbaum 2010, p. 44).

Regardless of the approach taken, when the various accounts are contradictory or simply do not cohere, the report writer must arbitrate these differences without sowing confusion (Buchanan and Norko 2011a, 2013). The report writer must also decide whether the relevant and important voices can be merged into a single story, or whether each of the various accounts must be given its turn. This choice is further complicated when informants' versions include moral judgments or when the factual reports differ in important ways.

A narrative understanding of evaluees' lives and circumstances has been a central feature of contemporary developments in forensic ethics (Candilis et al. 2001; Martinez and Candilis 2005) (see also Chapter 3, "Narrative and Ethics in Forensic Psychiatry"). It is also an important locus of attention for the current imperative that forensic mental health professionals more directly and responsibly address injustice and inequity in our dealings with the justice system (Candilis and Griffith 2021; Martinez and Candilis 2020). Questions related to narrative and voice await further development and elaboration in the evolution of forensic ethics (Martinez and Candilis 2020).

The Report's Formulation and Conclusion

The sections in which data are synthesized to reach a medical or psychiatric opinion, the formulation and conclusion, represent the crux of the report. Here the narrative shifts from what is generally a fairly objective description of historical information to a formulation in which authors insert their own ideas and explanations. This practice has been conceptualized as an effort to find meaning in the search for truth (Norko 2018); it can also be viewed as an area prone to subjectivity or bias. Thus, it is here that forensic psychiatrists must place particular attention on the process by which they arrived at conclusions; through transparent presentation, the reader should have a reasonable understanding as to how the conclusions were ultimately reached.

One specific challenge concerns the certainty with which an opinion is formed. When offering an opinion in a legal matter, evaluators are often asked that it be made with a reasonable degree of medical certainty (RMC). In part because it is a phrase not used in clinical medicine, there has been much disagreement about the meaning of RMC (Leong et al. 2011; Lewin 1998). At times, it simply equates to "more likely than not" (Anfang et al. 2018), but this definition is hardly universal. Jonas Rappeport famously described the ambiguity around such terminology while noting his own definition to be "that level of certainty which a physician would use in making a similar clinical judgement" (Rappeport 1985, p. 9). Seymour Pollack thought that a higher level of proof was required in forensic psychiatry (Pollack 1974).

Bernard Diamond disagreed and stressed that the expert's level of certainty may vary depending on the question being answered (Diamond 1985). Experts should be clear about how they are using RMC in any particular situation, and their reports should make clear the basis for and the process by which they reached their conclusions.

An additional area of controversy involves the use of and adherence to diagnoses as described in DSM-5 (American Psychiatric Association 2022). Psychiatric diagnoses may be required in certain legal and administrative situations (Wills and Gold 2014), but concerns have been raised about their use outside of clinical treatment (Buchanan 2005). DSM-5 offers a cautionary statement regarding its use in forensic settings, specifying that it is not intended to meet "the technical needs of the courts and legal professionals" (American Psychiatric Association 2022, p. 29). Consequently, forensic psychiatrists may face situations in which limiting their opinions to the production of DSM-5 diagnoses seems overly restrictive, including times in which a particular diagnosis does not apply yet psychiatric expertise could still assist the legal process through its understanding of interpersonal dynamics or the psychological underpinnings of behavior.

Technical Aspects of Report Writing

Along with the actual writing of a forensic report, a variety of other issues must be considered. One such issue involves whether to provide the retaining attorney with a draft of a report before submitting the finalized version. This practice can have distinct advantages, such as providing an opportunity for the attorney to identify potential factual inconsistencies, but it can also lead to attempts at reshaping the structure or content. If the choice is made to provide a draft, it is essential to clarify its purpose, as well as carefully consider what types of feedback can be accommodated and what could alter the integrity of the report.

In some situations, forensic evaluators may be asked to limit their reports to an abbreviated format. Although such a product may accurately convey the ultimate conclusions, it risks being less transparent about the deliberative process. Regardless of length, it is essential that the report contain enough data to support the opinion reached. Additionally, the goals of transparency and thoroughness must be weighed against the potential consequences of information disclosed in the report, some of which may be unintended or unforeseen by the writer (Buchanan and Norko 2011b). Thus, in deciding on the appropriate length and content, it is essential to consider the impact on the overarching goals of the report and their relation to the underlying search for truth as balanced with respect for involved parties.

Many forensic evaluators participate in a peer-review process. This may be through a forensic case conference, as often occurs in fellowship programs (Buchanan et al. 2016); formalized discussion with colleagues, as may happen in a group private practice; or a specific process offered by professional organizations, such as the AAPL Peer Review of Psychiatric Testimony Committee. These different models offer what may be important opportunities for consultation and supervision, often serving to further the search for truth and the goal of objectivity, but they also raise important questions about the discussion of privileged and confidential information, which has the potential to conflict with the evaluator's obligations concerning nonmaleficence and respect for persons. Additionally, in the course of expert testimony, psychiatrists must often disclose with whom they spoke about a case, and thus careful consideration should be given to how to best address such inquiries.

Although significant emphasis has been placed on using quality improvement principles to optimize the delivery of clinical care (Georgiou and Townsend 2019; Sunderji et al. 2017; Young et al. 2016), less progress has been made in their application to forensic assessments (Wettstein 2005). The limited attempts to examine the quality of forensic reports have identified significant deficiencies in quality across report types (Fuger et al. 2014; Nguyen et al. 2011; Robinson and Acklin 2010). The quality of the report is not always synonymous with that of the assessment (Wettstein 2010), but it must be remembered that the report serves as the window through which the assessment is viewed and understood.

Working in a System of Inequities

Historically, forensic psychiatric ethics focused on two principles: truth-telling and respect for persons (Appelbaum 1997). More recent literature recommends that these principles be expanded to include factors such as culture (Griffith 1998), professionalism (Candilis et al. 2001), compassion (Norko 2005), and respect for individual dignity (Buchanan 2015). By focusing on more humanistic principles, these formulations have stressed the importance of fairness and how individuals are ultimately affected by forensic evaluations. However, these effects cannot be fully understood without taking into account the profound inequities present within the criminal justice system. The question of how to perform fair and ethical evaluations within a system characterized by prominent disparities requires further development; there is a growing concern about the need to address these issues (Chaimowitz and Simpson 2021; Martinez and Candilis 2020).

More and more data point to multiple areas of inequity affecting forensic evaluations. Black and Latinx individuals face adversity at many levels of the criminal justice process: policing (Federal Bureau of Investigation 2020), pretrial detention (Jones 2013), sentencing (Carson 2020), and parole (Huebner and Bynum 2008). Discriminatory effects are not limited to the judicial system, with studies suggesting that ethnicity has a significant effect on the psychiatric diagnosis an individual receives (Gara et al. 2019). In the context of a forensic report, these various inequities may have a significant impact on the ultimate formulation and conclusion. This is in part because of the prominent role of historical factors in assessing for things such as risk and mitigation, which serves to further amplify the effects of factors such as targeted policing and disparate sentencing (see also Chapter 20, "Structural Racism and Ethics").

To address these concerns, Candilis and Griffith (2021, p. 3) have written about the importance of a culturally sensitive narrative, suggesting that an evaluator can combat certain structural inequities through examining cases "from the nondominant perspective, through the lens of implicit bias, and in the historical context." They go on to suggest that this narrative approach, which may describe issues such as the disadvantaged neighborhood in which an individual grew up or the impacts of mass incarceration on an individual's community, can have the effect of opposing systemic racism and should be part of every evaluation.

Conclusion

In a different arena of the critical appraisal of historical text, Carroll reminds us that "[t]here is no such thing as history undistorted" (Carroll 2015, p. 243). As an exercise in both history and interpretation, the written forensic report is a demanding example of ethics as praxis, consistent with the view advocated by Alan Stone that ethical choices of physicians are context bound and part of the "moral adventure of one's life" (Stone and MacCourt 2008, p. 619). Even agreeing to produce a report involves moral and ethical judgments on the part of an evaluator (Buchanan 2006). Forensic experts who do take on this task confront multiple challenges in narrating a history as undistorted as possible by the potential hazards discussed in this chapter. The interpretation of that history, which underlies the expert opinion, adds further complexity to the ethics demands of report writing. For the ethics of forensic report writing to contribute to the fuller realization of equity and justice, forensic experts not only need to understand current principles, constraints, and practice but also to design and implement appropriately focused empiric research and attend to the further evolution of professional ethics guidelines that address systemic inequity and injustice.

References

American Academy of Psychiatry and the Law: Ethics Guidelines for the Practice of Forensic Psychiatry. Adopted May 2005. Bloomfield, CT, American Academy of Psychiatry and the Law, 2005. Available at: https://www.aapl.org/ethics-guidelines. Accessed October 1, 2020.

American Psychiatric Association: The Principles of Medical Ethics With Annotations Especially Applicable to Psychiatry. Arlington, VA, American Psychiatric Association, 2013

American Psychiatric Association: Diagnostic and Statistical Manual of Mental Disorders, 5th Edition, Text Revision. Washington, DC, American Psychiatric Association, 2022

Anfang SA, Gold LH, Meyer DJ: AAPL Practice Resource for the forensic evaluation of psychiatric disability. J Am Acad Psychiatry Law 41:S1–S47, 2018

Appelbaum KL: Commentary: the art of forensic report writing. J Am Acad Psychiatry Law 38(1):43–45, 2010 20305073

Appelbaum PS: The parable of the forensic psychiatrist: ethics and the problem of doing harm. Int J Law Psychiatry 13(4):249–259, 1990 2286491

Appelbaum PS: A theory of ethics for forensic psychiatry. J Am Acad Psychiatry Law 25(3):233–247, 1997 9323651

Atwood M: MaddAddam. New York, Anchor Books, 2014

Buchanan A: Descriptive diagnosis, personality disorder and detention. Journal of Forensic Psychiatry and Psychology 16(3):538–551, 2005

Buchanan A: Psychiatric evidence on the ultimate issue. J Am Acad Psychiatry Law 34:14–21, 2006 16585230

Buchanan A: Respect for dignity and forensic psychiatry. Int J Law Psychiatry 41:12–17, 2015 25888501

Buchanan A, Norko MA: Conclusion, in The Psychiatric Report: Principles and Practice in Forensic Writing. Edited by Buchanan A, Norko MA. Cambridge, UK, Cambridge University Press, 2011a, pp 264–269

Buchanan A, Norko MA: Report structure, in The Psychiatric Report: Principles and Practice in Forensic Writing. Edited by Buchanan A, Norko MA. Cambridge, UK, Cambridge University Press, 2011b, pp 93–97

Buchanan A, Norko M: The forensic evaluation and report: an agenda for research. J Am Acad Psychiatry Law 41(3):359–365, 2013 24051588

Buchanan A, Norko M, Baranoski M, et al: A consultation and supervision model for developing the forensic psychiatric opinion. J Am Acad Psychiatry Law 44(3):300–308, 2016 27644862

Candilis PJ, Griffith EEH: Thoughtful forensic practice combats structural racism. J Am Acad Psychiatry Law 49(1):12–15, 2021 33246987

Candilis PJ, Martinez R, Dording C: Principles and narrative in forensic psychiatry: toward a robust view of professional role. J Am Acad Psychiatry Law 29(2):167–173, 2001 11471782

Carroll J: Christ Actually: Reimagining Faith in the Modern Age. New York, Penguin Books, 2015

Carson EA: Prisoners in 2019. Washington, DC, Office of Justice Programs, U.S. Department of Justice, NCJ 255115. October 2020. Available at: https://bjs.ojp.gov/redirect-legacy/content/pub/pdf/p19.pdf. Accessed July 18, 2024.

Chaimowitz GA, Simpson AIF: Charting a new course for forensic psychiatry. J Am Acad Psychiatry Law 49(2):157–160, 2021 34131057

Ciccone JR, Clements CD: The ethical practice of forensic psychiatry: a view from the trenches. Bull Am Acad Psychiatry Law 12(3):263–277, 1984 6478069

Diamond BL: Reasonable medical certainty, diagnostic thresholds, and definitions of mental illness in the legal context. Bull Amer Acad Psychiatry Law 13:121–128, 1985

Federal Bureau of Investigation: Crime in the United States, 2019. Washington, DC, Government Printing Office, 2020

Fuger KD, Acklin MW, Nguyen AH, et al: Quality of criminal responsibility reports submitted to the Hawaii judiciary. Int J Law Psychiatry 37(3):272–280, 2014 24326082

Gara MA, Minsky S, Silverstein SM, et al: A naturalistic study of racial disparities in diagnosis at an outpatient behavioral health clinic. Psychiatr Serv 70(2):130–134, 2019 30526340

Georgiou M, Townsend K: Quality network for prison mental health services: reviewing the quality of mental health provision in prisons. J Forensic Psychiatry Psychol 5(10):794–806, 2019

Goodman-Delahunty J, Dhami MK: A forensic examination of court reports. Aust Psychol 48:32–40, 2012

Griffith EEH: Ethics in forensic psychiatry: a cultural response to Stone and Appelbaum. J Am Acad Psychiatry Law 26(2):171–184, 1998 9664254

Griffith EEH, Baranoski MV: Commentary: the place of performative writing in forensic psychiatry. J Am Acad Psychiatry Law 35(1):27–31, 2007 17389341

Griffith EEH, Stankovic A, Baranoski MV: Writing a narrative, in The Psychiatric Report: Principles and Practice in Forensic Writing. Edited by

Buchanan A, Norko MA. Cambridge, UK, Cambridge University Press, 2011, pp 68–80

Gutheil TG, Bursztajn HJ, Brodsky A, et al: Decision Making in Psychiatry and the Law. Baltimore, MD, Williams and Wilkins, 1991

Huebner B, Bynum T: The role of race and ethnicity in parole decisions. Criminology 46:907–938, 2008

Jones CE: "Give us free": addressing racial disparities in bail determinations. NY Univ J Legis Public Policy 16:919–962, 2013

Kohut H: Introspection, empathy and psychoanalysis: An examination of the relationship between mode of observation and theory, in The Search for the Self: Selected Writings of Heinz Kohut: 1950–1978 (Vol 1). Edited by Ornstein PH. London, Karnac, 2011, pp 205-232

Leong G, Silva JA, Weinstock R: Reasonable medical certainty, in The Psychiatric Report: Principles and Practice in Forensic Writing. Edited by Buchanan A, Norko MA. Cambridge, UK, Cambridge University Press, 2011, pp 214–223

Lewin JL: The genesis and evolution of legal uncertainty about "reasonable medical certainty." MD Law Rev 57:380–504, 1998

Martinez R, Candilis PJ: Commentary: toward a unified theory of personal and professional ethics. J Am Acad Psychiatry Law 33(3):382–385, 2005 16186204

Martinez R, Candilis P: Ethics in the time of injustice. J Am Acad Psychiatry Law 48(4):428–430, 2020 32900819

Nguyen AH, Acklin MW, Fuger K, et al: Freedom in paradise: quality of conditional release reports submitted to the Hawaii judiciary. Int J Law Psychiatry 34(5):341–348, 2011 21920604

Norko MA: Commentary: compassion at the core of forensic ethics. J Am Acad Psychiatry Law 33(3):386–389, 2005 16186205

Norko MA: What is truth? The spiritual quest of forensic psychiatry. J Am Acad Psychiatry Law 46(1):10–22, 2018 29618531

Norko MA, Buchanan A: Introduction, in The Psychiatric Report: Principles and Practice in Forensic Writing. Edited by Buchanan A, Norko MA. Cambridge, UK, Cambridge University Press, 2011, pp 1–9

Norko MA, Buchanan MA: The forensic psychiatric report. J Psychiatr Pract 21(1):67–71, 2015 25603453

Pollack S: The role of psychiatry in the rule of law. Psychiatric Ann 4(8):16–31, 1974

Rappeport JR: Reasonable medical certainty. Bull Am Acad Psychiatry Law 13(1):5–15, 1985 3995190

Redding RE, Floyd MY, Hawk GL: What judges and lawyers think about the testimony of mental health experts: a survey of the courts and bar. Behav Sci Law 19(4):583–594, 2001 11568962

Robinson R, Acklin MW: Fitness in paradise: quality of forensic reports submitted to the Hawaii judiciary. Int J Law Psychiatry 33(3):131–137, 2010 20483159

Stone AA, MacCourt DC: Ethics in forensic psychiatry: re-imagining the
    wasteland after 25 years. J Psychiatry Law 36:617–643, 2008

Sunderji N, Ion A, Ghavam-Rassoul A, Abate A: Evaluating the
    implementation of integrated mental health care: a systematic review to
    guide the development of quality measures. Psychiatr Serv 68(9):891–898,
    2017 28502244

Swinton J: Beyond kindness: the place of compassion in a forensic mental
    health setting. Health and Social Care Chaplaincy 1(1):11–21, 2013

Wettstein RM: Quality and quality improvement in forensic mental health
    evaluations. J Am Acad Psychiatry Law 33(2):158–175, 2005 15985658

Wettstein RM: Commentary: conceptualizing the forensic psychiatry report. J
    Am Acad Psychiatry Law 38(1):46–48, 2010 20305074

Wills CD, Gold LH: Introduction to the special section on DSM-5 and forensic
    psychiatry. J Am Acad Psychiatry Law 42(2):132–135, 2014 24986338

Young AS, Cohen AN, Miotto KA: Improving the quality of care for serious
    mental illness, in Quality Improvement in Behavioral Health. Edited by
    O'Donohue W, Maragakis A. Cham, Springer, 2016, pp 275–288

6

Ethical Challenges While Testifying

Gregory B. Leong, M.D.
Mendel Feldsher, M.D.

Ethical challenges have been present ever since psychiatrists first offered testimony in a legal proceeding as psychiatric expert witnesses. The *hired gun* first comes to mind when thinking about unethical behavior among expert witnesses. Hired gun experts testify in favor of the side who paid them, regardless of the truth. The hired gun conjures up the image of a mercenary who is similarly primarily concerned with making money at the expense of ethics. However, other situations when testifying may pose similar and more frequent ethical challenges for forensic psychiatrists. Before further exploring the hired gun and related ethical challenges, we explore the contours of psychiatric expert witness testimony.

The adversarial nature of the legal system is the foremost feature from which ethical challenges arise for the psychiatric expert witness. Depending on the stakes and the parties involved (the litigants and their respective attorneys), the degree of desire to be the prevailing party may vary. In its extreme, one or both parties would want to exhaust every option, including those which appear legally or ethically dubious, to prevail. The psychiatric expert witness enters a case against this backdrop and is subject to powerful influences from this setting.

Ideally, the psychiatric expert witness would be immune to the adversarial nature of the case in which they have been retained.

Beyond the adversarial nature of legal proceedings, the legal system has adopted a set of rules to regulate what the expert witness can convey in court. What expert testimony is permissible varies by jurisdiction. Broadly speaking, jurisdictions are guided by either the *Frye* (1923) or *Daubert* (1993) case, both of which in theory impose standards for the admissibility of expert witness opinions based on the quality of the science used in arriving at those opinions. Moreover, additional jurisdiction-specific evidentiary rules guide what testimony expert witnesses are permitted to offer. Some jurisdictions also require psychiatric expert witnesses to offer their opinions with *reasonable medical certainty* or *reasonable medical probability*.

The legal framework is not absolute, because the judicial gatekeeper is not infallible; reasonable medical certainty and reasonable medical probability generally lack a clear definition (Leong et al. 2011). So despite the current backdrop of the judicial gatekeeper and the requirement to offer psychiatric-legal opinions with reasonable medical certainty or probability, there remains a gap through which clearly partisan psychiatric-legal opinions can be offered that would not violate these legal or clinical procedures and processes. The development of ethical guidelines for the practice of forensic psychiatry by the American Academy of Psychiatry and the Law (AAPL) (2005) includes *honesty* and *striving for objectivity* as its two core fundamental ethical underpinnings, with the goal of limiting ethical transgressions such as the hired-gun expert witnesses who offer partisan psychiatric-legal opinions. In fact, forensic psychiatrist Bernard Diamond offered an idealistic notion that organizational oversight, which included an ethics code and peer review, could mitigate the hired-gun problem (Diamond 1990).

Although the cornerstone of the practice of forensic psychiatry is the forensic assessment (Glancy et al. 2015), regardless of the specific psychiatric-legal issue, the findings of the forensic assessment subsequently need to be communicated by the forensic psychiatrist to the legal system. This is done by preparing a written report of the forensic assessment and testifying in a legal proceeding. The forensic report may be the precursor to testifying, but in most cases, the forensic report is sufficient to answer the psychiatric-legal issues raised. Therefore, many of the ethical challenges for report writing would also apply to oral testimony (see Chapter 5, "Ethical Report Writing"). However, there are important differences between these two communication processes. For forensic psychiatric cases that are resolved with only a forensic psychiatric report, the inference would be that the opposing parties (e.g., prosecutor and defendant in criminal cases; plaintiff and respondent/defendant in civil cases) have reached an agreement as to what to do with the report's findings, including whether to accept or reject them. If so, the report's author does not need to appear at the legal proceeding. However, when enough disagreement remains between the opposing parties, forensic psychiatrists who have prepared reports can be asked to testify in court or other legal proceedings to permit the trier of fact to decide. At that point, the testifying psychiatric expert witness enters the explicitly adversarial proceeding.

Attorneys take a case to trial with the goals of attempting simultaneously to demonstrate that their position is superior to that of the opposing side and to discredit the opposing side's position, including that of any psychiatric expert witness holding a psychiatric-legal opinion favorable to the opposing side. Unlike the world of medicine, in which there is an attempt to map out a therapeutic course for the clinical benefit of a patient, the stakes in the legal arena can involve extreme results, such as imposition of capital punishment in a criminal case, considerable loss of capital or property in a civil case, or loss of custody or visitation rights for a child. It is against this potentially tumultuous adversarial backdrop that ethical challenges can become amplified.

The hired-gun problem has been a focus of professional discourse by Diamond (1959, 1973, 1990), who highlighted a starting point for hired-gun and related ethical challenges. Diamond offered a dichotomous conceptualization in which the presence of honesty separates an honest advocate (expert witness) from a hired gun. Diamond also specifically rejected the concept of impartiality in the legal setting. The AAPL forensic psychiatric ethical guidelines contain the concept of honesty but not impartiality, suggesting Diamond's influence. Diamond offers specific examples of the hired gun: the Texas psychiatrist James Grigson, known as "Dr. Death," and a California psychiatrist hired by the prosecution in criminal cases near where Diamond practiced.

Diamond died before Grigson was expelled from the American Psychiatric Association and the associated district branch (Texas Society of Psychiatric Physicians) in 1995 for violation of the organizational ethical guidelines (Tolson 2004). The testimony of Dr. Death had become available for all to see in the U.S. Supreme Court decisions in *Estelle v. Smith* (1981) and *Barefoot v. Estelle* (1983). Even years after his own death in 2004, Grigson's professional testimony long continued to be the subject of appellate challenge (see, e.g., Court of

Criminal Appeals of Texas 2018). Grigson has been the subject of several professional and popular articles and represents an extreme case of a hired gun.

In Diamond's other example, he described a California psychiatrist as testifying that a criminal defendant was neither psychotic nor legally insane because such a person would not have been able to sleep soundly (the psychiatrist's examination consisted of having observed the defendant sleeping at the jail, with no attempt to awaken the defendant). Diamond wrote that the prosecutor stated privately that he knew

> [the] psychiatrist was an ignoramus and was sure the jury knew it as well. But by allowing his own expert to be exposed as foolish and ridiculous, this would cause the jury to disregard all psychiatric evidence as foolish and implausible. (Diamond 1990, p. 77)

Conversely, Diamond gave examples of an honest expert witness, including the case of a psychiatric expert witness who hopes "that his testimony will expose legal procedures that are archaic, unjust, and detrimental to a free society" (Diamond 1990, p. 78). Diamond continued that as long as the forensic psychiatrist was "competent, scrupulously honest, and does not give false evidence" (Diamond 1990, p. 79), this would distinguish the hired gun from the honest advocate.

Although the hired-gun problem was considered the number one concern in a survey of forensic psychiatrists (Weinstock 1986), Diamond would arguably be the most visible forensic psychiatrist who throughout his professional career consistently addressed the honest advocate versus hired gun as a dichotomous choice rather than along a continuum (Diamond 1959, 1973, 1990). In between these two poles, there would appear to be an ambiguous zone of psychiatric expert witnesses who would be considered neither solely honest nor solely dishonest.

Identifying the expert witness who deliberately distorts data when testifying to arrive at a desired psychiatric-legal opinion may be a difficult, if not impossible, undertaking. It is within this ambiguous zone that ethical ambiguities are most likely to appear, rather than at the extreme position of dishonesty such as Dr. Death (who is considered unethical both within and outside of psychiatry).

In the ethically ambiguous zone, what constitutes distortion of data to support the expert witness opinion—or just outright distortion of an expert witness opinion—may not be readily evident. Consider the case of *U.S. v. Gigante* (1997a), which involved a high-profile criminal defendant, Vincent Gigante, who presented with cognitive impairment;

Gigante's attorney sought to have him adjudicated incompetent to stand trial. This case is often used when teaching forensic psychiatric fellows about malingering in the context of competence-to-stand-trial evaluations. Although it has not been considered a case containing ethical challenges for psychiatric expert witnesses, we reexamine it here for heuristic purposes.

In *U.S. v. Gigante,* mental health expert witnesses supported both the prosecution and defense positions (namely, competent to stand trial for the prosecution and not competent to stand trial for the defense). Several well-known psychiatrists and psychologists with impressive academic and professional credentials, including former AAPL presidents, served as expert witnesses. At the close of the hearings, the defendant was found to have continuously feigned mental illness. He was ruled physically and mentally competent to be tried (*U.S. v. Gigante* 1997b).

Although there has been no suggestion of data distortion or other ethical transgressions, the large number of expert witnesses with divergent opinions raises the possibility of unrecognized biases or tendencies among them, even if the opinions were all offered with reasonable medical (or psychological) probability and all met the striving-for-objectivity threshold. Confirmation bias, which has been shown to lead to inaccurate diagnostic decisions by psychiatrists (Mendel et al. 2011), may also have been a factor. Although there is considerable academic literature on cognitive science and the subtopic of cognitive bias, there do not appear to be data-driven studies that can be applied to minimizing potential bias in forensic psychiatric and psychological testimony, just surveys among forensic mental health evaluators recognizing the presence of bias, especially in other evaluators (Commons et al. 2004, 2012; Zapf et al. 2018).

So far, little has been said about financial incentives, which is the correlation implied by the hired-gun ethical transgression. Clearly, money can be a prime motivator. For a single case, it may be difficult to discern whether money or other motivations may be the driving force behind a professional psychiatric-legal opinion. Rather, a series of cases from the same attorney or set of attorneys, testifying solely for the defense or the prosecution for criminal cases or testifying solely for the plaintiff or the defense in civil cases, can raise suspicion of a less-than-honest psychiatric-legal opinion or a lack of effort in striving for objectivity, whether for financial benefit or other, less-visible motivations. As *U.S. v. Gigante* suggests, arriving at an ethical transgression would require an extraordinary amount of proof. Perhaps only in the repeated instances at the extreme pole of a lack of honesty or lack of striving for objectivity can the ethical transgressions be definitively identified. Of course, testifying an equal number of times for the plaintiff/prosecution and defense sides does not necessarily reflect a forensic psychiatrist reaching the ethical threshold for honesty and striving for objectivity.

Psychiatric expert witnesses can encounter a variety of ethical challenges besides the testimony itself: for example, when asked to assist the retaining attorney with cross-examination of the expert witness testifying in support of the opposing party. How ethically acceptable would this activity be? Another example is a psychiatric expert witness not waiting for a request for assistance but rather offering to perform these services. Does acting in this manner place the psychiatric expert witness in the adversary role beyond that of an expert witness? Examples may concern even more aspirational ethics goals, such as when an expert hired by the prosecution says nothing if an evaluee says, "I know you are trying to help me, doctor." Does this place an ethical demand on the expert to reeducate the evaluee regarding the nonclinical role of the forensic evaluator, and that the evaluator has been retained by the prosecution? Entering into the adversarial legal arena as a testifying psychiatric expert witness increases the likelihood of encountering a myriad of ethical questions by which honesty and striving for objectivity can be challenged.

The fact that Diamond's dichotomous ethical framework regarding the psychiatric expert witness appeared in the first issue of the *Journal of Psychiatry & Law* in 1973, and was revisited in commentary by forensic psychiatrist Robert Sadoff in what would turn out to be the journal's final issue in 2012 (Weiss and Sadoff 2012), would suggest the significance of Diamond's contribution, although Sadoff recognized Diamond's uniqueness. Even another decade out, we started here with Diamond's model for ethical behavior for the testifying psychiatric expert witness but found more complexities than Diamond might have envisioned. In the limited exploration of this chapter, we have not included internal personal vulnerabilities (Gutheil and Simon 2005) or unprocessed emotions (Goldenson and Gutheil 2023) of the psychiatric expert witnesses that could adversely affect honesty or striving for objectivity, although expert witnesses need to be mindful of the multiple potential sources of bias.

Conclusion

The ethical goal of achieving honesty and striving for objectivity with regard to forensic psychiatric testimony can be considered aspirational, as it is difficult to accomplish and involves more than simply staying out of trouble. There may be instances in which consultation with other forensic psychiatrists or psychologists, along with being vigilant about the various sources of bias and external and internal pressures, may assist in keeping one's ethical compass pointed in the direction of honesty and striving for objectivity.

References

American Academy of Psychiatry and the Law: Ethics Guidelines for the Practice of Forensic Psychiatry. Adopted May 2005. Bloomfield, CT, American Academy of Psychiatry and the Law, 2005. Available at: https://www.aapl.org/ethics-guidelines. Accessed March 1, 2021.

Barefoot v Estelle, 463 U.S. 880 (1983)

Commons ML, Miller PM, Gutheil TG: Expert witness perceptions of bias in experts. J Am Acad Psychiatry Law 32(1):70–75, 2004 15497632

Commons ML, Miller PM, Li EY, et al: Forensic experts' perceptions of expert bias. Int J Law Psychiatry 35(5–6):362–371, 2012 23046867

Court of Criminal Appeals of Texas: No. WR-45, 500–02, Unpublished Opinion From 2/21/2018 on the Application for Writ of Habeus Corpus for Jeffrey Lee Wood. February 21, 2018. Available at: https://www.supremecourt.gov/DocketPDF/18/18A820/87394/20190207113949344_2019.02.06%20WOOD%20Exhibit%201.pdf. Accessed July 31, 2021.

Daubert v Merrell Dow, 509 U.S. 579 (1993)

Diamond BL: The fallacy of the impartial expert. Archives of Criminal Psychodynamics 3(2):221–236, 1959

Diamond BL: The psychiatrist as advocate. J Psychiatry Law 1(1):5–21, 1973

Diamond BL: The psychiatric expert witness: honest advocate or "hired gun"? in Ethical Practice in Psychiatry and the Law. Edited by Rosner R, Weinstock R. New York, Plenum, 1990, pp 75–84

Estelle v Smith, 451 U.S. 454 (1981)

Frye v U.S., 293 F. 1013 (D.C. Cir. 1923)

Glancy GD, Ash P, Bath EP, et al: AAPL Practice Guideline for the forensic assessment. J Am Acad Psychiatry Law 43(2 Suppl):S3–S53, 2015 26054704

Goldenson J, Gutheil T: Forensic mental health evaluators' unprocessed emotions as an often-overlooked form of bias. J Am Acad Psychiatry Law 51(4):551–557, 2023 37748917

Gutheil TG, Simon RI: Narcissistic dimensions of expert witness practice. J
        Am Acad Psychiatry Law 33(1):55–58, 2005 15809240

Leong GB, Silva JA, Weinstock R: Reasonable medical certainty, in The
        Psychiatric Report: Principles and Practice of Forensic Writing. Edited by
        Buchanan A, Norko MA. New York, Cambridge University Press, 2011,
        pp 214–233

Mendel R, Traut-Mattausch E, Jonas E, et al: Confirmation bias: why
        psychiatrists stick to wrong preliminary diagnoses. Psychol Med
        41(12):2651–2659, 2011 21733217

Tolson M: Effect of "Dr. Death" and his testimony lingers. Houston Chronicle,
        June 17, 2004. Available at: https://www.chron.com/news/houston-texas
        /article/Effect-of-Dr-Death-and-his-testimony-lingers-1960299.php.
        Accessed August 5, 2024.

U.S. v Gigante, 996 F. Suppl 140 (E.D.N.Y. 1997a)

U.S. v Gigante, 996 F. Suppl 194 (1997b)

Weinstock R: Ethical concerns expressed by forensic psychiatrists. J Forensic
        Sci 31(2):596–602, 1986 3711835

Weiss KJ, Sadoff RL: From the Journal of Psychiatry & Law archives: Bernard
        L. Diamond, M.D. on "The Psychiatrist as Advocate." J Psychiatry Law
        40(2):121–133, 2012

Zapf PA, Kukucka J, Kassin SM, et al: Cognitive bias in forensic mental health
        assessment: evaluator beliefs about its nature and scope. Psychol Public
        Policy Law 24(1):1–10, 2018

7

Ethical Implications for the Use of Neuroscience, Neuroimaging, and Artificial Intelligence in the Courtroom

Michael R. MacIntyre, M.D.
Richard G. Cockerill, M.D.
R. Ryan Darby, M.D.

Understanding of neuroscience has advanced dramatically in the twenty-first century. Advancements in neuroimaging have led to earlier detection and better understanding of disease processes such as dementia and multiple sclerosis. Advances in computing power have ignited rapid developments in artificial intelligence (AI) and machine learning, leading to increasingly specific models of human behavior prediction, such as suicide and violence risk. These newer tools have helped researchers to study the relationship between brain function, neuropsychiatric disease, and human behavior. Despite the promise of these novel developments, however, psychiatrists must be aware of the ethical concerns that arise when new technology is applied in different contexts, such as a legal arena.

When using neuroscience in the clinical setting, a psychiatrist's primary ethical concern is maximizing the welfare of the patient. In the majority of situations, the guiding principles of autonomy, beneficence, and nonmaleficence will help the clinician achieve the most ethical action (Beauchamp and Childress 2013). The limitations of new research or techniques may be acceptable, as long as patient outcomes are improved through better diagnosis, more effective treatment options, and increased stratification of important health outcomes. Similarly, a researcher has a primary duty to advance scientific knowledge and may ethically use new technologies to their advantage, assuming they obtain informed consent and work to minimize potential harm to research subjects (Darby and Weinstock 2018). Once a psychiatrist enters a forensic role, however, the duties change, and the ethics decision-making shifts.

When applied in a legal context (such as civil, criminal, correctional, regulatory, or legislative matters), neuroscience evidence may have serious potential to cause harm or negative consequences for an individual. New research may be misrepresented, with attorneys or expert witnesses making definitive claims inconsistent with the current state of science. AI-powered algorithms may be construed as absolute truth when defining an individual's risk for future behavior. Evaluees may be coerced to undergo testing they would have otherwise refused in medical settings, with unforeseen or poorly understood consequences. Finally, groundbreaking science has the potential to confuse and mislead the trier of fact, potentially distorting the search for truth and justice in a courtroom.

Advanced techniques are currently used in limited clinical settings when there is enough evidence that the tests could ultimately benefit the patient, but in the courtroom, neuroimaging evidence has greater potential to harm, and the ethical considerations are very different. Machine learning may help clinicians better anticipate the disease course for a patient and make appropriate treatment adjustments, but when used for decisions such as prolonged incarceration versus release, a limited understanding and lack of human oversight in how computers arrive at a decision may cause concern.

Neuroscientific explanations for human behavior and personal responsibility have a "seductive allure" to the trier of fact that may not be fully supported by the current literature (Weisberg et al. 2008). The legal system may turn to neuroscience to help explain issues such as culpability, liability, intentionality, truth, and punishment. The expert witness does not use neuroscience to benefit an individual patient but rather attempts to answer questions regarding a defendant's mental state at the time of an offense, whether a witness is lying, or whether a witness is overly biased. Prominent neurologist Helen Mayberg boldly stated that the use of neuroimaging in courtrooms is "a dangerous distortion of science that sets dangerous precedents for the field" (Hughes 2010, p. 340). Although this concern has some validity, we should not ignore significant progress solely for fear of potential risk. Other scientific advances, such as DNA evidence, have been able to address controversies while revolutionizing forensic science and benefiting the legal system. Rather than ignore neuroscience, forensic psychiatrists should embrace the field while consciously weighing the risks and benefits of using new developments in the courtroom. When appropriate, forensic psychiatrists should take steps to thoughtfully and ethically incorporate neuroscience into their opinions and reasoning and strive to present these findings in a manner understandable and usable by the legal system.

Use of Neuroimaging in Forensic Psychiatry

Neuroimaging techniques are increasingly used in legal settings. Mainstays such as MRI and computed tomography are regularly introduced as evidence, and advanced techniques such as positron emission tomography, single-photon emission computed tomography, diffusion tensor imaging (DTI), and quantitative electroencephalography have all been accepted by courts (Farahany 2016; Moriarty 2008). Neuroimaging has three major functions in legal proceedings. First, it can be used as evidence of a clinical diagnosis in a defendant accused of a crime. Neuroimaging findings are a major component of the diagnostic criteria for conditions such as stroke, dementia, and multiple sclerosis. Other neuropsychiatric diagnoses, such as concussions or schizophrenia, are not directly impacted by neuroimaging findings, although some research suggests that differences may be detectable on imaging. Neuroimaging never allows a clinician to make a diagnosis in the absence of related clinical symptoms or findings on neuropsychiatric examination.

A diagnosis alone is insufficient for any meaningful forensic determination. A diagnosis must also be shown to result in the specific behavioral impairment that diminishes responsibility for a crime. This leads to the second use of neuroimaging: providing a neurologic mechanism to support claims that a defendant had impaired behavioral capacities. For example, a defendant's lesion in a specific brain region may match the neuroanatomical localization of specific behavior found through research. The presence of a behavioral symptom together with a lesion scientifically associated with that symptom provides evidence of a neurological basis for the behavior in question.

When analyzing impaired behavioral capacities as a potential excuse for a crime, courts also require a temporal link between the neurologic injury and the behavior. Experts commonly err when they suggest the presence of an altered mental state based solely on an abnormal image, an inaccurate and inappropriate conclusion known as *reverse inference* (Scarpazza et al. 2018). Experts must avoid equating neuroimaging findings associated with impaired behavioral capacities to one's specific mental state at the time of a crime. Although neuroimaging evidence may help infer a mental state at the time of a criminal act, it can do so only indirectly. Temporal inferences become more difficult with insidious or progressive conditions such as dementia or fluctuating conditions such as epilepsy or psychosis. Additionally, neuroimaging in a legal case often is not obtained until years after a crime is committed, significantly limiting the ability to make a temporal inference. These limitations have led some legal scholars to question any application of neuroimaging for determining criminal intent, causation, criminal responsibility, or future risk (Morse 2011, 2014). Conversely, a close temporal relationship between documented neuropsychiatric behavioral syndromes and specific neuroimaging changes strengthens an argument that a brain injury or disease process affected behavioral capacities and contributed to a criminal act. Neuroimaging data may improve causal inferences by providing convergent evidence (Darby 2018; Darby et al. 2016; Scarpazza et al. 2018).

The third use of neuroimaging is to infer an individual's mental state at the actual time the imaging is performed. For example, neuroimaging has the potential to form the basis of a lie detector test, to determine the credibility of eyewitnesses, and to examine implicit biases in court participants. When it is used for this purpose, the expert must be aware of the state of the subject because acute factors such as sleep deprivation, caffeine use, and mental effort may cause distinct changes in functional neuroimaging.

The Current State of Neuroscience

Despite the advances in our understanding of human behavior, the brain is incredibly complex, and our knowledge remains in its infancy relative to many other medical fields. Any expert using neuroimaging must be aware of the current state of the science and its limitations. Neuroimaging studies often have limited reproducibility because of varying methodology, small and poorly representative samples, differences in computer software processing, and variations in statistical analysis (Moriarty et al. 2013). Certain clinical diseases or symptoms may localize better to a brain network than a specific region, resulting in further inconsistency across studies (Darby and Fox 2019; Darby et al. 2019). To avoid distorting the truth, the expert witness must use results that have been replicated (or be able to understand and clearly articulate the reasons for the lack of replication). It is always prudent for an expert to understand the details of any scientific methods that influence an opinion because, depending on the jurisdiction, any neuroimaging evidence introduced by an expert may be subject to an admissibility challenge based on *Kelly-Frye* (scientific evidence must be "generally accepted" by the relevant scientific field [*Frye v. United States* 1923]) or *Daubert* (sound research "illustrative factors" must be demonstrated [*Daubert v. Merrell Dow* 1993]).

Scientists study average differences in brain and behavior over multiple subjects and trials. These population-based variations provide incredibly useful information for scientists and clinicians, but when an expert introduces such research, courts must figure out how to apply group data to an individual, a challenge termed *group-to-individual inference* or *G2i inference* (Faigman et al. 2013). Although group data may provide a likelihood that an individual's behavior is related to a brain insult, imaging alone cannot directly provide a conclusion in that individual's case with any reasonable certainty. For example, although changes in the frontotemporal region of the brain are associated with behavioral disinhibition, the presence of frontotemporal changes on a defendant's MRI does not offer any conclusive information about that individual's behavioral capacities. Many studies focus on a specific population (such as the elderly or combat veterans), further limiting generalizability of results to any individual.

The expert must address two issues when applying imaging to a single subject: 1) the validity of a detected neuroimaging abnormality and 2) the likelihood that the neuroanatomical location of the abnormality relates to a specific behavioral change. For certain structural abnormalities, such as stroke or tumor, the likelihood of being a true abnormality is high, and validity is less of a concern. In other instances, the validity of a single-subject abnormality is less clear. As an example, brain atrophy in single subjects may be measured using voxel-based morphometry and cortical thickness; patient MRIs are then compared to those of subjects with no underlying neurologic or psychiatric disease (Scarpazza et al. 2013, 2016; Tetreault et al. 2020). Depending on analysis methods, these approaches may have false-positive rates (i.e., tending to suggest brain damage in a normal person) unacceptable to a criminal court.

Despite limitations, quantitative approaches remain superior to unaided clinician interpretation of images in a forensic setting, which is subject to bias. For instance, radiologists are more likely to detect lesions when informed of a clinical abnormality; this situation would be the norm in a courtroom, because expert testimony on imaging is required only after inappropriate behavior has occurred (Hugh and Dekker 2009).

Cutting-edge research suggests that the regional location of a brain lesion may be less important than its effect on specific neural networks. Darby et al. (2018a) systematically examined the relationship between focal brain lesions and antisocial changes in behavior, including criminal behavior. After reviewing 17 cases with a clear temporal association between lesion onset and behavioral change, they found that lesions occurred in several different locations, and no single brain region was affected in all cases. Clinical symptoms do not necessarily stem from a brain lesion directly and may arise from other locations connected to the lesion. This finding allowed the authors to use a new method called lesion network mapping to identify regions functionally connected to each of the specific lesions and demonstrate that all lesions were connected to the same common brain network. Furthermore, connectivity to this network was highly specific, and lesions outside of the network were less likely to result in criminal behavior (Darby et al. 2018a). The authors replicated the results in a second group of 23 patients who had antisocial behavioral changes suspected to result from brain lesions, although the temporal relationship was less clear. Finally, the identified criminal behavior network was shown to be involved in moral- and value-based decision-making, cognitive processes that are impaired in antisocial behavior (Darby et al. 2018b). The study took a significant step toward determining the likelihood that a neuroimaging abnormality is related to acquired antisocial behavior. However, a forensic psychiatrist must be aware of the limitations before using this research in a forensic setting.

Neuroimaging and Individual Autonomy

It is not settled whether courts can mandate neuroimaging or whether a defendant's consent is required. Compelled neuroimaging would present issues related to respect for persons and their autonomy. For example, if a person elected against neuroimaging in clinic but was forced to undergo a study for a trial, what if the results showed a structural abnormality they did not want to know about? Additionally, the findings may have genetic implications for people not even involved in the case, such as children or siblings. The ethical calculus would become even more complicated if a court wished to use neuroimaging for someone not a party in the case (i.e., potential jury members to assess for biases or witnesses to detect lying). Neuroimaging in the courtroom has the potential to violate basic constitutional rights. Some have argued that as technology advances, forced neuroimaging could infringe on individual privacy or violate search-and-seizure protections (Boundy 2012; Shen 2013). If used to detect guilt or innocence in a defendant, neuroimaging used for lie detection may interfere with Fifth Amendment protections against self-incrimination (Kraft and Giordano 2017).

Lie Detection

The ultimate goal of a trial can be considered to determine the truth of a legal matter. However, it is exceedingly difficult to consistently and accurately detect intentional deception from a defendant, the prosecution, or a witness. People attempting to detect deception perform barely above chance (Vrij et al. 2000), and those with professional investigative training and experience perform no better than the average layperson (Mann et al. 2004). Researchers have long attempted to find a scientific way to detect lying. Recent efforts to use functional MRI (fMRI) for lie detection serve as a cautionary tale.

fMRI attempts to determine truth-telling by measuring blood flow to and from regions of the brain associated with the act of lying. Studies do not directly examine lying, however; rather, they assess blood flow in the brain after a subject is instructed to lie. This requires multiple tasks of executive functioning such as processing the instruction, remembering the command, determining the true statement, coming up with a lie, and then stating the lie. The totality of processes may involve neural networks of executive control highly overlapping with or distinct from neural networks responsible solely for lying (Farah et al. 2014). Additionally, fMRI cannot distinguish between misremembering events, a biased recollection of events, or intentional lying. To this point, fMRI studies show brain activation patterns when an individual recognizes a face similar to those when they simply believe they recognize a face (Rissman et al. 2010). Thus, when fMRI research studies are applied to a defendant, the imaging results may not actually suggest what the expert implies or what the court wants. Given these significant limitations, any forensic psychiatrist using fMRI for lie detection introduces a serious potential for harm to a defendant without a compelling justification, because the evidence does not increase the honesty of the evaluation. The Supreme Court has not yet commented on fMRI for lie detection, but the Court of Appeals for the Sixth Circuit refused to admit fMRI evidence because there are no real-life error rates for lie detection and no standards for how images are obtained (*United States v. Semrau* 2012).

Effect of Neuroimaging on the Trier of Fact

Neuroimaging may create bias in a judge or jury, resulting in decisions of guilt based on a defendant's abnormal imaging rather than the individual's behavior. However, it remains unclear how neuroimaging evidence affects any individual judge or court. In general, research has found that the presence of a neuroimage makes a neuroscientific claim more compelling (McCabe and Castel 2008), but others have questioned the empirical evidence for this conclusion (Farah and Hook 2013). Studies have shown that the presence of neuroimaging evidence can tilt a judge's decisions either way. The decision to present neuroimaging evidence can be a double-edged sword for an attorney. It could suggest reduced culpability, resulting in a lesser sentence; it could also suggest an untreatable, structural cause of criminal behavior necessitating prolonged incarceration for public safety.

Juries consist of a cross-section of the general population, and the typical understanding of science varies enormously within the United States. Expert witnesses must be particularly cautious of the potential for jury members to misunderstand, misinterpret, or overinterpret neuroimaging. Various visual representations of data may confuse a jury member inexperienced with interpreting neuroimages. For example, DTI fiber-tracking maps may lead a jury to believe they are looking at an actual picture of neural connections (Feigl et al. 2014). Brain images with strong, bright coloring may be prejudicial to juries (Brown and Murphy 2010). Experts and researchers may even "dial-a-defect," where they use computer processing and varied statistical analysis to result in a colored image that appears more compelling for their legal argument (Brown and Murphy 2010). Although an expert must be careful not to oversimplify or overstate research, the opposite problem may occur. If the scientific explanation presented is too complex or detailed, jurors may be confused about the relevant points and potentially ignore the information altogether.

The expert must strive to explain neuroscience honestly and objectively, and also in a way that the trier of fact can understand and appropriately use to come to a conclusion. The expert should focus on how a neuroimage directly strengthens the expert's ultimate opinion and reasoning. To do this, the expert should provide a descriptive diagnosis of the evaluee, clearly assess causal links between behavioral symptoms and criminal behavior, describe how the neuroimaging findings support the link, and use the neuroimage only if it provides an accepted anatomical correlation to clinical findings. Several experts have proposed ethical guidelines for using neuroimaging in a legal setting (Meltzer et al. 2014; Scarpazza et al. 2018).

Artificial Intelligence in Forensic Psychiatry

AI plays an increasingly central role across a broad swath of industries. From self-driving cars to recommendation engines, sophisticated AI algorithms make predictions that affect people's lives more each year. In January 2020, a landmark paper was published in *Nature* describing an AI algorithm that consistently outperformed six experienced radiologists in the evaluation of thousands of screening mammograms across multiple institutions in two countries, with significant improvements in both sensitivity and specificity, all the while completing the task in a fraction of the time (McKinney et al. 2020). Such powerful algorithms can also learn forensic psychiatry. In particular, they can perform risk assessments, one of the core functions of the forensic psychiatrist. If machines do such work, there is no doubt ethical concerns will arise.

AI and Machine Learning: The Basics

To understand the basics of AI and its potential applications, we must first understand a few key terms. *Artificial intelligence* is a broad umbrella term describing the use of automated processes to perform cognitive tasks. *Machine learning* is a subset of AI that describes the process by which machine processes, or algorithms, improve their predictive power as they are exposed to more data over time. *Deep learning* is a subset of machine learning that mimics the way the human brain learns by using *artificial neural networks*.

With deep learning, the idea is to build an algorithm that learns naturalistically, with minimal human input or supervision required. For example, say we want to design an intelligent algorithm to identify dogs. One way to start might be to tell the algorithm what features make a dog, such as a tail, characteristic facial features, and fur. Then, the algorithm uses these features to identify dogs. Although this is an intuitive approach on its face, it is not difficult to think of the problems it may lead to. Some dogs have cropped tails, some have atypical facial features, and some lack fur. An alternative approach is to give the algorithm minimal initial guidance but expose it to enormous amounts of data. Each time it makes a guess, it is given feedback on whether it was correct or incorrect. Each time, the algorithm makes adjustments to its model for "dog." In other words, it constructs, for itself, the features that make a dog a dog. This is deep learning in a nutshell.

If exposed to enough data, an algorithm trained in this way can be incredibly accurate. Machine image recognition is a problem computer scientists have been working on for decades. In 2010, when few leading computer scientists used deep learning, the average algorithm was wrong more than half the time when asked to identify an unknown object from an image—even the absolute best were incorrect a quarter of the time. By 2017, when deep learning and neural networks had been widely adopted, the error rate for the average algorithm had plunged to 5% (Gershgorn 2017). This is where the magic of deep learning lies: once the system gains basic competency in some discipline, it can self-improve at an astonishing rate. The same basic principles apply to the mammography study described earlier. When the study was published, the algorithm (compared with radiologists) had absolute reductions of 5.7% for false positives and 9.4% for false negatives (McKinney et al. 2020). If these results could be generalized, such algorithms would have the potential to save thousands of lives each year.

The Potential Role of Algorithms in the Courtroom

How might such powerful technology be used in forensic psychiatric settings? AI can be deployed safely only when it consistently and significantly outperforms human comparators. For example, in the cases of autonomous driving and breast cancer screening, the existing human comparators (drivers and radiologists, respectively) are already quite proficient. What about applying AI technology to something much more challenging for human practitioners: psychiatric risk assessment?

The assessment of suicide or violence risk is an essential component of the practice of forensic psychiatry, yet existing assessment tools for these purposes are imprecise. A 2017 systematic review of 15 suicide risk assessment instruments found that none met the minimum benchmarks for accuracy—sensitivity > 80% and specificity > 50% (Runeson et al. 2017). The story is similar for violence risk assessments: the best available instruments, such as the Violence Risk Appraisal Guide (VRAG), perform only modestly better than chance (Douglas et al. 2017). Deep learning may be the best method for these types of problems. Suicide and violent behaviors are both relatively infrequent events affected by countless variables. Artificial neural networks can consider orders of magnitude more factors in their assessments than traditional tools or individual practitioners. And like all applications of deep learning, the algorithms can continually improve themselves, as they analyze more and more data.

The earliest applications of deep learning to these problems are encouraging. In a 2020 study, an algorithm using artificial neural networks was trained to assess suicide risk with a large population of patients in a major U.S. health system. By examining clinical data available in the electronic medical record (EMR), such as a doctor's progress notes, the algorithm risk-stratified patients into four suicide risk groups, from low to very high. Those in the "very high" risk group had a relative risk of suicide of 59.02 compared with the lowest risk group (Zheng et al. 2020). If extrapolated, this method would represent a dramatic improvement over traditional assessments, which, when pooled, had an OR of < 5 for predicting suicide (Runeson et al. 2017). Similar progress has been made in violence risk assessment. An AI algorithm used clinical notes in the EMR to predict violent behavior among psychiatric inpatients at two psychiatric institutions in the Netherlands. The predictive validity of the algorithm was 0.80 at the first site and 0.76 at the second (Menger et al. 2019); this compares quite favorably to existing tools—the VRAG, for example, has a predictive validity of about 0.72 in pooled data for making similar predictions (Douglas et al. 2017).

So, based on two recent examples, AI algorithms are already outperforming existing prediction instruments. With their ability to continually self-improve, the performance difference will only grow. Considering their efficiency, ease of use, and potential accessibility, it is almost inconceivable that AI algorithms will not be widely adopted in forensic psychiatric settings. As such, practitioners in this arena must be familiar with the technology and aware of the ethical concerns raised by its use. Some of the most important are identified and described next.

Informed Consent

The ability to give informed consent is a bedrock principle of biomedical ethics, flowing from the principle of respect for persons. When a procedure is necessary, especially if it is new or experimental, proper education must be provided to allow those receiving the procedure to make informed choices. As medical technology has advanced, this has become increasingly difficult. It is much easier to comprehend the risks and benefits of an appendectomy than it is to understand the consequences of proton beam therapy—and artificial neural networks represent an even higher level of complexity. If they are to be used in clinical or forensic psychiatric settings, methods must be developed to properly inform those who will be subject to their assessments. In forensic settings, future defendants may be required by law to undergo assessments that use AI algorithms. If such a defendant or their counsel does not understand how the assessment works, their ability to challenge its findings is extremely limited. Thus, before AI-powered tools are widely implemented, it is essential that policymakers consider their complexity and potential impacts on the autonomy of psychiatric patients or forensic evaluees.

Moral Responsibility

When high-stakes decisions are made about an individual's life, especially those that involve deprivation of liberty, traditionally there exists a responsible party accountable for those decisions. If a judge applies an unreasonably harsh sentence for a defendant, the ruling can be appealed. If this is a pattern of behavior, that judge can be removed from office by various mechanisms. When an algorithm is making the call, however, who is to blame for bad outcomes? Violence risk assessment algorithms are increasingly used in sentencing decisions. When an algorithm imposes a sentence a defendant believes is unreasonably harsh, how can the decision be rectified? The decision could be appealed, but judges are not computer scientists. It is much easier to review the decision-making of another judge than it is to dissect the decisions made by a sophisticated algorithm. If an algorithm is consistently unfair, it cannot be sanctioned in the same way an erring human would be. These issues implicate the ethical principles of justice and striving to treat fairly each person who encounters the justice system. Before algorithms are widely implemented in this regard, it is critical that processes are developed to preserve accountability for the decisions that result from their use.

Justice and Equity Concerns

AI algorithms do have the potential to reduce bias and improve objectivity. Computers, unlike humans, do not have implicit biases. However, there is significant risk of human biases slipping into AI software. Sentencing algorithms, which use risk assessment to recommend sentences for criminal defendants, are particularly susceptible. Although the algorithm may be blinded to a defendant's race, if police reports, probation officer documentation, policing practices, and an individual's conviction history all are subject to preexisting biases, and the underlying algorithms being used rely on those data to generate assessments, then those assessments will further propagate such systemic biases, even if the system does not explicitly "know" an individual's race. Thus, the sheen of objectivity provided by these tools conceals the propagation of inequity in the justice system. This has been seen with facial recognition tools, with one study showing that deep learning applied to facial recognition had lower verification accuracy for females, younger subjects, and Black persons (Khiyari and Wechsler 2016). To strive to reach the ethical principle of justice, such tools need to be analyzed repeatedly to ensure they are a force for equity, rather than inequity, in the justice system (van Eijk 2017).

Conclusion

Advances in technology provide new tools for forensic psychiatrists that may potentially revolutionize the field. However, new technology also brings novel ethical challenges. Forensic psychiatrists must understand any technology they use while constantly reexamining the risks and benefits of its implementation in the courtroom. When used cautiously and vigilantly with regard to limitations and biases, techniques such as neuroimaging and artificial intelligence can be useful tools to improve a forensic psychiatrist's ability to provide an honest, objective opinion and minimize harm.

References

Beauchamp TL, Childress JF: Principles of Biomedical Ethics, 7th Edition. New York, Oxford University Press, 2013

Boundy M: The government can read your mind: can the constitution stop it? Hastings Law Journal 63(6):1627–1643, 2012

Brown T, Murphy E: Through a scanner darkly: functional neuroimaging as evidence of a criminal defendant's past mental states. Stanford Law Rev 62(4):1119–1208, 2010 20429137

Darby RR: Neuroimaging abnormalities in neurological patients with criminal behavior. Curr Neurol Neurosci Rep 18(8):47, 2018 29904892

Darby RR, Fox MD: Reply: Heterogeneous neuroimaging findings, damage propagation and connectivity: an integrative view. Brain 142(5):e18, 2019 30907402

Darby WC, Weinstock R: Prescribing stimulants in college populations: clinical and ethical challenges. Adolesc Psychiatry (Hilversum) 7(3):179–189, 2018

Darby RR, Edersheim J, Price BH: What patients with behavioral-variant frontotemporal dementia can teach us about moral responsibility. AJOB Neurosci 7(4):193–201, 2016

Darby RR, Horn A, Cushman F, et al: Lesion network localization of criminal behavior. Proc Natl Acad Sci USA 115(3):601–606, 2018a 29255017

Darby RR, Joutsa J, Burke MJ, et al: Lesion network localization of free will. Proc Natl Acad Sci USA 115(42):10792–10797, 2018b 30275309

Darby RR, Joutsa J, Fox MD: Network localization of heterogeneous neuroimaging findings. Brain 142(1):70–79, 2019 30551186

Daubert v Merrell Dow, 509 U.S. 579 (1993)

Douglas T, Pugh J, Singh I, et al: Risk assessment tools in criminal justice and forensic psychiatry: the need for better data. Eur Psychiatry 42:134–137, 2017 28371726

Faigman DL, Monahan J, Slobogin C: Group to individual (G2i) inference in scientific expert testimony. University of Chicago Law Review 81(2):417–480, 2013

Farah MJ, Hook CJ: The seductive allure of "seductive allure." Perspect Psychol Sci 8(1):88–90, 2013 26172255

Farah MJ, Hutchinson JB, Phelps EA, et al: Functional MRI-based lie detection: scientific and societal challenges. Nat Rev Neurosci 15(2):123–131, 2014 24588019

Farahany NA: Neuroscience and behavioral genetics in US criminal law: an empirical analysis. J Law Biosci 2(3):485–509, 2016 27774210

Feigl GC, Hiergeist W, Fellner C, et al: Magnetic resonance imaging diffusion tensor tractography: evaluation of anatomic accuracy of different fiber tracking software packages. World Neurosurg 81(1):144–150, 2014 23295636

Frye v United States, 293 F. 1013 (D.C. Cir. 1923)

Gershgorn D: The Data That Transformed AI Research and Possibly the World. Quartz, July 26, 2017. Available at: https://qz.com/1034972/the-data-that-changed-the-direction-of-ai-research-and-possibly-the-world. Accessed July 8, 2024.

Hugh TB, Dekker SWA: Hindsight bias and outcome bias in the social construction of medical negligence: a review. J Law Med 16(5):846–857, 2009 19554863

Hughes V: Science in court: head case. Nature 464(7287):340–342, 2010 20237536

Khiyari H, Wechsler H: Face verification subject to varying (age, ethnicity, and gender) demographics using deep learning. J Biom Biostat 7:323, 2016

Kraft CJ, Giordano J: Integrating brain science and law: neuroscientific evidence and legal perspectives on protecting individual liberties. Front Neurosci 11:621, 2017 29167633

Mann S, Vrij A, Bull R: Detecting true lies: police officers' ability to detect suspects' lies. J Appl Psychol 89(1):137–149, 2004 14769126

McCabe DP, Castel AD: Seeing is believing: the effect of brain images on judgments of scientific reasoning. Cognition 107(1):343–352, 2008 17803985

McKinney SM, Sieniek M, Godbole V, et al: International evaluation of an AI system for breast cancer screening. Nature 577(7788):89–94, 2020 31894144

Meltzer CC, Sze G, Rommelfanger KS, et al: Guidelines for the ethical use of neuroimages in medical testimony: report of a multidisciplinary consensus conference. AJNR Am J Neuroradiol 35(4):632–637, 2014 23988754

Menger V, Spruit M, van Est R, et al: Machine learning approach to inpatient violence risk assessment using routinely collected clinical notes in electronic health records. JAMA Netw Open 2(7):e196709, 2019 31268542

Moriarty JC: Flickering admissibility: neuroimaging evidence in the U.S. courts. Behav Sci Law 26(1):29–49, 2008 18327830

Moriarty JC, Langleben DD, Provenzale JM: Brain trauma, PET scans and forensic complexity. Behav Sci Law 31(6):702–720, 2013 24132788

Morse SJ: The future of neuroscientific evidence, in The Future of Evidence: How Science and Technology Will Change the Practice of Law. Edited by Henderson C, Epstein J. Chicago, IL, American Bar Association, 2011, pp 137–163

Morse SJ: Brain imaging in the courtroom: the quest for legal relevance. AJOB Neurosci 5(2):24–27, 2014

Rissman J, Greely HT, Wagner AD: Detecting individual memories through the neural decoding of memory states and past experience. Proc Natl Acad Sci U S A 107(21):9849–9854, 2010 20457911

Runeson B, Odeberg J, Pettersson A, et al: Instruments for the assessment of suicide risk: a systematic review evaluating the certainty of the evidence. PLoS One 12(7):e0180292, 2017 28723978

Scarpazza C, Sartori G, De Simone MS, et al: When the single matters more than the group: very high false positive rates in single case Voxel Based Morphometry. Neuroimage 70:175–188, 2013 23291189

Scarpazza C, Nichols TE, Seramondi D, et al: When the single matters more than the group (II): addressing the problem of high false positive rates in single case voxel based morphometry using non-parametric statistics. Front Neurosci 10(6):6, 2016 26834533

Scarpazza C, Ferracuti S, Miolla A, et al: The charm of structural neuroimaging in insanity evaluations: guidelines to avoid misinterpretation of the findings. Transl Psychiatry 8(1):227, 2018 30367031

Shen FX: Neuroscience, mental privacy, and the law. Harvard J Law Public Policy 36(2):653–713, 2013

Tetreault AM, Phan T, Orlando D, et al: Network localization of clinical, cognitive, and neuropsychiatric symptoms in Alzheimer's disease. Brain 143(4):1249–1260, 2020 32176777

United States v Semrau, 693 F.3d 510 (6th Cir. 2012)

van Eijk G: Socioeconomic marginality in sentencing: the built-in bias in risk assessment tools and the reproduction of social inequality. Punishm Soc 19(4):463–481, 2017

Vrij A, Edward K, Roberts KP, et al: Detecting deceit via analysis of verbal and nonverbal behavior. J Nonverbal Behav 24(4):239–263, 2000

Weisberg DS, Keil FC, Goodstein J, et al: The seductive allure of neuroscience explanations. J Cogn Neurosci 20(3):470–477, 2008 18004955

Zheng L, Wang O, Hao S, et al: Development of an early warning system for high-risk patients for suicide attempt using deep learning and electronic health records. Transl Psychiatry 10(1):72, 2020 32080165

8

Ethical Issues in the Forensic Psychiatric Use of Psychological and Neuropsychological Testing

Daniel A. Martell, Ph.D.

This chapter explores the ethical contours of psychological testing in forensic settings, what it entails, and what criteria need to be met to undertake it. Psychological testing is traditionally the bailiwick of clinical psychologists who have completed specialized graduate-level coursework and training; received supervision in the proper administration, scoring, and interpretation of specific tests; and mastered the fundamentals of the underlying psychometric and statistical principles required to analyze the test results and correlate them with a patient's history, mental status examination, and clinical presentation. Hence, clinical psychologists—particularly those with forensic specialization—can be a significant resource for the forensic psychiatrist.

Types of Psychological Testing

Psychodiagnostic Testing

Psychodiagnostic testing involves the use of empirical psychological instruments to aid in the assessment of psychopathology and psychiatric differential diagnosis. These tests are generally considered to fall into two camps. *Objective* psychodiagnostic tests rely on answers to numerous questions that are assigned to scales. Those scale scores are compared to norms to generate a diagnostic profile that shows how the client's responses compare with known clinical groups. Examples of such tests include Personality Assessment Inventory (PAI) and Minnesota Multiphasic Personality Inventory (MMPI). In contrast, so-called *projective* psychological tests are more subjective in both their administration and interpretation. Tests such as the Rorschach test or Thematic Apperception Test (TAT) rely on the client responding to vague test stimuli by describing what they see in an inkblot or telling a story about a picture, respectively. The resulting stories or descriptions are then scored by the test administrator using various interpretive rubrics to determine personality features and reality testing operations.

Neuropsychological Testing

Neuropsychology is a specialty area within clinical psychology that studies the relationships between brain functioning and human behavior. Neuropsychologists use a large battery of tests tapping various neurocognitive domains, including intellectual functioning, academic achievement, memory, language, attention, concentration, visual organization, speed of information processing, sensory perception, and pure motor functioning. The resulting data help to inform findings from techniques such as brain imaging (e.g., computed tomography, MRI, positron emission tomography, and single-photon emission computed tomography) by providing qualitative and quantitative data regarding the cognitive, psychiatric, and neurobehavioral correlates of brain diseases and specific brain lesions.

Specialized Forensic Testing

Finally, numerous tests have been developed to assess various forensic issues, including 1) assessment of psychiatric malingering; 2) symptom validity testing; 3) susceptibility to interrogative suggestibility; 4) comprehension of Miranda rights; 5) assessment of adaptive functioning in intellectual disability cases; 6) assessment of competency to stand trial; 7) assessment of mental state at the time of the offense; 8) suicide risk assessment; 9) testamentary capacity; 10) future dangerousness risk assessment; and 11) psychopathy.

Professional Ethical Standards for Forensic Psychological Testing

Professional and ethical standards for psychological testing flow primarily from general professional standards that are provided in several authoritative volumes. *Standards for Educational and Psychological Testing* is published by the American Educational Research Association (2014) in conjunction with the American Psychological Association and the National Council on Measurement in Education. This volume describes 1) the foundations for psychological testing (i.e., expectations for test reliability and validity, precision and errors of measurement, and cultural fairness); 2) appropriate methods for test design and development, including development of scales and scoring, normative populations, and the establishment of cut scores; 3) standards for test administration, scoring, application of norms, and interpretation; and 4) testing applications in various settings including user qualifications, test selection, administration, interpretation, reporting, and maintaining test security. These standards can be directly relevant in evaluating the admissibility of any particular psychological tests in the context of a *Daubert* or *Kelly-Frye* proceeding (*Daubert v. Merrell Dow* 1993; *Frye v. United States* 1923).

Turning to published professional ethical standards that address psychological testing, the American Psychological Association's (2017) Ethical Principles of Psychologists and Code of Conduct (EPPCC) contains the following:

9.02 Use of Assessments

(a) Psychologists administer, adapt, score, interpret, or use assessment techniques, interviews, tests, or instruments in a manner and for purposes that are appropriate in light of the research on or evidence of the usefulness and proper application of the techniques.

(b) Psychologists use assessment instruments whose validity and reliability have been established for use with members of the population tested. When such validity or reliability has not been established, psychologists describe the strengths and limitations of test results and interpretation.

(c) Psychologists use assessment methods that are appropriate to an individual's language preference and competence, unless the use of an alternative language is relevant to the assessment issues.

9.09 Test Scoring and Interpretation Services

(a) Psychologists who offer assessment or scoring services to other professionals accurately describe the purpose, norms, validity, reliability, and applications of the procedures and any special qualifications applicable to their use.

(b) Psychologists select scoring and interpretation services (including automated services) on the basis of evidence of the validity of the program and procedures as well as on other appropriate considerations.

(c) Psychologists retain responsibility for the appropriate application, interpretation, and use of assessment instruments, whether they score and interpret such tests themselves or use automated or other services. (p. 13, cross-references deleted)

EPPCC standards are further addressed in the specific context of forensic work by the American Psychological Association's (2011) *Specialty Guidelines for Forensic Psychology* (SGFP):

10.02 Selection and Use of Assessment Procedures

Forensic practitioners use assessment procedures in the manner and for the purposes that are appropriate in light of the research on or evidence of their usefulness and proper application. This includes assessment techniques, interviews, tests, instruments, and other procedures and their administration, adaptation, scoring, and interpretation, including computerized scoring and interpretation systems.

Forensic practitioners use assessment instruments whose validity and reliability have been established for use with members of the population assessed. When such validity and reliability have not been established, forensic practitioners consider and describe the strengths and limitations of their findings. Forensic practitioners use assessment methods that are appropriate to an examinee's language preference and competence, unless the use of an alternative language is relevant to the assessment issues.

Assessment in forensic contexts differs from assessment in therapeutic contexts in important ways that forensic practitioners strive to take into account when conducting forensic examinations. Forensic practitioners seek to consider the strengths and limitations of employing traditional assessment procedures in forensic examinations. Given the stakes involved in forensic contexts, forensic practitioners strive to ensure the integrity and security of test materials and results.

When the validity of an assessment technique has not been established in the forensic context or setting in which it is being used, the forensic practitioner seeks to describe the strengths and limitations of any test results and explain the extrapolation of these data to the forensic context. Because of the many differences between forensic and therapeutic contexts, forensic practitioners consider and seek to make known that some examination results may warrant substantially different interpretation when administered in forensic contexts.

Forensic practitioners consider and seek to make known that forensic examination results can be affected by factors unique to, or differentially present in, forensic contexts including response style, voluntariness of participation, and situational stress associated with involvement in forensic or legal matters.

10.03 Appreciation of Individual Differences

When interpreting assessment results forensic practitioners consider the purpose of the assessment as well as the various test factors, test-taking abilities, and other characteristics of the person being assessed, such as situational, personal, linguistic, and cultural differences that might affect their judgments or reduce the accuracy of their interpretations. Forensic practitioners strive to identify any significant strengths and limitations of their procedures and interpretations.

Forensic practitioners are encouraged to consider how the assessment process may be impacted by any disability an examinee is experiencing, make accommodations as possible, and consider such when interpreting and communicating the results of the assessment. (pp. 15–16, references deleted)

Professional Competence and Knowing When to Seek a Referral

Training in forensic psychiatry rarely provides the degree of training and experience required to conduct psychological testing independently. Unless a forensic psychiatrist has pursued a rigorous course of graduate study and obtained additional supervision and experience in psychological testing, they would be well advised to develop collaborative relationships with well-qualified forensic psychologists and neuropsychologists in their community whom they can consult for particular cases in which psychological testing is indicated (or would be helpful) in reaching informed forensic opinions.

Sections 2 and 5 of the Principles of Medical Ethics With Annotations Especially Applicable to Psychiatry (American Psychological Association 2013) emphasize the importance of having proper qualifications for practicing within one's specialty areas and of seeking a referral when needed:

[Section 2]

A physician shall uphold the standards of professionalism, be honest in all professional interactions, and strive to report physicians deficient in character or competence, or engaging in fraud or deception to appropriate entities. (p. 4)

3. A psychiatrist who regularly practices outside his or her area of professional competence should be considered unethical. Determination of professional competence should be made by peer review boards or other appropriate bodies. (p. 5)

[Section 5]

A physician shall continue to study, apply, and advance scientific knowledge, maintain a commitment to medical education, make relevant information available to patients, colleagues, and the public, obtain consultation, *and use the talents of other health professionals when indicated.*

2. In the practice of his or her specialty, the psychiatrist consults, associates, collaborates, or integrates his or her work with that of many professionals, including psychologists, psychometricians, social workers, alcoholism counselors, marriage counselors, public health nurses, and the like. Furthermore, the nature of modern psychiatric practice extends his or her contacts to such people as teachers, juvenile and adult probation officers, attorneys, welfare workers, agency volunteers, and neighborhood aides. In referring patients for treatment, counseling, or rehabilitation to any of these practitioners, the psychiatrist should ensure that the allied professional or paraprofessional with whom he or she is dealing is a recognized member of his or her own discipline and is competent to carry out the therapeutic task required. The psychiatrist should have the same attitude toward members of the medical profession to whom he or she refers patients. Whenever he or she has reason to doubt the training, skill, or ethical qualifications of the allied professional, the psychiatrist should not refer cases to him/her. (p. 8, emphasis added)

This emphasis on competence is further reinforced in Section V of the American Academy of Psychiatry and the Law's (2005) *Ethics Guidelines for the Practice of Forensic Psychiatry,* which also establishes guidelines regarding limiting one's practice to those areas in which the forensic psychiatrist has proper qualifications:

V. Qualifications
Expertise in the practice of forensic psychiatry should be claimed only in areas of actual knowledge, skills, training, and experience.

COMMENTARY
When providing expert opinion, reports, and testimony, psychiatrists should present their qualifications accurately and precisely. As a correlate of the principle that expertise may be appropriately claimed only in areas of actual knowledge, skill, training and experience, there are areas of special expertise, such as the evaluation of children, persons of foreign cultures, or prisoners, that may require special training or expertise. (p. 4)

Special Ethical Concerns in Forensic Psychological Testing

Any forensic mental health professional undertaking psychological testing should be careful to observe ethical best practices. These include the following.

Test Selection and Administration

Cultural Sensitivity and Test Selection

It is critical to select only those psychological tests and procedures that are culturally appropriate for the individual being evaluated. For example, it would be inappropriate to administer a test in English to an individual who is not fluent in English. On-the-fly translations of psychological tests should be avoided because of variations in the skill level and approach taken by individual translators; rather, tests that have been translated and made available by the test publisher help standardize the process. Similarly, intelligence testing that relies on questions about American culture (for example, naming past U.S.

presidents) could place an individual from Uganda or China at a disadvantage and potentially result in an unreliable IQ score.

Obtaining Informed Consent

In any forensic context, it is imperative to obtain and document the informed consent of the individual being examined before administering psychological testing. This ensures that the test-taker is aware of the nature and purpose of the examination and the limitations of confidentiality in the specific forensic context.

Arranging for Proper Testing Conditions to Maximize Test Validity

Forensic mental health settings, particularly jails, prisons, and psychiatric treatment centers, often lack optimal conditions for undertaking psychological (and particularly neuropsychological) testing. Noisy and distracting correctional or psychiatric hospital settings can interfere with the validity of the test data obtained. Deviations from standardized administration conditions (e.g., having the test-taker in handcuffs or having others in the examination room) are obviously a threat to test validity. Recent advances in telehealth permit remote testing in some circumstances, but often this is impossible in correctional settings because of unavailable equipment and other security and practical constraints. Prearrangements to avoid such problems are the preferred method for maximizing the reliability and validity of the test data in a manner that best protects the ultimate opinions offered.

Test Interpretation and Reporting

Detailing the Impact of Test Conditions on Data Reliability and Validity

In situations where optimal conditions cannot be arranged, the forensic mental health professional should consider postponing the examination until they can. If suboptimal conditions are unavoidable, it would be the examiner's ethical duty to describe in detail the deviations from optimal testing conditions and the resulting impact on the reliability and validity of the test data in their reports and testimony.

Overreliance on Computer-Based Test Interpretation

Many psychodiagnostic tests have associated computerized "interpretive" programs that can be used both to score the test and to provide descriptive interpretative language. However, reliance on the interpretive statements provided by such programs is fraught with concerns in the forensic context. Schulenberg and Yutrzenka (2004) discussed the ethical contours of this issue. The primary concern is the lack of transparency from the test publisher about the underlying algorithms that are used to associate test responses and patterns with interpretive statements. Because of this lack of transparency, the end user is unable to explain in court the basis for the interpretive statements generated by the "black box," creating concerns for *Daubert* admissibility. For this reason, overreliance on such narrative reports presents a significant ethical dilemma for forensic mental health professionals and is best avoided.

Selecting a Normative Data Set That Provides the Best Fit for the Person Being Tested

Fairness in testing requires cultural sensitivity and careful consideration of cultural invalidity. In many cases, more than one set of norms might be applied to a particular individual's test results to interpret the findings (comparing the person to someone of a similar age, sex, or educational background). This is particularly true in neuropsychological testing, where there may be multiple sets of norms available for a particular test. Most norms currently in use reflect data collected from the general U.S. population; such norms may be problematic if applied to foreign-born, non-native English speakers, for example. Recent years have also seen the development of separate norms for African American and Hispanic populations, which (while seemingly intuitive) have raised a host of concerns about errors in identifying the presence of brain pathology. The concerns have been thoughtfully addressed in studies (e.g., Brickman et al. 2006; Gasquoine 2009; Manly and Echemendia 2007); the researchers argue that race serves as a proxy for other sociocultural and educational factors and that adjusting scores for race may ultimately deny minority group members needed services. Gasquoine (2022) recently proposed performance-based alternatives to using race norms as one alternative to deal with this issue.

Interpreting Invalid Test Results

Many psychological tests have validity scales built in to detect individuals who are either underreporting or exaggerating impairment. Freestanding tests of effort are also routinely administered in the course of neurocognitive testing. When there are indications that a test result is invalid because of manipulation by the test-taker, it would not be appropriate to provide interpretations of those data.

Protection of Test Security and the Release of Test Data

Duty to Prevent Psychological Tests From Falling Into the Public Domain

It is important to recognize the ethical duty to prevent psychological tests from falling into the public domain, because the years of research and investment that the test publishers put into test development can be damaged if the tests suddenly appear online—for example, allowing individuals to prepare in advance for upcoming testing and corrupting the reliability and validity of the test results. There are also issues of copyright protection. These concerns are addressed in EPPCC (American Psychological Association 2017, p. 14), which makes a critical distinction between *test materials* and *test data*:

> **9.11 Maintaining Test Security**
> The term *test materials* refers to manuals, instruments, protocols, and test questions or stimuli and does not include test data as defined in Standard 9.04, Release of Test Data. Psychologists make reasonable efforts to maintain the integrity and security of test materials and other assessment techniques consistent with law and contractual obligations, and in a manner that permits adherence to this Ethics Code.

Duty to Comply With Court Orders and Resolving Conflicts Between Professional Ethics and Legal Requirements

The SGFP (American Psychological Association 2011, p. 14) notes the importance of complying with court orders:

8.01 Release of Information

Forensic practitioners are encouraged to recognize the importance of complying with properly noticed and served subpoenas or court orders directing release of information, or other legally proper consent from duly authorized persons, unless there is a legally valid reason to offer an objection. When in doubt about an appropriate response or course of action, forensic practitioners may seek assistance from the retaining client, retain and seek legal advice from their own attorney, or formally notify the drafter of the subpoena or order of their uncertainty.

Distinguishing Test Data From Test Materials in Releasing Psychological Testing

Because of the adversarial nature of American justice systems, there is typically a duty to produce psychological test data along with other material that forms the basis for one's opinions for independent scrutiny by the opposing side. Here, the distinction between *test materials* and *test data* is of paramount importance. There remains a duty to protect proprietary *test materials* (i.e., test questions, manuals, and stimulus materials) from falling into the public domain. However, *test data* (e.g., the subject's answers and scores) may be disclosed. This is directly addressed in EPPCC (American Psychological Association 2017, p. 13):

9.04 Release of Test Data

(a) The term *test data* refers to raw and scaled scores, client/patient responses to test questions or stimuli, and psychologists' notes and recordings concerning client/patient statements and behavior during an examination. Those portions of test materials that include client/patient responses are included in the definition of test data. Pursuant to a client/patient release, psychologists provide test data to the client/patient or other persons identified in the release. Psychologists may refrain from releasing test data to protect a client/patient or others from substantial harm or misuse or misrepresentation of the data or the test, recognizing that in many instances release of confidential information under these circumstances is regulated by law.

In situations where a court orders the release of test materials via discovery rules, seeking the use of protective orders to seal the test materials is recommended to discharge one's duty to protect them.

Conclusion

Best ethical practices for forensic psychiatrists considering the use of psychological testing involve a careful assessment of the boundaries of one's own competence, recognizing when consultation with a forensic psychologist is in the best interest of the client, the case, and one's ethical duties. Using cultural sensitivity in test selection, obtaining informed consent, and optimizing testing conditions in correctional and maximum-security settings are all important factors to consider. Being cognizant of the limitations of reliance on computer-based interpretive reports and of appropriate normative data for test interpretation are key to providing valid opinions based on forensic behavioral science to inform judicial decision-making.

References

American Academy of Psychiatry and the Law: Ethics Guidelines for the Practice of Forensic Psychiatry. Adopted May 2005. Bloomfield, CT, American Academy of Psychiatry and the Law, 2005. Available at: https://www.aapl.org/ethics-guidelines. Accessed January 29, 2022.

American Educational Research Association, American Psychological Association, National Council on Measurement in Education: Standards for Educational and Psychological Testing. Washington, DC, American Educational Research Association, 2014. Available at: https://www.testingstandards.net/uploads/7/6/6/4/76643089/9780935302356.pdf. Accessed January 29, 2022.

American Psychiatric Association: The Principles of Medical Ethics With Annotations Especially Applicable to Psychiatry. Arlington, VA, American Psychiatric Association, 2013

American Psychological Association: Ethical Principles of Psychologists and Code of Conduct Including 2010 and 2016 Amendments. Washington, DC, American Psychological Association, 2017. Available at: https://www.apa.org/ethics/code. Accessed January 29, 2022.

American Psychological Association: Specialty Guidelines for Forensic Psychology. Washington, DC, American Psychological Association, 2011. Available at: https://www.apa.org/practice/guidelines/forensic-psychology. Accessed January 29, 2022.

Brickman AM, Cabo R, Manly JJ: Ethical issues in cross-cultural neuropsychology. Appl Neuropsychol 13(2):91–100, 2006 17009882

Daubert v Merrell Dow, 509 U.S. 579 (1993)

Frye v United Statess, 293 F. 1013 (D.C. Cir. 1923)

Gasquoine PG: Race-norming of neuropsychological tests. Neuropsychol Rev 19(2):250–262, 2009 19294515

Gasquoine PG: Performance-based alternatives to race-norms in neuropsychological assessment. Cortex 148:231–238, 2022 35033337

Manly JJ, Echemendia RJ: Race-specific norms: using the model of hypertension to understand issues of race, culture, and education in neuropsychology. Arch Clin Neuropsychol 22(3):319–325, 2007 17350797

Schulenberg SE, Yutrzenka BA: Ethical issues in the use of computerized assessment. Comput Human Behav 20(4):477–490, 2004

9

How to Interpret the Role of the Forensic Psychiatrist to Promote Ethical Work

Jennifer Piel, M.D., J.D.
Drew Calhoun, M.D.

In recent decades, interest in and use of forensic mental health services have grown, as evidenced by the number of specialty training programs in forensic psychiatry and forensic psychology, the number of scientific journals dedicated to psycholegal topics, and the volume of mental health evaluations performed for legal cases. Forensics, a recognized subspecialty for both psychiatry and psychology, has prompted leaders in these fields to develop specialty and practice guidelines, including those that address forensic ethics. The American Psychological Association's (2013) *Specialty Guidelines for Forensic Psychology* was developed and first published in 1991; the American Academy of Psychiatry and the Law's *Ethics Guidelines for the Practice of Forensic Psychiatry* was first adopted in 1988 and most recently revised in 2005 (American Academy of Psychiatry and the Law 2005). These resources recognize that the knowledge, skills, and practice of forensic mental health have unique aspects and differ in important ways from traditional clinical practice for psychiatrists and psychologists, including ethical considerations that uniquely arise in the setting of forensic mental health services.

The American Academy of Psychiatry and the Law (AAPL) (2005, p. 1) defined forensic psychiatry as a "subspecialty of psychiatry in which scientific and clinical expertise is applied in legal contexts involving civil, criminal, correctional, regulatory, or legislative matters, and in specialized clinical consultations in areas such as risk assessment or employment." From this general definition, one can see that the scope and variety of forensic services are vast and that forensic mental health clinicians may serve in a variety of roles. This chapter highlights several roles for forensic mental health clinicians and discusses some of the ethical considerations they may encounter in these roles. When working in this field, it is important to understand the specific role being served by the forensic clinician, recognize ethical considerations likely to arise in the specific context, and know how to move forward in addressing ethical challenges.

Identifying the Forensic Role

Professional guidelines commonly recognize the importance of ethical decision-making. This is true of the AAPL's (2005) *Ethics Guidelines for the Practice of Forensic Psychiatry*. The guidelines can help resolve most ethical dilemmas that arise in forensic psychiatry, but much like the law, they serve as the floor, not the ceiling (Weinstock 2013). Ethical guidelines can be invaluable tools in guiding mental health professionals confronted with ethical challenges. But situations that are not directly or clearly addressed by guidelines require mental health professionals to consider alternative ethical frameworks and approaches. These complex ethical dilemmas—which may encompass competing duties and responsibilities, and even conflicting rules without clear guidance on prioritization—have no easy solutions.

In applying ethical frameworks to a complex ethical situation, a prudent place for health care professionals to start is to think about their role and the responsibilities, relationships, and ethical duties that arise from that role. General psychiatrists may take on different roles within the course of their professional work, such as working as a health care administrator with responsibilities to manage resources; teaching roles with obligations to the trainees that work with them; and clinical responsibilities toward the patients they treat. The responsibilities and relationships inherent in these roles differ. In contrast to a clinician who decides to advocate for their patient in a treatment role, an administrator may have additional considerations such as managing staff and other resources that could conflict with a particular patient's wishes.

Like general psychiatrists, forensic psychiatrists may hold different roles within the vast subspecialty, often with different obligations and stakeholders involved. Added to the challenge for forensic psychiatrists is that these roles interface with the legal system, which has its own professional and ethical standards; at times, professionals working at the intersection of psychiatry and law may find that the interests of the disciplines cause confusion, do not align, or both. It is not uncommon for a forensic psychiatrist to experience tension between responsibilities owed to a person (a patient or an evaluee) and the service owed to the justice system.

Notwithstanding that forensic psychiatrists serve in vast roles, the American Bar Association (ABA) (2016) has defined roles of mental health professionals who serve the criminal justice system. Among these, the ABA identifies those who evaluate and offer psycholegal expert opinions and testimony, as both evaluators and scientific experts; those who provide consultation relevant to prosecution or defense strategy; those who provide treatment to people in secure settings; and those who consult with policymakers in efforts to improve responses for people with mental illness who are involved in the criminal justice system. The ABA specifically recognizes that these roles can involve conflicting obligations, stating that "the nature and limitations" of these roles and obligations "should be clarified" and the services provided be consistent with the professional's ethical principles (American Bar Association 2016, p. 3).

To that end, Robert Weinstock and William Darby have proposed dialectical principlism as a method to determine the most ethical course of action in the approach toward complex ethical dilemmas (see Chapter 2, "Dialectical Principlism") (Weinstock 2015). Weinstock and Darby's approach specifically prioritizes an understanding of the role of a professional and what duties stem from that role. In this method, one begins with the specific context such as the *setting* and the *specific role,* and then determines the *proximal* and *distal duties* for that particular role. The competing duties and principles are balanced, and the proximal duties are weighed against the distal duties. After an attempt to resolve the conflicts in a way that minimizes their impingement on each other, the weighed principles can be applied to the specific situation, with those of less weight or import perhaps appropriately being removed from the decisional equation.

Forensic psychiatrists use our knowledge and training in both psychiatry and law to help the legal system and promote just and equitable outcomes. By identifying and understanding our role, we are in a better position not only to recognize ethically complicated situations likely to manifest in that role but also to analyze and best address the ethical dilemmas that do arise. As mentioned previously, forensic psychiatrists may serve in many different roles. For the purposes of this chapter, the following roles will be discussed in more detail: expert evaluation, scientific expertise, consultation, treatment, and policymaking.

Forensic Evaluator Role

Forensic evaluator has long been viewed as the primary role for forensic psychiatrists, the role that essentially defined the field of forensic psychiatry. This role can come in many forms. The ABA, with respect to mental health clinicians working in the criminal justice system, defines the evaluator as someone who assesses and offers "legally relevant expert opinions and testimony about a particular person's past, present, or future mental or emotional condition, capacities, functioning, or behavior, and about the effects of interventions, treatments, services, or supports on the person's condition, capacities, functioning, or behavior" (American Bar Association 2016, p. 3).

It is useful to think of this definition because Seymour Pollack, who established one of the earliest forensic psychiatry fellowships in 1965 at the University of Southern California, emphasized the forensic evaluator role. He argued that forensic psychiatry should be distinguished from the broader category of psychiatry and the law. The latter he considered to be the broad, general field of psychiatry as applied to legal matters; he defined forensic psychiatry more narrowly, limiting it to psychiatric evaluations done for legal purposes, in service of the legal system, and primarily legal objectives (namely justice), separating it from the primary therapeutic objective of the medical system (Weinstock et al. 2017). Others have shared the sentiment that so long as forensic psychiatrists clearly indicate that they are not the evaluee's personal physician, they can ethically function outside their role as physicians (Weinstock et al. 2017).

Although Bernard Diamond, another stalwart in the field of forensic psychiatry, agreed that forensic psychiatry entails the application of psychiatry for legal purposes, he thought that psychiatrists should retain medical and psychiatric ends even in their forensic role, and that the forensic psychiatrist should not blindly accept all legal ends. He believed that the forensic psychiatrist has a fiduciary responsibility to the legal system much the same as the treating psychiatrist owes a fiduciary responsibility to a patient (Diamond 1992)—that is, doing what is best based on professional judgment rather than simply what is demanded by the evaluee or any other interested party. Diamond (1992, p. 123) argued that "the psychiatrist is no mere technician to be used by the law as the law sees fit, nor is the science, art, and definitions of psychiatry and psychology to be redefined and manipulated by the law as it wishes." Diamond believed that by retaining medical and psychiatric ends, a forensic psychiatrist may work toward making the legal system more therapeutic and less vengeful, consistent with a concept of therapeutic jurisprudence.

Both Diamond and Pollack agreed that they had an obligation to adequately explain their reasoning so that others understood the basis for their opinion and detect potential biases. Pollack believed it important to give an impartial, objective opinion in the forensic role and diligently tried to overcome biases, including "therapeutic bias," as best he could, refusing to participate in cases in which he could not overcome strong bias (Weinstock et al. 2017). In contrast, Diamond held truth and honesty in highest regard and believed that because impartiality and objectivity were impossible, in strict adherence with his goal of complete honesty, he would participate only in cases in which he could expect the attorney to allow him to present the whole psychiatric truth (Diamond 1992).

Tenets of the priorities of both Diamond and Pollack are reflected in the ethical principles that have been described for the modern forensic psychiatrist in the years since. Paul Appelbaum has emphasized for the forensic psychiatrist the primacy of the ethical principles of truth-telling, respect for persons, and promoting justice (Appelbaum 1997). When the AAPL Ethics Guidelines were last revised in 2005, they advised similar priorities for psychiatrists in a forensic role, that they "should be bound by underlying ethical principles of respect for persons, honesty, justice, and social responsibility" (American Academy of Psychiatry and the Law 2005, p. 1).

Although Pollack's approach was historically a dominant one in forensic psychiatry, Diamond offered an alternative approach that, according to survey results (Weinstock et al. 1991), may have better reflected the predominant forensic psychiatrist perspective. That is, most psychiatrists functioning within a forensic role do not see themselves as doing so completely divorced from their medical and psychiatric roles.

Further, many contemporary forensic psychiatrists would argue that the retention of medical values by physicians practicing within the legal system is also a societal expectation. Ezra Griffith proposed a narrative approach that takes cultural considerations into account (Griffith 1998), whereas Philip Candilis and colleagues suggested an approach that integrates both the individual's personal narrative and traditional medical values, emphasizing the importance of professional integrity (Candilis et al. 2001). Weinstock (2001) agreed that the duty to the legal system is primary in the forensic evaluator role, but he also suggested that this duty should be balanced by secondary duties, including that owed to the evaluee, and that forensic psychiatrists should strive to balance potentially conflicting ethical considerations.

In the evaluator role, the forensic mental health clinician is asked to opine on psycholegal issues by performing an evaluation and providing opinions in legal and regulatory matters. Although a treating clinician could provide information to the court about their patients, the scope of information typically available to the treating clinician, the skills and knowledge needed to make the psycholegal assessment, and the nature of the relationship with the clinician differ in meaningful ways between forensic and clinical roles. The "purposes and uses of forensic evaluations differ qualitatively from the purpose and uses of evaluations developed for treatment purposes" (Melton et al. 2018, p. 10).

The treating clinician's duty is to their patient. The forensic evaluator's responsibilities are to the legal decision-maker, rather than the patient or evaluee. Although there may be some exceptions, the examinee is not a patient of someone in a forensic evaluator role. In contrast to clinical encounters for treatment purposes, in which clinicians often rely heavily on the examinee's self-report, forensic opinions call on clinicians to strive for a fuller, more accurate account of the relevant information. In contrast to clinician encounters in which therapeutic relationships are built over time and the clinician becomes invested in supporting (and even advocating for) the interests of the patient, the forensic evaluator's duty is to the trier of fact and aims to promote a truthful and objective presentation of information. As such, the assessments and opinions offered by the forensic evaluator are not offered for the purpose of helping the examinee—at times, they can actually run counter to the examinee's wishes. Given this reality, one can see that ethical and professional dilemmas are bound to arise in the evaluator role. Table 9.1 lists some examples of issues that may present ethical challenges for the evaluator.

Table 9.1 Examples of ethical issues in the forensic evaluator role

---

- Professional preparation/competency for the type of assessment
- Relationships/conflicts of interest
  - Relationship to examinee
  - Relationship to retaining counsel
- Informed consent for the evaluation
- Privacy and confidentiality notifications
- Bias/impartiality
- Methodology and scope of data
  - Beyond examinee self-report
  - Third-party observers
  - Opinions without personal examination
- Documentation
  - Sufficient to "show your work"
  - Inclusion of potentially embarrassing or irrelevant information

---

Forensic Scientific Expert Role

Much like the forensic evaluator, the forensic scientific expert offers opinions and testimony to the court and has a primary obligation to assist the trier of fact. In contrast to the forensic expert evaluator, whose expert opinion is primarily derived from the forensic evaluation of a specific examinee, the primary basis for the testimony offered by the scientific expert is their scientific or clinical knowledge. In this role, the scientific expert has been instructed to function impartially within their area of expertise to educate the court about scientific knowledge relevant to the case (American Bar Association 2016).

The majority of opinions offered by forensic evaluators would be expected to follow their evaluations, but in a minority of cases, forensic scientific experts may offer a strict scientific opinion that is not based on an evaluation. In this role, practitioners may be asked to serve as a *case-blind didactic expert* with the specific purpose of presenting research relevant to the case without actually having reviewed any case-related documents (Gould et al. 2011). By employing this strategy adeptly, an attorney may enhance the perceived objectivity and credibility of the expert, reducing any assertions of case-related bias, by allowing them to focus only on the science.

A retaining attorney may also request that a forensic psychiatrist review the professional work product of a peer and testify as to their opinions about it in court (e.g., the scientific validity of assessment tools used by an opposing expert to form their opinion). Forensic experts serving in this role are advised to limit their opinions to matters specifically relating to the work reviewed, or at least to broader psychological principles, and to avoid opining on the specific psychological issues in question without performing their own evaluations (Gould et al. 2011). Answering hypothetical questions may be acceptable, because the opposing counsel has an opportunity to object when they believe the hypotheticals as framed assume or misrepresent facts in evidence.

Scientific experts asked to review a peer's work product should aim to minimize biased or advocacy-based testimony and make sure the comments reflect an objective appraisal of the methods and procedures used and the comprehensiveness of the literature reviewed, as well as a fair analysis of the relationship between the data used and the opinion proffered by the expert (Gould et al. 2011).

It is important to note that when an attorney enters into an initial contract with a forensic psychiatrist, asking them to review a work product, the request, in and of itself, does not define the psychiatrist's ultimate role (if any) in the case. After the initial review, the forensic expert is advised to orally communicate their impressions to the attorney. If the attorney believes that the forensic expert could be useful to the case, they are encouraged to enter into a second contract, with well-defined parameters about roles, including whether the forensic expert will be expected to testify, and if so, whether they should conduct an evaluation or limit testimony to scientific expertise relevant to the legal matter (Gould et al. 2011). Figure 9.1 depicts a method for distinguishing roles and suggests the possible use of two contracts.

Experts who testify in an evaluator or scientific role are most effective when they are perceived as having a genuine interest in educating the court. The forensic evaluator should be careful to use sound methodology in arriving at their opinions; otherwise they face potential challenges to the credibility of their work from scientific experts asked to testify about their work. Scientific experts should similarly take care to protect their credibility and the validity of the scientific knowledge they present. In many situations, it would be wise for the testifying

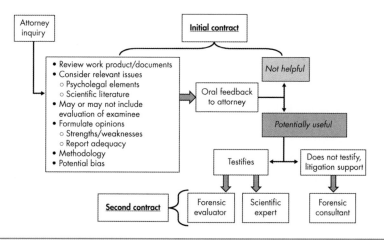

Figure 9.1 Method for distinguishing roles and contracts in forensic neuropsychiatry

scientific expert to minimize contact with interested parties of either side in a case, as such communications are at best unnecessary and, even worse, may impair their objectivity and open them up to (likely avoidable) challenges to their credibility.

It is worth emphasizing the distinction between whether an expert's knowledge will be used to educate the court by testimony or simply to educate the retaining lawyer. In the latter situation (when the expert is not expected to provide any written or oral testimony for the court), they have no obligation to the court (instead, their role would be considered to be a consultative one [see next section], with a primary duty owed to the retaining attorney and, accordingly, not subjected to the same rules of discovery; ethical priorities shift). Although not exhaustive, listed in Table 9.2 are some examples of ethical issues discussed in this section and relevant to the forensic scientific expert role.

Forensic Consultant Role

In *Ake v. Oklahoma* (1985), the U.S. Supreme Court ruled that a state must provide an indigent criminal defendant with free psychiatric assistance in preparing an insanity defense when the defendant's sanity at the time of the offense is seriously in question. In dicta, the court specified that the psychiatrist should be provided not only to examine the defendant

Table 9.2 Examples of ethical issues in the forensic scientific expert role

- Professional preparation/competency in the subject
- Bias/impartiality
- Methodology
- Risk of self-promotion

but also to "assist in evaluation, preparation, and presentation of the defense," highlighting tasks that may be required of psychiatrists beyond those of evaluation and testimony.

The forensic psychiatrist as trial consultant has been increasingly recognized as a distinctly separate role from the testifying forensic expert, with different duties and responsibilities and, accordingly, some unique ethical considerations. In this role, the forensic psychiatrist provides consultative services to help with the legal strategy of the prosecution or defense (American Bar Association 2016), sometimes described as litigation support services.

Trial or case consultants may be asked to help the retaining side strategize and prepare for events at various stages of the case process, including depositions and trials, in any number of ways. Possible tasks that have been described include assistance with the following (Dale et al. 2021; Gould et al. 2011):

- Reviewing, evaluating, and critiquing work product (e.g., medical records, police reports, forensic reports);
- Drafting direct and cross-examination questions;
- Identifying psychological elements pertinent to the legal strategy;
- Conceptualizing, preparing, and presenting the case;
- Identifying appropriate expert witnesses;
- Preparing witnesses;
- Assessing case strengths/weaknesses including feedback on client strengths/liabilities;
- Predicting and responding to possible strategies of opposing counsel;
- Monitoring in-court testimony to aid in the evolving legal strategy of direct and cross-examination; and
- Organizing, presenting, and summarizing relevant scientific literature.

The field of trial consultation has grown considerably over the last several decades, yet there is relatively little professional consensus on the primary ethical principles that should guide forensic trial consultants. Certainly, it remains advisable to uphold generally accepted standards of professionalism and to be honest in all professional interactions, as advised by the American Medical Association (AMA) (2001) and supported by the American Psychiatric Association (APA) (2002). One should also consider the underlying ethical principles advised of those serving in a forensic role as described in the AAPL Ethics Guidelines revision from 2005, including respect for persons, honesty, justice, and social responsibility (American Academy of Psychiatry and the Law 2005). However, it should be noted that these guidelines do not specifically address the consultative role for forensic psychiatrists, despite the unique differences in duties and responsibilities—and accordingly, ethical obligations—for those practicing in a trial consultant role.

The absence of a universally accepted code of ethics for consultants has led some to propose the establishment of such a code (Mental Health Articles 2021). The proposed code of ethics for consultants initially arose out of principles discussed in the available consultation literature. The work emphasized that a consultant's clients are the agencies that hire them, and that a consultant's responsibility is to the welfare and interests of their consultees and client organizations. Consultants are advised to accurately present their professional qualifications, note the potential risks of consultation activities, and disclose any relationships, biases, or values that are likely to affect their work, so that clients may make informed decisions about using their services. They are advised to avoid multiple roles or relationships that may create conflicts and jeopardize their effectiveness. They are advised to establish contracts with well-defined parameters and to enter into contracts only when they are reasonably sure the client will benefit from their services. The code also advises mental health consultants to behave in a way that protects the reputation of their profession (Mental Health Articles 2021).

Discussion in the literature of the ethical considerations specific to the trial consultant role has been relatively limited. In the highly contentious arena of child custody evaluations, Jonathan Gould and colleagues have written extensively. They have described several key differences between testifying experts and nontestifying trial consultants, and they advise forensic mental health professionals to keep the roles separate, to enhance the effectiveness of both (Gould et al. 2011). They reiterated previous sentiments that although the testifying expert has an obligation to assist the court, the nontestimonial consultant (specifically hired for litigation support services and to help prepare the attorney for trial) has a primary responsibility to the retaining side, namely the retaining attorney—further advising that the consultant insist that the attorney, not the litigant, be identified as the client, because communications within an attorney-consultant relationship are not subject to discovery demands and ordinarily are protected from disclosure by attorney work product privilege (Gould et al. 2011).

In the course of a legal case, attorneys may not recognize the role distinctions between testifying experts and nontestifying expert consultants, or they may seek to have the forensic expert change roles. Some attorneys and legal advisors will turn to forensic mental health experts to support them in multiple ways to achieve success in their case (Casey 2020). Some attorneys will assume that a consultant role is inherently part of the services of any retained forensic mental health expert, even one who will be testifying. Forensic mental health professionals typically see this as a dual role, that is, serving in two roles that each can have separate responsibilities and ethical considerations. Although an expert's role may change in the course of a case, conflicts can be minimized when experts perform "one role at a time" to the extent possible. The distinction is not always easy to appreciate, whether for attorneys or for forensic mental health experts. For example, in providing a rebuttal opinion as a forensic evaluator, the expert is likely also providing the attorney with some tips and information to challenge the opposing expert's methodologies or opinions. The mental health expert can explore their own motives to determine whether they are engaging in a new or dual role. In this example, it should be noted that an expert providing the rebuttal information to better inform the trier of fact of the relevant issues and opinions is different from an expert providing the rebuttal to advocate for the trial position of the retaining attorney as an extension of the legal team. Figure 9.1 depicts one possible method for distinguishing roles and (where appropriate) making two separate contracts.

Testifying experts that simultaneously provide litigation support services are arguably more prone to bias and certainly more vulnerable to accusations of bias and attacks on the objectivity and credibility of their testimony. As stated in Gould et al. (2011, p. 40), "One cannot advocate for the data if at the same time one is being asked to advocate for a legal position." Testifying experts have a primary obligation to assist the trier of fact and are expected to provide objective, honest information to educate the court. When an expert in this role is also observed to be providing litigation support, "it is likely that the judge will conclude that the earlier testimony was not as neutral and free of bias as it may have appeared" (Gould et al. 2011, p. 40).

While serving in a consultant role to the prosecution or defense, forensic psychiatrists generally have the same obligations and immunities as any member of the prosecution or defense, except as may be limited by the law (American Bar Association 2016). As it is the ethical responsibility of the attorney to "zealously advocate" for the litigant's legal position, the forensic consultant who is assisting an attorney through their consultative activities, by extension, can be reasonably argued to be assisting in the advocacy of a specific litigant's position. Functioning in this role requires the consultant to adopt an adversarial mindset and help the retaining side, becoming a part of the legal team and helping with the legal strategy in an effort to win the case. This is distinctly different from the role of a testifying evaluator or scientific expert, even one hired by a specific side, because their primary concern is to communicate relevant information and their opinions to the court (Gould et al. 2011).

It is worth emphasizing that although the nontestifying trial consultant retained for that express purpose has an obligation to help the attorney, their effectiveness in assisting the attorney is arguably only enhanced when they maintain their objectivity and honesty. Part of a consultant's effectiveness relies on their ability to openly and honestly communicate their opinions, including about the weaknesses of the case, to the retaining attorney, which is precisely why keeping this role separate from that of testifying expert is advisable. Expert-attorney communications are often discoverable, whereas consultant-attorney communications are not.

Just as sound methodology aids expert witnesses (both evaluators and scientific experts) in establishing the validity of their tests, and accordingly their opinions, sound methodology as employed by a trial consultant similarly enhances the effectiveness of their advice regarding legal strategy. Forensic trial consultants would be well advised to avoid advising attorneys of legal strategies with dubious or limited evidence to support their utility (for example, advising on jury selection based on the reading of nonverbal cues of prospective jurors) (Myers and Arena 2001). Conversely, the application of empirically tested psychological or social science methods to support recommended legal strategies would be both acceptable and recommended. Table 9.3 illustrates some of the ethical issues that may arise in the forensic consultant role.

Table 9.3 Examples of ethical issues in the forensic consultant role

• Professional preparation/competency in subject

• Bounds of partisan role

• Shifting roles during the case

• Serving as both consultant and examining or testifying expert

• Conflicts of interest

Treatment Role in Forensic Settings

As modern definitions of forensic psychiatry have expanded to more broadly recognize the several areas in which psychiatry and the law interface, including the care of patients in forensic settings, it is essential to consider the distinct ethical priorities that differentiate the forensic evaluator role from the treatment role.

Forensic settings can include correctional facilities (e.g., jails, prisons, juvenile detention halls), state hospital forensic wards, and other secure or custodial settings including those mandated by terms of a person's probation, parole, and conditional release. By and large, as much as is reasonable and feasible, the psychiatric treatment of patients seen in forensic settings—and accordingly, the ethical foundations that guide such treatment—should mirror that of other treatment settings. But some unique challenges and differences warrant attention.

Pollack separated the forensic evaluator role, with its legal ends, from other psychiatric involvement, which he agreed better aligned with the more traditional ends of psychiatry, that is, helping the patient (Weinstock et al. 2017). The AAPL Ethics Guidelines also specifically delineate the ethical priorities of "psychiatrists practicing in a forensic role" from those expected "when a treatment relationship exists [in which] the usual physician-duties apply" (AAPL 2005, p. 1). Separately, the guidelines specify that they are meant to "supplement the Annotations Especially Applicable to Psychiatry of the American Psychiatric Association to the Principles of Medical Ethics of the American Medical Association" (AAPL 2005, p. 1).

Historically, biomedical ethics emphasized the primacy of care in the benefit of the patient and the concepts of nonmaleficence and beneficence. The AMA Principles of Medical Ethics advises physicians to "regard responsibility to the patient as paramount," reminding us that the ethical principles were "developed primarily for the benefit of the patient" (American Medical Association 2016). Other ethical principles emphasized include compassion, respect for human dignity and rights, honesty, and the safeguarding of patient confidences and privacy (American Psychiatric Association 2013).

Psychiatrists practicing in both forensic evaluator roles and treatment roles have been advised of the importance of honesty and respect for persons. The ethical priority for those practicing in a treatment role, however, is the duty owed to the patient, specifically geared to their benefit; the primary ethical priority of the forensic evaluator may lean more toward social responsibility and justice.

As such, it is important to recognize the unique circumstances of forensic settings that may inherently interfere with the treating physician's responsibility to the patient. In many of these settings, the facility or the court has a special interest in the progress of the person's psychiatric treatment (e.g., competency restoration) or changes in their violence risk factors to ensure the safety of the facility's staff, their peers, and the community. In their Annotations to the AMA Principles of Medical Ethics, the APA recognized that the psychiatrist may have relationships and duties to multiple other entities that may affect their interactions with patients (American Psychiatric Association 2013). It is recommended that the psychiatrist first consider the impact of these relationships and resolve the conflicts in a way "likely to be beneficial to the patient" (American Psychiatric Association 2013). For significant relationships that conflict with a patient's clinical needs, it is recommended to inform the patient of these relationships, the potential conflicts, and their treatment options and to assist them in making an informed treatment decision (American Psychiatric Association 2013).

The policies and procedures that govern many forensic settings are often quite rigid and restrictive. Sometimes patient interviews cannot be performed in the absence of other personnel such as correctional officers. Not infrequently, documentation—even for medical or psychiatric treatment—can be readily viewed by persons involved with the legal system, including lawyers and judges. In these settings, it is essential that psychiatrists are familiar with the institutional policies regarding confidentiality and that they clearly communicate any limitations on confidentiality to the patient (AAPL 2005).

Similarly, the capacity threshold needed to consent to a forensic evaluation is typically quite different from that required for consenting to treatment. Whenever possible, obtaining a patient's informed consent is recommended. It is recommended that psychiatrists practicing in the treatment role be familiar with the regulations of their specific jurisdictions in regard to the patient's rights to consent to or refuse treatment.

In some situations, such as when recommending the involuntary administration of medication over objection, the treating psychiatrist may be thrust into a dual role, as both treating clinician and testifying expert—for example, by taking on the additional role of forensic psychiatric expert in a Sell hearing (opining on the appropriateness of involuntary medication for the purposes of trial competency restoration [*Sell v. United States* 2003]) or civil commitment proceedings. A treating provider may be put in a dual role in other circumstances, such as providing forensic evaluator services in geographic regions with provider shortages, military court-martials, and some circumstances around psychiatric emergencies in which there is a blending of roles in an effort to provide for the welfare of the patient or protection of certain members of the community.

As with other dual roles, when providing expert testimony, the mental health professional's obligation is primarily to the legal system, not to the patient, requiring the expert to provide objective and truthful information. For the patient, such testimony may go against their wishes and may result in a legal outcome with significant impact to their liberty, such as when the opinion results in civil detention or criminal punishment. "A dual clinical and forensic relationship with a single patient risks compromising relationships between clinicians and patients and can compromise quality patient care" (Gordon 2016, p. 1345). In these situations, it is important to balance conflicting duties as much as is possible. A recognition of the psychiatrist's fiduciary responsibility—that is, to use their professional judgment to guide decisions in the best interests of the patient, even those against the patient's wishes—may be especially helpful in approaching these complex situations. Table 9.4 provides some examples of topics that can raise ethical issues for individuals in treatment roles in forensic settings.

Policy Role

As the field of forensic psychiatry has developed, one core element that has remained constant over the years is the application of psychiatric knowledge in the legal context. It is commonplace for the forensic psychiatrist to serve in a consultative role to the legal system. As discussed previously, such consultation is frequently afforded to attorneys for specific legal cases in both criminal and civil matters, but it need not

Table 9.4 Examples of ethical issues in treatment in forensic settings

- Professional preparation/competency in working with justice-involved persons
- Responsibilities to community (e.g., safety considerations)
- Dual roles
- Conflicts of interest
- Confidentiality

be limited to the individual level. Consultation with the courts, legislatures, and other stakeholders involved in the advancement of mental health policy for justice-involved individuals, as well as other regulatory and clinical matters that affect the delivery of mental health services, is another essential role mental health professionals may play, more broadly, on a societal level (American Bar Association 2016). Forensic mental health professionals, by nature of their training and experience with the legal system, reading statutes and case law, and testifying in court proceedings, have developed skills that naturally align with serving in policy roles (Piel 2018).

In defining the subspecialty of forensic psychiatry, the AAPL Ethics Guidelines describe the role forensic psychiatrists have involving "regulatory and legislative matters" (AAPL 2005, p. 1). The AMA Principles of Medical Ethics, also adopted by the APA, highlight a policy role, noting that physicians have "a responsibility to participate in activities contributing to the improvement of the community and betterment of public health," to "support access to medical care for all people," and to both "respect the law and also recognize a responsibility to seek changes in those requirements which are contrary to the best interests of the patient" (American Medical Association 2016). In the APA's Annotations Especially Applicable to Psychiatry of the AMA Principles of Medical Ethics, psychiatrists are "encouraged to serve society by advising and consulting with the executive, legislative, and judiciary branches of the government" (American Psychiatric Association 2013).

Indeed, multiple organizations have encouraged physician participation in health advocacy. The position of the AMA, and promulgated by the APA, calls physicians to "advocate for the social, economic, educational, and political changes that ameliorate suffering and contribute to human well-being" (American Medical Association 2001; American

Psychiatric Association 2002). The Accreditation Council for Graduate Medical Education (2020a, 2020b) milestones for general and forensic psychiatry have identified advocacy as an important competency for professional development and education in advocacy as a program requirement for general psychiatry residents.

Physicians often advocate for their patients on the individual level, but promoting the advancement of health care policy can affect a larger stakeholder group and may impact society broadly. Forensic mental health professionals can participate in advocacy at a broader level in a number of ways, such as promoting legislative changes through local and federal policymaking, contributing to elections through political campaigns, assisting the courts by way of expert testimony that may have implications beyond the case at issue or working on amicus briefs on a topic with broader impact than a single case, and participating in social movements through education such as by writing op-eds or providing media consultation on issues that affect mental health services.

One of the most common ways for forensic psychiatrists to get involved in societal advocacy and policymaking is through legislative advocacy. For forensic psychiatrists working in this space, it is prudent to get to know system leaders and administrators such as court administrators and health services directors who have familiarity with the legal regulation of mental health services within their communities; advocacy groups and nonprofit organizations whose mission or constituents align with their interests; and local legislators and their aides, especially those who have sponsored or supported related mental health topics previously.

Legislative advocacy refers to efforts to introduce, enact, or modify legislation at a local or federal level; for example, the development and application of mental health legislation (Piel 2018). Because forensic psychiatrists operate at the interface of psychiatry and the law and are acutely aware of the legislative and regulatory processes that affect the profession and patients, they may be uniquely qualified for legislative advocacy roles. In addition to a duty to the legal system in this regard, Bloom (2011) has argued that forensic psychiatrists even owe a responsibility to fellow psychiatrists to be aware of the laws and proposed changes that may affect psychiatric practice in that state.

It is important to delineate again how role affects ethical priorities. In the current AAPL Ethics Guidelines, striving for objectivity is encouraged (American Academy of Psychiatry and the Law 2005). Advocacy, specifically advocating for the side of the hiring party, can be seen as a source of bias, in conflict with one's best efforts for objectivity.

Table 9.5 Examples of ethical issues in policy roles

• Professional preparation/competency in subject

• Consent if speaking about any particular case or identifiable person

• Individual position versus position of larger mental health community

• Reputation of professional discipline

• Reflection of current scientific understanding

• Honest delivery of information

Although advocating for one's opinion is acceptable, advocating for one side is typically discouraged (Piel and Resnick 2016). To be clear, legislative advocacy—advocating for policy change, in a policy role on a societal level (vs. an individual level)—is distinctly different, and highly encouraged.

As in other areas of forensic mental health practice, one should not speak or present information on topics outside one's competencies or knowledge base. It is not uncommon to present some examples when testifying before the legislature or contributing to an amicus brief to better illustrate and personalize the concepts or problems at hand. But in a policy role, the forensic clinician must be careful to protect any patient confidences and identifiable information, unless given explicit consent for disclosure. As with other roles in forensic mental health, the clinician's voice should reflect current scientific standards; opinions that are not generally accepted or supported by evidence-based practices should be made known to the appropriate audience. Table 9.5 provides some examples of topics that can raise ethical issues for individuals in treatment policy roles.

Conclusion

Forensic mental health clinicians serve in many different roles, several of which have been described in this chapter. Roles not specifically discussed in this chapter include peer-to-peer consultation and peer supervision, administrative functions, and the teaching and research roles often expected in academic settings. All of these forensic roles serve justice-involved people (either patients or evaluees), the legal system, and, more broadly, society in different ways and are associated with different responsibilities, relationships, and ethical duties. While

Table 9.6 Forensic roles and primary duty/obligation

Forensic role	Primary duty	Primary duty owed to
Forensic evaluator	Provide expert opinions and testimony, based on forensic evaluation	Trier of fact/legal system
Scientific expert	Provide expert opinions and testimony of case-relevant knowledge, based on area of expertise	Trier of fact/legal system
Forensic consultant	Assist with legal strategy; provide litigation services	Client (i.e., retaining attorney)
Treating clinician	Provide therapeutic interventions and treatment	Patient (e.g., inmate with mental illness)
Policy/legislative	Advance mental health policy, especially related to justice-involved populations or regulation of mental health services	Societal stakeholders (e.g., population of patients or evaluees, community of mental health clinicians, public/community)

an initial recognition of one's setting is an important step in forensic role identification, it should be recognized that many settings expect one to function in multiple roles, often simultaneously. Developing an awareness of the likely roles one may be asked to take on in any practice setting, especially the dual roles that may be requested or obligated, is strongly encouraged. In each role, the professional may expect both primary and secondary duties and responsibilities, and with that, shifting (and potentially conflicting) primary and secondary ethical considerations. Identifying and understanding the specific role of the forensic mental health professional for any given situation helps to distinguish those responsibilities, the primacy of different ethical principles, and the ethical dilemmas that may reasonably be expected to arise in that role. Table 9.6 summarizes common forensic roles, the primary duty, and to whom that duty is owed.

In some ethically complex situations, even when the primary role and corresponding ethical priorities are clear, the potential impact of secondary ethical considerations may be significant and may outweigh the ethical considerations typically considered to be of primary importance when practicing in that role, which may change the most appropriate decision. Accordingly, mental health professionals are well advised not only to recognize the relevant primary and secondary ethical considerations but also to consider their weight and anticipate their potential impact in the decision-making process, so as to arrive at the most ethical course of action.

References

Accreditation Council for Graduate Medical Education: ACGME Program Requirements for Graduate Medical Education in Psychiatry, July 1, 2020. Deerfield, IL, Accreditation Council for Graduate Medical Education, 2020a. Available at: https://www.acgme.org/Portals/0/PFAssets/ProgramRequirements/400_Psychiatry_2020.pdf?ver=2020–06–19–123110–817. Accessed April 29, 2021.

Accreditation Council for Graduate Medical Education: Psychiatry Milestones, 2nd Revision. Deerfield, IL, Accreditation Council for Graduate Medical Education, 2020b. Available at: https://www.acgme.org/Portals/0/PDFs/Milestones/PsychiatryMilestones2.0.pdf?ver=2020-03-10-152105-537. Accessed April 29, 2021.

Ake v Oklahoma, 470 U.S. 68 (1985)

American Academy of Psychiatry and the Law: Ethics Guidelines for the Practice of Forensic Psychiatry. Adopted May 2005. Bloomfield, CT, American Academy of Psychiatry and the Law, 2005. Available at: https://www.aapl.org/ethics-guidelines. Accessed March 24, 2021.

American Bar Association: Criminal Justice Standards on Mental Health. Washington, DC, American Bar Association, 2016. Available at: https://www.americanbar.org/content/dam/aba/publications/criminal_justice_standards/mental_health_standards_2016.authcheckdam.pdf. Accessed April 4, 2021.

American Medical Association: Declaration of Professional Responsibility: Medicine's Social Contract With Humanity. Adopted December 4, 2001. Chicago, IL, American Medical Association, 2001. Available at: https://www.ama-assn.org/system/files/2020–03/declaration-professional-responsibility. Accessed April 14, 2021.

American Medical Association: Code of Medical Ethics. AMA, 2016. Available at: https://code-medical-ethics.ama-assn.org/. Accessed October 1, 2024.

American Psychiatric Association: Association News: Declaration of Professional Responsibility. Psychiatric News, July 19, 2002. Available at: https://psychnews.psychiatryonline.org/doi/10.1176/pn.37.14.0004a. Accessed April 14, 2021.

American Psychiatric Association: The Principles of Medical Ethics with Annotations Especially Applicable to Psychiatry. Arlington, VA, American Psychiatric Association, 2013. Available at: https://www.psychiatry.org/psychiatrists/practice/ethics. Accessed April 4, 2021.

American Psychological Association: Specialty guidelines for forensic psychology. Am Psychol 68(1):7–19, 2013 23025747

Appelbaum PS: A theory of ethics for forensic psychiatry. J Am Acad Psychiatry Law 25(3):233–247, 1997 9323651

Bloom JD: Forensic psychiatry, statutory law, and administrative rules. J Am Acad Psychiatry Law 39(3):418–421, 2011 21908761

Candilis PJ, Martinez R, Dording C: Principles and narrative in forensic psychiatry: toward a robust view of professional role. J Am Acad Psychiatry Law 29(2):167–173, 2001 11471782

Casey C: The many roles of an expert witness during a legal case. The Expert Institute, October 1, 2020. Available at: https://www.expertinstitute.com/resources/insights/the-many-roles-of-an-expert-witness-during-a-legal-case. Accessed April 27, 2021.

Dale MD, Gould JW, Levine A: Cross-examining experts in child custody: the necessary theories and models…with instructions. J Am Acad Matrimonial Law 33:327–389, 2021

Diamond BL: The forensic psychiatrist: consultant versus activist in legal doctrine. Bull Am Acad Psychiatry Law 20(2):119–132, 1992 1633333

Gordon S: Crossing the line: Daubert, dual roles, and the admissibility of forensic mental health testimony. Cardozo Law Rev 37(4):1345–1390, 2016

Gould JW, Martindale DA, Tippins TM, et al: Testifying experts and non-testifying trial consultants: appreciating the differences. J Child Custody 8:32–46, 2011

Griffith EEH: Ethics in forensic psychiatry: a cultural response to Stone and Appelbaum. J Am Acad Psychiatry Law 26(2):171–184, 1998 9664254

Melton GB, Petrila H, Poythress NG, et al: Psychological Evaluations for the Courts: A Handbook for Mental Health Professionals and Lawyers, 4th Edition. New York, Guilford, 2018

Mental Health Articles: Mental Health Professional Consultant's Code of Ethics. Mental Health Articles, 2021. Available at: http://www.mentalhealthmy.com/articles/a-mental-health-professional-consultants-code-of-ethics.html. Accessed April 15, 2021.

Myers B, Arena M: Trial consultation: a new direction in applied psychology. Prof Psychol Res Pr 32(4):336–391, 2001

Piel J: Legislative advocacy and forensic psychiatry training. J Am Acad Psychiatry Law 46(2):147–154, 2018 30026391

Piel J, Resnick P: Psychiatrist as expert witness. Dir Psychiatry CME J 36(3):165–178, 2016

Sell v. United States, 539 U.S. 166 (2003)

Weinstock R: Commentary: a broadened conception of forensic psychiatric ethics. J Am Acad Psychiatry Law 29(2):180–185, 2001 11471784

Weinstock R: Commentary: the forensic report: an inevitable nexus for resolving ethics dilemmas. J Am Acad Psychiatry Law 41(3):366–373, 2013 24051589

Weinstock R: Dialectical principlism: an approach to finding the most ethical action. J Am Acad Psychiatry Law 43(1):10–20, 2015 25770274

Weinstock R, Leong GB, Silva JA: Opinions by AAPL forensic psychiatrists on controversial ethical guidelines: a survey. Bull Am Acad Psychiatry Law 19(3):237–248, 1991 1777687

Weinstock R, Leong G, Piel J, et al: Defining forensic psychiatry: roles and responsibilities, in Principles and Practice of Forensic Psychiatry, 3rd Edition. Edited by Rosner R, Scott C. Boca Raton, FL, CRC Press, 2017, pp 7–13

10

Is Impartiality Attainable in Forensic Work?

Managing Bias and Subjectivity in Psychiatric Expert Testimony

Aryeh Goldberg, M.D., M.A.

In the year 1959, 10 years before the founding of the American Academy of Psychiatry and the Law, forensic psychiatry was less a subspecialty than an accidental foray into the strange and foreign land of the American court system. It was precisely then that Bernard Diamond set out to debunk what he had seen as this budding field's greatest myth: the fallacy of the impartial expert. He opined that the impartial psychiatric expert neither existed nor ought to. He shed light on the fact that a psychiatric expert forms "a close operational identification with one side of the conflict" (Diamond 1959, p. 218) and ultimately becomes an advocate—if not for a particular legal party, then for his own "particular prejudiced point of view" (Diamond 1959, p. 221).

These modest, yet groundbreaking, reflections on a specialty in its infancy laid the groundwork for the questions that would shape the field for decades. Can a forensic psychiatric expert be impartial? Is impartiality even a desired goal? Is forensic psychiatric testimony inherently subjective, or does it strive for a modicum of objective truth? Finally, if Diamond is right that impartiality is impossible, then what are we, as forensic psychiatrists, to do?

It is worth taking a moment to expand on Diamond's concerns of partiality, some of which he himself explicated in multiple writings over the half-century to follow. The charge of partiality and subjectivity landed pointedly and equally on the message and the messenger—namely, on the psychiatric expert and their testimony. Diamond effectively highlighted the contrast with matters that other medical consultants are asked. An orthopedic surgeon, for example, is to "supply particular, specialized information to the court…derived both from his direct observation…and from his fund of general professional knowledge about the structure and mechanics of the human body" (Diamond and Louisell 1965, p. 1336). To be sure, a psychiatric expert is often used for much the same purpose. When asked to opine on the presence of a mental disorder at the time of a criminal offense, or the presence or absence of emotional distress, a psychiatric expert similarly draws on qualified observations and consensus knowledge within the field.

This sort of testimony is not, per se, what kept Diamond up at night. He found himself particularly concerned with what he saw, in the 1960s, as a changing tide, whereby new legal questions were posed to "new" experts (psychoanalysts). (The twenty-first-century psychiatrist might find odd the reference to a Freudian analyst as "new." As Diamond himself explained, psychiatric illness historically fell under the domain of neurologists, who had prided themselves on their precision and heavy reliance on objectively demonstrable, observable data points. The rise of psychoanalysis, which caused a shift in the treatment of many behavioral problems to the realm of psychiatry, did indeed introduce a new sort of expert into the legal domain, one who prioritized subjective interpretation and individualized experiences of transference over quantifiable data points.) Diamond noted a changing focus in American law, which had begun to understand the purpose of the justice system as rehabilitative, rather than strictly punitive. To this end, he felt that psychiatry—and psychodynamic psychiatry, in particular—fit nicely into such humanitarian aspirations. What was now requested, however, was a different kind of expert and a different kind of expertise. The psychiatric expert was called on not merely to observe and then quantify observable data but rather to infer, interpret, and reframe data in a way that other legal parties either would not or could not do alone. Therein lies the rub. As Diamond explained, "his inferences, as well as his observations, are strongly colored by the qualities of his observing instrument: that is, his own personality, experience, and theoretical training" (Diamond and Louisell 1965, p. 1341).

Note that Diamond's recognition of the psychiatric expert's subjectivity is borne entirely from the known characteristics inherent in the work itself. The problem deepens considerably when one reflects on the biases inherent in any expert as a human. Griffith (1996) later addressed such issues of bias, including racial bias, through his seminal work on cultural connectedness. He emphasized the influence of culture on a forensic evaluation, and consequently on a forensic opinion. This includes the pitfalls of an expert's positive cultural identification with an evaluee, as well as the challenge of an expert whose own culture conflicts with (or is at least dissimilar to) that of the person evaluated. He rightly pointed out the gravity of this problem regarding any and all varieties of cultural identity, including religion, gender, and age, to name but a few.

Diamond's assessment of the problem was more nuanced than many have perceived. He had no qualms about impartiality being a farce, and he was similarly not bothered by its purported unattainability. The difficulty, as Diamond saw it, was in our continued operations under the guise of impartiality when, realistically, it was nowhere to be found. The solution is therefore not to become impartial. Doing so would not be possible or, in Diamond's opinion, even desired. The answer is for the forensic psychiatrist and the justice system to embrace the subjectivity of the psychiatric expert and configure the rules of evidence in accordance. This would involve a number of changes enacted by both the expert and the courts (Diamond 2013). First, the expert and professional organizations ought to clearly delineate the limitations and boundaries of legitimate psychiatric testimony. Second, standards applied by the courts on qualifications of a psychiatric expert should be more rigorous. Third, courts should insist that the expert remain abreast of the relevant scientific literature and that any deviations from consensus opinion be noted and justified. Fourth, an expert ought to be granted leeway in how they choose to present their opinion without the limitations and constraints set forth by direct and cross-examination. (In Diamond and Louisell [1965], Diamond clarified what he envisioned here. He described the psychiatric expert presenting his opinion in an unabridged, uninterrupted narrative form. A cross-examination would still take place, which would serve the primary purpose of ironing out the kinks and addressing inconsistencies in the formulated expert opinion.)

Fifth, one cannot rely on simply the adversarial battle to expose the dishonest or unqualified expert; expert standards and a vetting process ought to play a role. Sixth, the law ought to forfeit its "naive" pursuit of certainty in science. As Diamond put it, "Scientific knowledge is always approximate, tentative, and subject to revision as knowledge grows" (Diamond 2013). Seventh, the expert's role, however partisan, should be fully and unabashedly revealed to the trier of fact. Finally, eighth, professional organizations must take an active role and responsibility in setting out these guidelines. (Note that other systems-based solutions to the problem of impartiality have been suggested as well, for instance, court-appointed mental health panels or team-based approaches to forensic assessments [Smith 1966–1967].)

Diamond's ideal solution, as he very well understood, was simply aspirational at the time he presented it. It remains aspirational to this day. It offers little guidance to the struggling forensic psychiatrist who is operating within the justice system in its present iteration. So how must psychiatry confront the magnitude of this problem? Broadly, three general approaches have emerged. The first approach is to abstain entirely from this dicey line of work. The second considers a path toward advocacy and unabashed partiality from within the forensic practice. The third is to continue practicing forensic psychiatry with the aspirational goal of objectivity despite inevitable bias, and with concrete steps to further that aspirational aim. We consider each of these approaches independently.

An Argument for Early Retirement

If Diamond's treatment of the "impartiality myth" was a tectonic foreshock to forensic psychiatry, then Stone's 1984 Presidential Address was a groundbreaking earthquake (Stone 1984). Stone went beyond Diamond's observations, raising the overarching concern that a forensic psychiatrist is caught between two contradictory worlds. As he put it, "psychiatrists are immediately over the boundary when they go into court" (Stone 1984). He stepped away from this challenge entirely, concluding that "it will be impossible to sweep the ethical problems of psychiatry under the rug of intelligible adversarial ethics" (Stone 1984).

Faced with a perceived binary choice between "adjust[ing] to the adversarial system [and] remain[ing] true to your calling as a physician," Stone forfeited the former and clung to the latter. This seminal speech set off a ripple—no, a wave—throughout the field. Many interpreted Stone's speech as challenging forensic psychiatrists to establish a system of ethics that would guide their work. That response, in no small part, is the seed that flourished into this very book on ethics.

Despite the consternation that Stone's address wrought, some have come to agree with him. Edward Colbach similarly stopped doing forensic work, concluding that the whole field of forensic psychiatry was suspect if there was indeed no such thing as an impartial expert witness (Colbach 1997). He conditioned his return to the courtroom on much of the ambitious change that Diamond suggested, including the open recognition and acceptance by courts of law that experts are, indeed, subjective and partial partisans.

The Forensic Psychiatrist as Advocate

Another approach to the problem of impartiality is quite simply to embrace the professional bias of the psychiatric expert and to be, unapologetically, an advocate. Such advocacy can be done in two ways, which I term *selective participation* and *advocacy from within*.

Selective participation involves the conscientious and intentional choosing of cases such that the expert only accepts a case (and only for the particular side) that comports with their personal and professional values. This is the pragmatic compromise that Diamond himself adopted (personal letter from B.L. Diamond to R. Weinstock, July 1988). Diamond, in fact, was so careful in this regard that he ultimately participated in only 10% of cases that sought to retain him (Weinstock et al. 1992). He was scrupulously honest and in no way a hired gun. For instance, he was known to reject cases in which defense attorneys used legal technicalities to exclude any relevant evidence. He was, however, quick to acknowledge the difficulty of such a practice for the career forensic psychiatrist. As he concluded in the same letter, "It is very hard to be an idealistically honest expert if it means your children will go hungry."

Others, such as Weinstock, suggested that a forensic psychiatrist ought to be selective only with regard to cases that most strongly conflict with the Hippocratic tradition in cases of capital punishment

(Weinstock et al. 1992). Even so, he encouraged a form of activism from within, rather than abstinence. Weinstock challenged the false choice between abstaining from capital cases and participating fully and equally with both prosecutors and defense. He argued that a forensic psychiatrist could participate for the prosecution at the early phases of a case (before a finding of guilt). But he proposed that when it came to the penalty phase (one at which death was an option considered), it would be contrary to the role of a physician to present solely aggravating factors to facilitate a death sentence. In such a circumstance at this phase of the trial, abstinence from cases for the prosecution would be warranted.

(A rare exception might have been if the prosecution was seriously interested in finding mitigating circumstances. A psychiatrist might take a case for the defense at this phase, to see whether the facts warranted it, or might otherwise choose to withdraw from such a case, after finding the facts would not legally support any mitigating circumstances [Weinstock et al. 1992]. Diamond considered it ethical to accept the case if the expert initially thought their findings might support life imprisonment [vs. death], but if it was too late to withdraw from the case when none were found, then the expert was still obligated to tell the truth. His view of the ethics is a subjective one to guide the expert based on their intent when undertaking the case. It rarely is possible for others to assess that.)

A concern similar to Weinstock's was voiced, in even stronger terms, by moral philosopher Philippa Foot: "Defendants facing the death penalty need psychiatrists, and the worst thing that could happen from their point of view would be a general exodus of those psychiatrists who oppose the death penalty on moral grounds" (Foot 2013, p. 216). Foot therefore found the forensic psychiatrist's advocacy from within to be palatable, but only when selectively participating on behalf of the defense.

Note that neither selective participation nor advocacy from within encourages (or even permits) a hired-gun mentality. Diamond (2013) addressed this very contention at great length, affirming that an honest advocate must never knowingly give false testimony, mislead, or conceal relevant evidence, even with a greater good in mind. To do so would be to operate as a hired gun, without allegiance to the forensic principles of honesty or truth-telling.

Aspiring for Objectivity and Toward Impartiality

Although Diamond's skepticism came to feature prominently in academic forensic scholarship, much of the field was unfailing in its continued aspirations toward impartiality. Pollack, a contemporary of Diamond's, led the way. He clearly understood (and taught) that the expectation of an expert witness was to avoid advocacy. He made no secret of the fact that bias interjects itself, purposely or unwittingly, obviously or discreetly. But such bias was a pitfall to be wary of, not a badge to be worn with honor (Pollack 1968). This perspective and its stark contrast with Diamond's approach had many practical ramifications. For instance, what should an expert do when the legal criteria are vague and ambiguous? Diamond might have modified or expanded his legal interpretations in ways that encouraged the most humanistic outcomes. Pollack, impartial and objective, saw himself strictly and solely responsible for ascertaining the law as intended by legislators and jurists, whatever the outcome may be (Weinstock et al. 1992).

Another question arises, whether the expert psychiatrist ought to limit their analysis to the threshold definitions of mental illness as legally conceived, or whether they ought to use the language of mental illness as a treating clinician would. Diamond, forever the clinician, would never cede ground to the courts. Pollack, a steward of the law, would happily concede to legally imposed thresholds of mental illness for the purposes of his expert opinion (Weinstock et al. 1992). Consensus ethics guidelines published by the American Academy of Psychiatry and the Law (2005) were modified to eliminate the ethical requirement to "remain unbiased." This has prudently been replaced with a requirement for "honesty." The guidelines do not explicitly distinguish between subjective and objective honesty but do elucidate an additional need to "strive for objectivity" (p. 3), suggesting that efforts to attain objective honesty are required.

Strict subservience to legal norms (and, therefore, objection to advocacy from within) does not necessarily imply being oblivious to the problems that Diamond raised. Guttmacher (1963), for example, wrote eloquently about the fallacy of impartiality and the problems inherent in the field. He offered many suggestions for improvement that mirrored those proposed by Diamond and that would have remedied much of the field's inherent bias. Specifically, he highlighted the benefits of a sort of court-appointed panel of experts, the need for an expert to be court-appointed rather than partisan, and the need for an expert to speak freely from the stand, without the limitations imposed by direct and cross-examination. Further, he suggested limitations placed on the content of a psychiatric testimony, particularly in the realm of insanity defenses. Briefly, he believed a psychiatrist ought to opine on the presence or absence of mental disorder and the degree of dysfunction it causes, but need not (maybe should not) render an opinion about the finding of insanity, which wanders too far off from the scientific methods with which they were trained. Diamond, however, objected to replacing the advocacy system with court-appointed experts in practice, based on his view that court-appointed experts often do not reach objective opinions, which would deprive the defense from having an opportunity to present an opposing point of view to the court.

Guttmacher strongly objected to advocacy from within, instead urging fierce advocacy through academic scholarship and the written word. As he put it, "the witness stand is not a soapbox from which to preach reform of the law" (Guttmacher 1963, p. 116). Be an advocate, he encouraged, but from the outside. Within this vein, he cautioned the forensic psychiatrist not to opine on the ultimate legal issue in a case. Interestingly, the community of trained forensic psychiatrists seem to have reached fairly broad consensus that such caution is unwarranted. The understanding is that a forensic psychiatrist is trained well enough in relevant legal areas to opine on the ultimate legal issue when needed. Doing so should not necessarily be considered an act of advocacy from within.

A View From the Bench

To address this topic fully without consulting legal precedent would be akin to marital counseling with a spouse who won't attend. If this odd and unusual marriage between psychiatry and the law is to thrive, it must be considered with both parties at the table. Does the court view the psychiatrist as a scientific expert in pursuit of objectivity (not unlike the orthopedist or pathologist)? Or do they serve a different function in the courtroom that champions their subjectivity and embraces their humanitarian advocacy?

The extensive discussion among forensic psychiatrists, prompted by Diamond's landmark paper, does indeed have a correlate in case law. As forensic psychiatrists struggled with their own legal identity, the courts openly, and with uncanny resemblance, debated their legal utility. This evolution can be tracked, in part, through use of the insanity defense in American law. Its advancement was largely driven by the very concerns made famous by Diamond, Guttmacher, and others. By no coincidence at all, Guttmacher was one of three expert psychiatrists serving on the committee of the American Legal Institute (ALI) that (for a brief period in American history) altogether reformed the criteria used for an insanity plea. Judge David Bazelon's 1954 decision in the case of *Durham v. United States* (1954) was largely influenced by the very works of Guttmacher that we've already discussed. He ruled in favor of what became known as the *Durham rule* (or the *product test* for insanity) on the basis of his belief that the traditional M'Naghten rule was scientifically inadequate and forced the expert witness to testify on matters beyond, and largely irrelevant to, their trained discipline (*Durham v. United States* 1954). In this light, Guttmacher served as a valuable, admirable, and historic example of successful advocacy from *without*.

Ironically, the thoughtfully crafted Durham rule itself became the object of a similar critique. Over time, insanity cases turned not on whether a defendant had a mental illness but on precisely whether the criminal act was a product of that mental illness. This question, a legal matter and the crux of the trial, fell into the lap of the expert psychiatric witness. In a sense, Guttmacher's dual concerns (that the expert would opine on legal matters and that the expert would supplant the trier of fact) had become the reality. This is precisely what prompted Bazelon to forbid the expert psychiatrist from opining on the product issue (*Thomas H. Washington, Jr., Appellant, v. United States of America, Appellee* 1967). And this is precisely what motivated Circuit Judge Harold Leventhal's decision to pivot away from Durham and toward the ALI standard, as he did in *United States v. Brawner* (1972). Bazelon's decision was intended expressly to "help the psychiatrists understand their role in court" (*Thomas H. Washington, Jr., Appellant, v. United States of America, Appellee* 1967). Leventhal quoted precedent from then–Circuit Judge Warren Burger, citing the "hazards in allowing experts to testify in precisely or even substantially the terms of the ultimate issue" (*United States of America v. Archie W. Brawner, Appellant* 1972). The evolution of the insanity defense is but one example of the ways in which the legal system grappled with the function of a psychiatric expert. It is worth considering how far the courts have gone to contemplate, accommodate, and delineate the amorphous existence of the psychiatrist in the courtroom.

The moral challenges that Diamond and Stone laid before the field of forensic psychiatry in its infancy perpetuated the ethical growth that was and is necessary. The forensic psychiatrist would be wise, first and foremost, to sit with the astuteness and profundity of these very challenging questions as they relate to one's personal practice. Doing so would similarly promote the necessary and fulfilling ethical growth of the individual, with all of its valuable growing pains.

Conclusion

Let's return to the questions we started with. Can a forensic psychiatric expert be impartial? Is impartiality even a desired goal? The likely answer is that impartiality cannot be obtained (and, according to some, ought not to be desired, either). This sentiment is now reflected in the ethical guidelines of the American Academy of Psychiatry and the Law (2005), which has extensive writings about striving for *objectivity*, without any mention of *impartiality* as a target. It is worth noting, even regarding objectivity, that the goal is to strive for it, without any promise of attaining it.

Finally, if Diamond is right, what are we, as forensic psychiatrists, to do? The purpose of this chapter was decidedly descriptive, rather than prescriptive. I hope that the forensic psychiatrist contending with these questions will know that many conscientious experts have faced this struggle before. I hope to have clearly laid out a map by which to navigate this intricate and nuanced debate. As the reader can see, the path forward has been trod in many directions, on the basis of varying practical, conceptual, personal, and ethical interests. The ethics guidelines of the American Academy of Psychiatry and the Law reflect broad, current consensus within our field and should be followed whenever possible. But there continue to be areas (such as cases of capital punishment) in which no consensus has been reached. My hope is not to tell you which path to follow; rather it is to assure you that, whichever of these paths you may choose, you walk on solid ground.

References

American Academy of Psychiatry and the Law: Ethics Guidelines for the Practice of Forensic Psychiatry. Adopted May 2005. Bloomfield, CT, American Academy of Psychiatry and the Law, 2005

Colbach EM: The trouble with American forensic psychiatry. Int J Offender Ther Comp Criminol 41(2):16–167, 1997

Diamond BL: The fallacy of the impartial expert. Arch Criminal Psychodyn 3(2):221–236, 1959

Diamond BL: The psychiatric expert witness: honest advocate or "hired gun"?, in Ethical Practice in Psychiatry and the Law. Edited by Rosner R, Weinstock R. Berlin, Springer, 2013, pp 75–84

Diamond BL, Louisell DW: The psychiatrist as an expert witness: some ruminations and speculations. Mich Law Rev 63(8):1335-1354, 1965

Durham v United States, 214 F.2d 862 (1954)

Foot P: Ethics and the death penalty: participation by forensic psychiatrists in capital trials, in Ethical Practice in Psychiatry and the Law. Edited by Rosner R, Weinstock R. Berlin, Springer, 2013, pp 207–217

Griffith E: Forensic psychiatrists and cultural connectedness. J Forens Psychiatry 7(3):477–479, 1996

Guttmacher MS: What can the psychiatrist contribute to the issue of criminal responsibility? J Nerv Ment Dis 136:103–117, 1963 13951477

Pollack S: Psychiatric consultation for the court, in The Psychiatric Consultation. Edited by Mendel W, Solomon P. New York, Grune and Stratton, 1968, pp 267–285

Smith S: The ideal use of expert testimony in psychology. Washburn Law J 6(2):300–306, 1966–1967

Stone AA: The ethical boundaries of forensic psychiatry: a view from the ivory tower. Bull Am Acad Psychiatry Law 12(3):209–219, 1984 6478062

Thomas H. Washington, Jr., Appellant, v United States of America, Appellee, 390 F.2d 444 (1967)

United States of America v Archie W. Brawner, Appellant, 471 F.2d 969 (1972)

Weinstock R, Leong GB, Silva JA: The death penalty and Bernard Diamond's approach to forensic psychiatry. Bull Am Acad Psychiatry Law 20(2):197–210, 1992 1633341

Death Penalty

Ethics Considerations for Participating in Capital Cases

Gregory B. Leong, M.D.

Michael Kanell, M.D.

Dustin B. Stephens, M.D., Ph.D.

In the practice of psychiatry, the entire population are potential patients, so in jurisdictions permitting capital punishment, psychiatric practice could intersect with those facing or potentially facing the death penalty. The ethical principles governing the practice of medicine adopted by the American Medical Association (AMA) (2021) include nine core principles (American Psychiatric Association 2013). The American Psychiatric Association (APA) adopted the AMA ethics principles for its membership and added annotations especially applicable to psychiatry.

The first AMA principle (Section 1) is, "A physician shall be dedicated to providing competent medical care with compassion and respect for human dignity and rights." APA's fourth annotation to the Section 1 ethical principle is, "A psychiatrist should not be a participant in a legally authorized execution." (The AMA [2021] has defined what constitutes such participation.) Although not all psychiatrists are AMA or APA members, these principles are used as the ethical measuring stick should there be a question about what constitutes ethically acceptable psychiatric practice.

At first glance, the practice of psychiatry itself would not appear to involve participation in a legally authorized execution (unless in the role of a physician to prepare or administer the drugs to be used in a lethal injection). Because of the unique nature of the death penalty, however, any professional contact with an individual facing or potentially facing the death penalty, whether as an evaluee or a patient, is subject to ethics inquiry.

Other than those providing direct psychiatric care in jails and prisons, forensic psychiatrists have the most professional psychiatric contact with people facing or potentially facing capital punishment, who can be divided into two broad categories: criminal defendants charged with a capital offense and those convicted of a capital offense and sentenced to death. The ethical challenges for each category are explored separately.

General Approach to Forensic Psychiatric Evaluation

Most professional forensic psychiatric involvement with capital defendants or death row inmates subject to ethical inquiry concerns the forensic psychiatric evaluation of these individuals. The exception will be encountered by a psychiatrist in the limited circumstance of treating a death row inmate found not competent to be executed. Otherwise, forensic psychiatrists will first encounter the usual ethical challenges of forensic evaluation. Because the end product of the forensic evaluation involves a forensic psychiatric report or courtroom testimony, the general ethical challenges for these professional activities are addressed elsewhere in this book (for example, see Chapter 5, "Ethical Report Writing," and Chapter 6, "Ethical Challenges While Testifying"). For the purposes of this chapter, the ethics guidelines are those adopted by the American Academy of Psychiatry and the Law (AAPL) (2005). Although all the AAPL guidelines are relevant, the ones most applicable to the evaluation of capital defendants or death row inmates involve honesty and striving for objectivity.

The irreversible nature of the death penalty gives rise to ethical challenges not encountered in usual professional practice; thus, the practitioner may benefit from using an ethical analysis that involves consideration of competing ethical values, such as dialectical princi700 (Weinstock 2015) (see Chapter 2). Before exploring ethical decision-making, we first describe the ethics and forensic landscape in capital cases. For the purposes of this chapter, we use the California model for capital trials, in which there is a guilt phase to determine whether the defendant is guilty of the charged capital offense; if the verdict is guilty, a penalty phase follows to determine whether the defendant receives the death penalty or an alternative disposition. (Other states may not have a separate penalty phase.) Psychiatrists can also establish unique ways of handling these ethical challenges. Bernard Diamond would testify only on behalf of the defense, and only if total honesty were permitted, in which the whole psychiatric truth can be revealed so that psychiatric facts are neither hidden nor distorted (Weinstock et al. 1992). Despite Diamond's stated view that impartiality or objectivity were not attainable (Weinstock et al. 1992), he would nonetheless be adhering to the current AAPL guidelines of honesty and striving for objectivity while preserving his secondary ethical value of working only for the defense side.

The Pretrial Phase

Maintaining honesty and striving for objectivity when participating in the evaluation of capital cases can take extra effort because of a forensic psychiatrist's personal convictions about capital punishment, which may also affect who elects to participate (Neal 2016). At multiple points during the pretrial capital proceedings, ethical concerns may arise when psychiatrists are asked to give an opinion. It could be argued that in capital cases, giving an opinion that the defendant is competent to stand trial or was not insane at the time of the act contributes to the death of the defendant. During the penalty phase of the trial, providing an opinion substantiating aggravating factors, including possibility for future dangerousness, may be seen as contributing to the defendant's death. At all stages, the question persists whether participation as an expert witness contributes to a death outcome that otherwise would not have occurred.

Preconviction Competencies and the Death Penalty

The most common attitude is that psychiatric participation in capital cases before a conviction is unproblematic, because death is just one of many possible outcomes, and multiple obstacles remain before a subject can be placed on death row, even if convicted of a capital offense (i.e., an actual execution is far removed temporally, procedurally, and ethically) (Bloche 1993; Scott 2006). Predisposition competencies do not address the question of the defendant's mental state during the offense and thus have minimal bearing on the ultimate question of the trial. As such, an argument that a forensic evaluator acted as the executioner's aide in opining that a defendant was competent to stand trial or capable of representing themselves pro se would be unconvincing. The reasoning in *Estelle v. Smith* (1981) seems to support this approach. The Supreme Court held that admission of a doctor's testimony, acquired for the purpose of competency to stand trial, at the penalty phase of the trial violated the defendant's Fifth Amendment privilege against self-incrimination. However, there is a potential pitfall for the concerned evaluator. The court implied that if the defendant were advised of his rights and knowingly waived them during the competency evaluation, the testimony might be admissible at other stages of the trial. Little analysis has been made surrounding the ethical danger of acquiring inculpating evidence in a predisposition competency evaluation of a capital case in jurisdictions that do not prohibit the use of such incriminating information at trial.

Mental State at the Time of the Offense

Evaluations of the defendant's mental status at the time of the alleged crime can play a major role in determination of the defendant's guilt. The arguments for symbolic distance from the ultimate outcome (applied to the various competencies discussed above) continue to be relevant here, because imposition of the death penalty does not occur at the guilt-finding stage of the trial, and the psychiatrist does not make the ultimate decision about the guilt of the defendant. More has been discussed surrounding the ethical impact of psychiatric testimony of insanity than of competency. Multiple studies have shown a correlation between unsuccessfully asserting an insanity defense and receiving the death sentence (Slobogin 2000). Given the elevated risk of death after a failed insanity defense, AAPL recommends discussing the high possibility of a death outcome with the defense attorney before undertaking a psychiatric evaluation (AAPL 2014).

Ethics After the Guilt Phase: Aggravating and Mitigating Circumstances

Once the defendant has been found guilty of a capital crime, a separate sentencing hearing follows to determine whether a death sentence is warranted. During this penalty phase of the trial, a forensic evaluator may be called on to provide testimony of mitigating or aggravating factors. Jurisdiction-specific rules define aggravating factors in each case. Various court cases (including decisions by the U.S. Supreme Court) have defined what could constitute mitigating factors (e.g., *Lockett v. Ohio* 1978; *Porter v. McCollum* 2009; *Wiggins v. Smith* 2003). Scott (2006) described a clinical approach to assessing mitigating factors.

Although the presentation of mitigating factors is intended to provide an opportunity for balance, to provide for all possible leniency when considering a death sentence, studies using interviews of actual capital jurors or mock jurors have found tendencies or trends in how certain factors are more likely to be viewed as aggravating or mitigating (Ellsworth et al. 1984; Garvey 1998; Jochnowitz 2011; Miley et al. 2020). A forensic expert witness who carries any preexisting biases or tendencies about the death penalty can use this research when presenting courtroom testimony, because how the aggravating or mitigating factors are presented may affect a jury's decision and not necessarily violate the ethical guideline of honesty and striving for objectivity.

Psychiatric testimony during the penalty phase of capital trials helps establish the presence of mitigating factors, and it can also help substantiate aggravating factors. At least one aggravating factor must be present to justify the death penalty. Each state has defined aggravating factors, and they commonly involve likelihood of future violence, degree of premeditation, cruelness of the crime, experience of the victim's family, and the defendant's criminal history (Scott 2006). The Supreme Court has ruled that a prediction of likely future violence as an aggravating factor was constitutional (*Jurek v. Texas* 1976). Their ruling a few years later, allowing admission of psychiatric testimony based not on a personal examination of a defendant but in response to hypothetical questions about predicting future violence (*Barefoot v. Estelle* 1983), heightens the ethical fragility of participating in evaluations when providing testimony in support of aggravating factors.

Given the high ethical stakes of a capital case, the forensic psychiatrist may have to look beyond the AMA, APA, and AAPL ethical guidelines before participating. To reduce ethical concerns in participating in capital cases, some practitioners might consider following the previously mentioned approach by Diamond and categorically limit participation: only for the defense, and only when the available facts support honest participation (Weinstock et al. 1992). Upon further reconsideration of the matter, Weinstock provided an ethical analysis guided by dialectical principlism on whether to accept a referral from the prosecution to examine and then testify in a capital case to address solely aggravating factors (and not both mitigating and aggravating factors as statutorily outlined) (Weinstock 2015). In Weinstock's analysis of competing ethical duties—which includes his view of the physician's appropriate societal role—the ethical course of action would be not to accept such a referral. Weinstock offers an aspirational ethical amendment that the "most ethical forensic psychiatrist should try to determine what is ethical for himself even if there is no consensus" (Weinstock 2015, p. 18).

Postconviction Ethical Conflict: Competence to Be Executed

The role of a forensic psychiatrist in a capital case after conviction primarily concerns competence to be executed, among the most difficult ethical dilemmas in the field. At this stage in the legal process, the court-ordered execution of a convicted defendant is highly proximate in both time and probability.

The principal landmark Supreme Court case in this area, *Ford v. Wainwright* (1986), legitimized competence to be executed as a viable question for forensic experts, but without establishing a clear legal standard beyond dicta suggesting that it involves the factual understanding of the impending execution. Twenty-one years later in *Panetti v. Quarterman* (2007), the Supreme Court cautiously advanced some semblance of a minimum standard ("floor") for competence to be executed, to include a rational understanding of the impending execution.

Although *Panetti* may provide some clarification, the competence-to-be-executed threshold seems readily satisfied, as few psychotic inmates sentenced to death would be expected to be found incompetent. Weinstock et al. (2010) raised concern that participating in such evaluations (especially in states where such evaluations are routine) without a specific doubt about competence having been raised could be viewed as inappropriate—as essentially trivializing a medical clearance. On balance, however, the authors concluded that providing competence-to-be-executed evaluations for the defense is not in itself unethical if doubt has been raised about a particular person's competence, and that it should be undertaken only with acknowledgment of the ethical concerns and biases of the individual expert, with honesty and striving for objectivity (Weinstock et al. 2010).

A forensic psychiatrist can generally decline to participate in a competence-to-be-executed case should there be any personal ethical dissonance. Even in the case where a psychiatrist is assigned to evaluate a death row inmate as an employee of the particular state or federal jurisdiction, there is no professional ethical prohibition by AAPL, APA, or AMA against performing competence-to-be-executed evaluations (in part to avoid having a less competent evaluator do so). Of course, forensic psychiatrists who are willing to perform such evaluations need to adhere to the ethical guidelines of honesty and striving for objectivity.

Should the death row inmate be found not competent to be executed, the ethical burden would then fall on their treating psychiatrist. Successful treatment of the mental illness would result in imposition of capital punishment, creating an ethical conundrum. Organized medicine has offered its guidance in the current AMA Medical Ethics Opinion 9.7.3 addressing capital punishment, which defines treatment of a death row inmate who has been found incompetent to be executed as participation in an execution, unless a commutation order is issued before beginning (or resumption) of treatment (American Medical Association 2021).

This AMA Ethics Opinion on capital punishment does not cover all possibilities. For example, in the protracted case of Arkansas death row inmate Charles Singleton (*Singleton v. Norris* 2003), the state attempted to continue the use of involuntary medications after an execution date had been set. The Eighth Circuit Court of Appeals held that the involuntary treatment of Singleton could continue under *Washington v. Harper* (1990) given prior evidence of his dangerousness, but the legal trail ended when the Supreme Court denied certiorari. He was executed by the state of Arkansas in 2004 (he had continued treatment voluntarily and declined further appeal). The *Singleton* case raises questions about the ethics of even the voluntary use of antipsychotic medication to maintain competence to be executed, specifically once an execution date is set, and whether the treating psychiatrist or other physician can decline to continue offering psychiatric treatment. Although forensic psychiatrists may not be directly involved in treatment decisions in a case like *Singleton,* they may be called on to consult about the ethical aspects of the psychiatric treatment of a death row inmate. In addition, depending on the jurisdiction, physicians may not be the only legally authorized prescribers. As *Singleton* demonstrated, the ethical questions can be complex but too subtle for a legal analysis; ethical analysis such as dialectical principlism may be useful in weighing the competing ethical values.

Conclusion

In this overview of forensic psychiatry in capital cases, we identify ethical quagmires through all stages of participation. When the death penalty is involved, competing ethical values are more likely to appear than in noncapital cases. The participating psychiatrist seeking resolution of ethical conundrums may benefit from ethical analysis to consider the competing proximal and distal ethical values and arrive at the most ethical course of action in a capital case (Weinstock 2015).

References

American Academy of Psychiatry and the Law: Ethics Guidelines for the Practice of Forensic Psychiatry. Adopted May 2005. Bloomfield, CT, American Academy of Psychiatry and the Law, 2005. Available at: https://www.aapl.org/ethics-guidelines. Accessed March 1, 2021.

American Academy of Psychiatry and the Law: AAPL Practice Guideline for forensic psychiatric evaluation of defendants raising the insanity defense. J Am Acad Psychiatry Law 42(4 Suppl):S3–S76, 2014 25492121

American Medical Association: Opinion 9.7.3 (Capital Punishment). Chicago, IL, AMA Code of Medical Ethics. Available at: https://www.ama-assn .org/delivering-care/ethics/capital-punishment. Accessed December 5, 2021.

American Psychiatric Association: The Principles of Medical Ethics with Annotations Especially Applicable to Psychiatry. Arlington, VA, American Psychiatric Association, 2013

Barefoot v Estelle, 463 U.S. 880 (1983)

Bloche MG: Psychiatry, capital punishment, and the purposes of medicine. Int J Law Psychiatry 16(3–4):301–357, 1993 8125676

Ellsworth PC, Bukaty RM, Cowan CL, et al: The death-qualified jury and the defense of insanity. Law Hum Behav 8:81–93, 1984

Estelle v Smith. 451 U.S. 454 (1981)

Ford v Wainwright, 477 U.S. 399 (1986)

Garvey SP: Aggravation and mitigation in capital cases: what do jurors think? Columbia Law Rev 98:1538–1576, 1998

Jochnowitz LD: How capital jurors respond to mitigating evidence of defendant's mental illness, retardation, and situational impairments: an analysis of the legal and social science literature. Crim Law Bull 47(5):839–892, 2011

Jurek v Texas, 428 U.S. 262 (1976)

Lockett v Ohio, 438 U.S. 604 (1978)

Miley LN, Heiss-Moses E, Cochran JK, et al: An examination of the effects of mental disorders as mitigating factors on capital sentencing outcomes. Behav Sci Law 38(4):381–405, 2020 32738090

Neal TM: Are forensic experts already biased before adversarial legal parties hire them? PLoS One 11(4):e0154434, 2016 27124416

Panetti v Quarterman, 551 U.S. 930 (2007)

Porter v McCollum, 558 U.S. 30 (2009)

Scott CL: Psychiatry and the death penalty. Psychiatr Clin North Am 29(3):791–804, 2006 16904512

Singleton v Norris, 319 F.3d 1018 (8th Cir 2003), cert. denied, 540 U.S. 832 (2003)

Slobogin C: Mental illness and the death penalty. Ment Phys Disabil Law Rep 24(4):667–677, 2000 10986859

Washington v Harper, 494 U.S. 210 (1990)

Weinstock R: Dialectical principlism: an approach to finding the most ethical action. J Am Acad Psychiatry Law 43(1):10–20, 2015 25770274

Weinstock R, Leong GB, Silva JA: The death penalty and Bernard Diamond's approach to forensic psychiatry. Bull Am Acad Psychiatry Law 20(2):197–210, 1992 1633341

Weinstock R, Leong GB, Silva JA: Competence to be executed: an ethical analysis post-Panetti. Behav Sci Law 28(5):690–706, 2010

Wiggins v Smith, 539 U.S. 510 (2003)

12

The Tarasoff Duty to Protect

Unintended Consequences and New Liability Concerns

Alexander C. Sones, M.D.

William C. Darby, M.D.

Robert Weinstock, M.D.

arasoff v. Regents of the University of California, a landmark case decided by the Supreme Court of California (1974, 1976), dramatically altered the relationship between mental health professionals, patients, and communities. According to the decision, a psychotherapist who believed a patient might represent a threat to others was expected to break confidentiality and attempt to protect the third party. Contemporary observers who were concerned with the denigration of confidentiality, the damage the decision could do to the therapeutic relationship, and the difficult nature of foreseeability of violence warned that the precedent could "destroy effective psychotherapeutic treatment" (Cohen 1978, p. 153). Similar duties, often conceptualized as a *duty to warn* or *duty to protect*, developed in many other states after

California. In this chapter, we discuss the ethical problems of this approach, focusing on the various interpretations of how psychotherapists are expected to protect third parties.

History of Tarasoff Duties

Tarasoff v. UC Regents

In the fall of 1968, Prosenjit Poddar, a 25-year-old graduate student in naval engineering at the University of California, Berkeley, met Tatiana Tarasoff while attending folk dancing classes (*People v. Poddar* 1974). Several months later, they shared a New Year's Eve kiss, which Poddar interpreted as a sign of their budding romance. Tarasoff, however, informed him that she was not interested in pursuing an intimate relationship with him. Poddar descended into a depressed emotional state: he neglected his appearance, did poorly in his studies, and was intermittently observed weeping and speaking disjointedly to himself. He met with Tarasoff a number of times during the next several months, was later found to have tape-recorded several of their conversations, and reportedly spent hours analyzing the taped conversations (Simone and Fulero 2005).

Persuaded by a friend, Poddar sought psychiatric care from student health services. On June 5, 1969, he was diagnosed with paranoid schizophrenia and was prescribed an antipsychotic medication at the campus-affiliated Cowell Memorial Hospital (Goodman 1985). His psychiatrist, Dr. Robert Gold, arranged for Poddar to obtain weekly psychotherapy from psychologist Dr. Lawrence Moore.

Moore and Poddar met weekly for a total of eight sessions; at the time, Tarasoff was on summer vacation in Brazil. During the sessions, Poddar shared information regarding his pathological attraction to Tarasoff. He described his fantasies of harming her and, ultimately, his plan to kill her once she returned from vacation. A friend of Poddar informed Moore that Poddar intended to buy a weapon. Moore was unable to dissuade Poddar from buying a pellet gun and later was unable to persuade him to dispose of it. On August 20, 1969, Poddar informed Moore that he intended to kill Tarasoff when she returned from Brazil. Although Poddar did not specifically identify Tarasoff by name, she was "readily identifiable" as Tatiana Tarasoff based on the information provided to Moore (Crocker 1985, p. 92).

Moore became concerned enough to consult with two psychiatrist colleagues. The three mental health providers determined that Poddar required involuntary hospitalization to prevent his potential danger-ousness toward Tarasoff. Moore contacted the campus police department by phone and hand-carried a letter to inform them of Poddar's need for hospitalization. The letter was quite explicit:

> At times he appears to be quite rational, at other times he appears quite psychotic.... [C]urrently the appropriate diagnosis for him is paranoid schizophrenic reaction, acute and severe. He is at this point a danger to the welfare of other people and himself. That is, he has been threatening to kill an unnamed girl who he feels has betrayed him and has violated his honor. He has told a friend of his... that he intends to go to San Francisco to buy a gun and that he plans to kill the girl. He has been somewhat more cryptic with me, but he has alluded strongly to the compulsion to "get even with" and "hurt" the girl. (Slovenko 1988, p. 148)

The police responded by bringing Poddar to the station for questioning and speaking with friends of Poddar's. Poddar denied intent to kill Tatiana Tarasoff and promised the police he would stay away from her. The police warned him to avoid Tatiana and concluded that involuntary commitment would not be necessary. Poddar never returned to psychotherapy with Moore, and neither Tatiana nor her parents were warned of the possible threat Poddar posed.

On October 27, 1969, 2 months after the police interrogated Poddar, he shot Tarasoff with his pellet gun and then stabbed her to death with a kitchen knife.

Tarasoff I

While Poddar's criminal case went through the courts, Tarasoff's parents filed a wrongful death civil lawsuit against the regents of the University of California, the psychotherapists involved in Poddar's case, and the campus police. They claimed that the defendants failed to warn Tarasoff or her parents of the impending danger, and that they failed to use reasonable care to confine Poddar under the Lanterman-Petris-Short Act (1967), which authorized involuntary psychiatric treatment in very limited circumstances. They also claimed that the therapists had a "duty to safeguard their patient and the public," and that Moore's actions in warning the campus police were insufficient. The psychotherapist defendants claimed that they did not owe a duty of care toward Tarasoff, as she was not their patient. The case was ultimately heard by the Supreme Court of California in 1974 and is now referred to as *Tarasoff I*. The court denied the defendants' arguments and issued their findings in the majority opinion authored by Justice Mathew Tobriner:

> When a doctor or a psychotherapist, in the exercise of his professional skill and knowledge, determines, or should determine, that a warning is essential to avert danger arising from the medical or psychological condition of his patient, he incurs a legal obligation to give that warning. (*Tarasoff v. Regents* 1974, p. 131)

The *duty to warn* was thus created. In *Tarasoff I*, the court concluded that

> the public policy favoring protection of the confidential character of patient-psychotherapist communications must yield in instances in which disclosure is essential to avert danger to others. The protective privilege ends where the public peril begins. (*Tarasoff v. Regents* 1974, p. 137)

To the psychotherapist community, the *Tarasoff I* decision was cataclysmic. An amicus curiae brief was filed on January 7, 1975, by numerous organizations representing psychotherapists and psychiatrists, including the American Psychiatric Association, the Northern California Psychiatric Society, the California State Psychological Association, and the National Association of Social Workers. The organizations argued that predicting violence is a notoriously difficult task, even for psychotherapists trained in violence risk assessment. Because violence is a relatively unlikely outcome, clinicians markedly overpredict violence; further, mental health professionals are not immune to racial, cultural, and other forms of bias in violence risk assessment (Venner et al. 2021). They maintained that therapy regularly entails "non-factual matters" and fantasies that sometimes involve violence, and the belief that these can be separated from true violent threats was in itself a fantasy. Confidentiality in the time of *Tarasoff I* was almost sacrosanct—if patients could not expect their psychotherapy sessions to remain confidential, therapists were concerned they might either not share their true feelings and desires or determine that engaging in therapy was not worth it at all.

The amicus brief went on to assert that the duty to warn placed therapists in an "impossible dilemma": liability if they fail to disclose violent patients, or liability if they invade their patient's privacy by warning potential victims of violence. The amicus curiae also argued that mandates to warn potential victims may paradoxically *increase* the chance for violence. If the patient learns of the therapist's belief that the patient's potential for violence merits a warning, the patient may be more inclined to act violently. Furthermore, the warned individual, fearing violence from the patient, might act out in violence toward the patient in a preemptive first strike against the perceived threat. Patients may refuse treatment if they believe their therapy sessions would not remain confidential and might then be more likely to act in violence if not under treatment (Weinstock 1988; Weinstock and Weinstock 1989). In fact, Prosenjit Poddar did discontinue his therapy sessions as soon as he was made aware of Moore's confidentiality breach in discussing his case with the campus police.

Because of the outpouring of criticism from the psychotherapy and psychiatry communities, the California Supreme Court granted defendants' petition to rehear the *Tarasoff* case in 1976, producing the case now commonly referred to as *Tarasoff II*.

Tarasoff II

The *Tarasoff II* decision differed from *Tarasoff I* in several ways. The campus police were exempted from liability, the court finding that their duties were fulfilled under the Lanterman-Petris-Short Act (1967). The therapists involved, however, remained liable under a newly established, redefined duty to *protect*, rather than the *duty to warn* described in *Tarasoff I*:

> When a therapist determines, or pursuant to the standards of his profession should determine, that his patient presents a serious danger of violence to another, he incurs an obligation to use reasonable care to protect the intended victim against such danger. The discharge of this duty may require the therapist to take one or more of various steps, depending upon the nature of the case. Thus it may call for him to warn the intended victim or others likely to apprise the victim of the danger, to notify the police, or to take whatever other steps are reasonably necessary under the circumstances. (*Tarasoff v. Regents* 1976, p. 431)

The court explicitly broadened the former *duty to warn* to the *duty to protect* in a nod to the psychotherapy community's concerns regarding the difficulty and potential damage delivering warnings could cause. The court also acknowledged the "difficulty that a therapist encounters in attempting to forecast whether a patient presents a serious danger of violence" (p. 438). The court again felt that there was a limit to which confidentiality must be respected, notably retaining the same language from *Tarasoff I*: "The protective privilege ends where the public peril begins" (p. 442). Unfortunately, the court did not elaborate further on the criteria on which psychiatrists should rely to predict when a patient "presents a serious danger of violence to another" or what "steps are reasonably necessary" to discharge the duty to protect—both areas that would later cause significant confusion and debate (Runck 1984). The reasoning in the decision also opened the door to confounding *confidentiality* with *privilege* in later "dangerous patient" exceptions for therapist-patient testimonial privilege (Aronson 2001). Confidentiality is an ethical requirement for mental health professionals and physicians that is sometimes also required by law. Privilege is a legal right of patients to keep information out of courtroom settings.

Post-*Tarasoff*

The *Tarasoff* ruling, in the words of Thomas Gutheil, "burst like a bomb over the clinical scene" (Gutheil 2001, p. 345). Therapists and psychiatrists felt the ruling to be an anomaly that would quickly be overturned by later decisions and legislation owing to its sharp detour from the standards of confidentiality between patients and their therapists. In 1976, Alan Stone, then professor of law and psychiatry at Harvard University, wrote that

> the imposition of a duty to protect, which may take the form of a duty to warn threatened third parties, will imperil the therapeutic alliance and destroy the patient's expectation of confidentiality, thereby thwarting effective treatment and ultimately reducing public safety. (Stone 1976, p. 368)

Justice William P. Clark, writing his dissent of the *Tarasoff II* opinion, agreed: "the duty to warn imposed by the majority will cripple the use and effectiveness of psychiatry" (*Tarasoff v. Regents* 1976, p. 460).

Nevertheless, the *Tarasoff* decision rapidly spread across different jurisdictions in the United States. Despite the initial resistance to the ruling, psychiatrists ultimately accepted its inevitable progression into the clinical field and have been reassured that *Tarasoff*-like encounters in clinical practice are rare (Beck 1985; Givelber et al. 1984; Wise 1978). In 1985, Paul Appelbaum described the *Tarasoff* ruling in frank terms: "Although problematic in many respects, it has become a factor that must be dealt with in routine clinical interactions" (Appelbaum

1985, p. 425). As of 2019, all but six states (Arkansas, Kansas, Maine, Nevada, New Mexico, and North Dakota) implemented a *Tarasoff*-type duty when an acute danger exists to protect victims or prevent violence against another person or place, although jurisdictions differ with regard to whether the duty is mandatory or permissive and on other principles (Johnson et al. 2019).

Duties in *Tarasoff*-Type Situations

There are numerous competing ethical and legal considerations for psychiatrists in the treatment role when a Tarasoff duty is triggered. The *Tarasoff* decision itself hinged on legal principles that ultimately balanced the interests of patients and public safety. The conceptual framework underlying these ethical principles can be better understood when they are divided into duties toward different entities: the patient, the potential victim of a patient's violence, society, and the therapist.

Duties to the Patient

The primary professional duty in the psychotherapist-patient relationship is the duty of the psychotherapist to the patient. The goal of psychotherapy and psychiatric care is to promote the welfare of the patient, primarily by alleviating mental illness. To accomplish this end, the therapist is guided by the first three of Beauchamp and Childress's four bioethics principles: autonomy, beneficence, nonmaleficence, and justice (Beauchamp and Childress 2013).

At the time of the *Tarasoff* decision, warning potential victims, notifying the police, and taking measures (such as involuntary hospitalization) to protect against violence when a patient communicates an imminent threat were seen as unprecedented and antithetical to the therapist's role. Patients at that time expected their psychotherapy sessions to be spaces in which they could divulge their most sensitive information and fantasies without risk of confidentiality ever being breached. Following *Tarasoff*, the psychotherapist-patient relationship would never be the same: consideration of third-party safety now needs to be weighed more heavily than before. The major concerns about how *Tarasoff*, and its offspring in other jurisdictions, would impact the practice of psychiatry, and more specifically psychotherapy, included that it would damage the rapport and trust necessary for therapeutic progress and also discourage people from starting or continuing treatment, including those who may have violent propensities that could be mitigated with therapy. Empirical analysis of violent behavior has lent some credence to the theory that Tarasoff duties may counterproductively increase violence by discouraging treatment. Griffin Edwards published data findings that suggest an increase in rates of teen suicide by 9% and homicide by 5% in states after enactment of *Tarasoff* statutes (Edwards 2013, 2014). In part for these reasons, the U.S. Supreme Court established a federal psychotherapist-patient privilege in the landmark 1996 *Jaffee v. Redmond* decision, granting patients the right to preclude court testimony about information that patients communicated to mental health professionals in confidence. This right has been adopted in some form by all 50 states (Aronson 2001).

Breaching psychotherapist-patient confidentiality for mandated duty to protect/warn purposes may have other unintended consequences. Consider a hypothetical patient who is venting and communicating extreme anger and frustration to his psychotherapist about his boss. The visibly upset patient states, "I'm so mad at my boss, I could kill him." The patient eventually calms down and retracts his statement and clarifies further that he has no intention, plan, or desire to kill or seriously harm his boss. Depending on the statute or case law in the therapist's jurisdiction, however, the patient's statement alone, regardless of the subsequent retraction and clarification, may be enough to trigger a mandated duty to notify the police or warn the boss, among other actions. The therapist would be in the predicament of being potentially liable for any future harm to the boss if the boss were not warned. This would be balanced against the potential serious harm to the patient if the therapist were to warn the boss in this case where the therapist strongly believed that there was no actual danger. Warnings can cause severe unintended consequences to patients, including job loss and potential prosecution for issuing violent threats.

Duties to Potential Victims of Patient Violence

The crux of the argument in the *Tarasoff* decision, and the biggest departure from pre-*Tarasoff* psychotherapy, is that psychotherapists have fiduciary duties toward potential victims of a patient's violence. The standard of care owed to others is determined in part by the existence of a "special relationship" and the "foreseeability" of a negative event occurring. Traditionally, common law has found that one person generally does not owe duty to control the conduct of another person— if an individual witnesses another running off a cliff, they have no duty to stop that person from doing so. However, if an individual has a *special relationship* to another individual, then they do have a duty to act. In *Carlsen v. Koivumaki* (2014), the California Court of Appeals defined *special relationship* as a situation in which "the plaintiff is particularly vulnerable and dependent upon the defendant who, correspondingly, has some control over the plaintiff's welfare" (p. 893).

The prototypical examples of special relationships include parents to children, teachers to students, innkeepers to guests, and therapists to patients. Before the *Tarasoff* case, lower courts had found no special relationship between psychotherapists and would-be victims of their patients. However, the California Supreme Court reversed this precedent, finding that "the therapist owes a legal duty not only to his patient, but also to his patient's would-be victim" (*Tarasoff v. Regents* 1976, p. 439). In essence, when the therapist acquires the unique knowledge that a third party might be in danger, an obligation to protect the third party is created.

Consider a scenario in which the duty to protect/warn third parties seems clear. A therapist is meeting with a student, and the student informs the therapist that he has purchased a gun and intends to kill his roommate the next day. A reasonable therapist would take one or more steps that serve to protect the roommate, such as involuntarily committing the patient, informing the police, arranging for the gun to be removed, or warning the roommate. Consider how the scenario might change if, after making his threat, the student storms out of the therapy session shouting, "I'm going to kill him right now!" The therapist, unable to hospitalize the patient, might inform the police and attempt to contact the patient's roommate. Warning the roommate in both cases would seem reasonable, and warning in the second scenario seems critical given the urgency of the situation.

Duties to Society

A separate secondary (or distal) duty in psychotherapy is to promote safety in society. Usually, this duty aligns with the primary (or proximal) duty of the therapist to advance the well-being of the patient. However, there are instances in which the therapist determines that breaching confidentiality for purposes of protecting third parties and society outweighs potential consequences and harm to the patient (Weinstock 2015).

The *Tarasoff* ruling attempted to balance the need for public safety with the privacy afforded to patients seeking psychotherapeutic treatment. The question of whether warning third parties is always the most protective action for promoting safety is not clear, as it is possible that warning third parties may actually increase potential violence in certain situations. For example, a potential victim may attack the patient who made threats, thereby increasing the overall risk of violence in the community. Patients are also unlikely to return to their psychotherapist for treatment, thereby increasing the risk of violence. These conclusions, which cannot be studied in a systematized and ethical way, are still up for debate.

Duties to Avoid Liability

All psychotherapists have duties to their own practice and to avoid liability. Personal liability can be a financial burden and a drain on time, and it can affect the therapist's ability to treat patients in the future. Unfortunately, the duties set forth in *Tarasoff* and subsequent legislation have not fully clarified how therapists may avoid liability. When presented with a patient who is making violent threats, all psychotherapists face liability from two sides: third parties can sue them if they do not sufficiently protect the third party from the patient's violence, and the patient can sue them if they breach confidentiality in the process of warning.

Codes of Ethics of Professional Societies

Given the conflicting duties and responsibilities of mental health providers to their patients and third parties in *Tarasoff*-like situations, organizational guidelines can be a useful tool in practice. The ethical guidelines of the American Psychological Association and the American Psychiatric Association both give considerable weight to the importance of confidentiality within the constraints of the law.

Section 4 of the American Psychological Association's Ethical Principles of Psychologists and Code of Conduct is devoted to privacy and confidentiality. Maintaining confidentiality is considered a "primary obligation" of psychotherapists; the code instructs psychologists to disclose confidential information without consent "only as mandated by law, or where permitted by law" for valid purposes such as to "protect the client/patient, psychologist, or others from harm" (American Psychological Association 2024, Section 4.05(b)).

The ethical guidelines of the American Psychiatric Association are published as the Principles of Medical Ethics With Annotations Especially Applicable to Psychiatry (American Psychiatric Association 2013). The guidelines do not specifically address prevention of violence, but they do esteem privacy of patients very highly: "Confidentiality is essential to psychiatric treatment. This is based in part on the special nature of psychiatric therapy as well as on the traditional ethical relationship between physician and patient.... A psychiatrist may release confidential information only with the authorization of the patient or under proper legal compulsion" (p. 6).

Conflicting Duties

New Frontiers in *Tarasoff*

The treating psychiatrist has proximal duty to the patient, but distal duties may overcome that duty when the risk is significant. When faced with a potentially violent patient, the treating professional must weigh the various proximal and distal duties before deciding on the most appropriate course of action. In many cases, proximal and distal duties will align. For example, preventing a patient from carrying out a dangerous action by warning the would-be victim may also be in the primary interest of the patient, as it may protect them from serious legal consequences. In cases in which there is misalignment between proximal and distal duties, the psychiatrist must weigh the importance of each duty as well as legal obligations. In extremely rare situations, a thoughtful, ethically aspirational approach may sometimes conflict with organizational guidelines or leave the treating psychiatrist vulnerable to legal liability.

Undermining of Therapist Protections

The original 1974 *Tarasoff* decision was reheard in 1976 in large part because the California Supreme Court recognized that the duty to warn was overly narrow. The *duty to warn* was thus replaced in the 1976 decision with the *duty to protect*, by which warning was one possible avenue of protecting the third party. The court did not elaborate on alternative methods that a therapist might take to protect the third party, nor did the court elaborate on what situations triggered the duty beyond the ambiguous "when a therapist determines, or pursuant to the standards of his profession should determine, that his patient presents a serious danger of violence to another" (*Tarasoff v. Regents* 1976, p. 431).

The American Psychiatric Association's Council on Psychiatry and Law in 1987 produced a model statute in an attempt to alleviate some of this confusion (Buckner and Firestone 2000). The model statute proposed expanding the potential avenues of obtaining immunity to include several options, only one of which had to be fulfilled: 1) communicating the threat to a potential victim, 2) notifying law enforcement, or 3) arranging for hospitalization of the potential offender. California legislators took a similar approach in 1985 in the adoption of Section 43.92 of the California Civil Code, which states that the duty to protect is triggered only when the patient communicates a serious threat of physical violence to a reasonably identifiable victim. The duty can be discharged by several avenues, including warning the potential victim and informing the police. Additionally, warning the potential victim and notifying the police would guarantee the therapist full immunity from liability.

Despite these rigorous efforts to clarify and limit the Tarasoff duty in California, there remains a lengthy, repetitive history of legislators, therapists, and even judges who misinterpret the duty and believe it is a duty to *warn* potential third parties, rather than *protect* (Sones et al. 2021; Weinstock et al. 2015). In the recent California case *Turner v. Rivera*, a patient (Mr. Turner) at a California Veterans Administration hospital communicated to his psychiatrist (Dr. Rivera) a plan to obtain a firearm and shoot his boss in the head. Rivera warned the patient's boss. When the patient was fired, he filed suit against Rivera, alleging that she negligently disclosed private health information. The *Turner* court denied Rivera's motion for summary judgment, and she was ultimately found liable to the patient for professional negligence in the wrongful disclosure of Turner's supposed threat to kill his supervisor. The United States Court of Appeals for the Ninth Circuit affirmed this judgment of the district court, citing the jury's finding that because Rivera did not actually believe Turner posed a serious threat, she was not entitled to immunity as a psychotherapist discharging a duty to warn, even though Turner communicated a serious threat (*Turner v. Rivera* 2021). This decision appears to have eliminated the statutory immunity for warning a potential victim after a serious threat has been made by a patient to an identifiable victim as stated in California Civil Code Section 43.92: "if the patient has communicated to the psychotherapist a serious threat of physical violence against a reasonably identifiable victim or victims." This interpretation of the statute creates greater confusion for psychotherapists who may be liable no matter what they do and unfairly punished if hindsight shows that an action led to a bad outcome. If a therapist warns, they may be liable to their patient; if they do not warn, they may be liable to the potential victim.

Tarasoff in College Mental Health

In March of 2018, the California Supreme Court held that universities have a special relationship with their students and a duty to protect them from foreseeable harm during curricular activities. When Damon Thompson was a student at the University of California, Los Angeles (UCLA), he began to hear voices and believe that students in his dormitory were making racist and critical comments toward him. After he wrote a letter to the Dean of Students warning that he might "end up acting in a manner that will incur undesirable consequences," he was referred to the school's mental health clinic and the Consultation and Response Team, a group of staff who assist students of concern (*Regents v. Superior Court of Los Angeles County* 2018, p. 26). He declined medications and ultimately withdrew from therapy in April 2009. Six months later, Thompson critically injured his classmate, Rosen, stabbing her in the cheek and neck with a kitchen knife during their chemistry laboratory in the belief that she was disparaging him. Rosen filed suit against Thompson, the Regents of the University of California, and several UCLA employees, including Thompson's psychologist, Nicole Green. The California Supreme Court held that colleges and universities have a "duty to use reasonable care to protect students from foreseeable acts of violence in the classroom or during curricular activities" (*Regents v. Superior Court of Los Angeles County* 2018, p. 14).

A similar special relationship and corresponding duty of care established between therapists and their patients in *Tarasoff* was extended to universities and their students in the Rosen case. And a problem similar to that created for therapists after the original *Tarasoff* decision now plagues universities, which are mandated to use reasonable care to protect students from foreseeable acts of violence but lack criteria or consensus defining reasonable care or what situations constitute a foreseeable act of violence. That is, the challenges created by this ruling echo those created in the original 1974 *Tarasoff* case, with no clear language on what specific situations trigger a duty and what specific actions discharge the duty. Rosen did not present any evidence that Thompson communicated a serious threat of violence against Rosen to any university employee, including psychologist Green. Although Section 43.92

provided immunity to Green in this case (because there was no evidence that Thompson triggered a Tarasoff duty), the university was found to have no such protection and was, in effect, held to a higher standard than the psychotherapist, who had more training and expertise to assess and manage violence risk stemming from psychotic disorders. Furthermore, the court created the duty without elaborating on the standard of care governing the triggering or the discharge of the duty for universities.

Nguyen v. Massachusetts Institute of Technology (2018), a Massachusetts Supreme Court wrongful death case arising out of the suicide of the plaintiff's son, faced similar challenges. As in the Rosen case before the California Supreme Court, the Massachusetts Supreme Court found that MIT has a duty to protect its students from harm related to mental illness. Unlike the ambiguity and confusion created with the Rosen decision, the Nguyen court established clear guidelines as to the situations that trigger a duty for universities to take reasonable measures to prevent student self-harm and suicide:

> where a university has actual knowledge of a student's suicide attempt that occurred while enrolled at the university or recently before matriculation, or of a student's stated plans or intentions to commit suicide. (*Nguyen v. Massachusetts Institute of Technology* 2018, p. 29)

Additionally, the *Nguyen* court outlined how universities discharge this duty:

> Reasonable measures by the university to satisfy a triggered duty will include initiating its suicide prevention protocol if the university has developed such a protocol. In the absence of such a protocol, reasonable measures will require the university employee who learns of the student's suicide attempt or stated plans or intentions to commit suicide to contact the appropriate officials at the university empowered to assist the student in obtaining clinical care from medical professionals or, if the student refuses such care, to notify the student's emergency contact. In emergency situations, reasonable measures obviously would include contacting police, fire, or emergency medical personnel. By taking the reasonable measures under the circumstances presented, a university satisfies its duty. (*Nguyen v. Massachusetts Institute of Technology* 2018, p. 35)

Taken together, the Rosen (UCLA) and Nguyen (MIT) state supreme court opinions suggest that universities need to be vigilant regarding students who are potentially suicidal or violent (Appelbaum 2019). Universities face liability for not "taking reasonable measures to protect and control their students" from "foreseeable" harm (suicide or violence). There is already precedent for college students being forced to take leaves of absence, not being allowed to live in dormitories, and in some cases not being allowed to even enter campus if they report suicidal ideation (Appelbaum 2006). In an effort to avoid liability, universities may be reluctant to admit students with known mental health problems, despite Americans With Disabilities Act protections, or may be incentivized to dismiss students who are psychiatrically hospitalized or experience psychotic symptoms. The Rosen decision may have the unintended consequence of discouraging students from seeking out mental health services. Psychiatrists working in college mental health settings must now pay special attention to the shifting duties of care for universities and standards of care owed to patients, as universities may face extreme liability for bad outcomes that may only have been seen in hindsight.

Conclusion

The landmark *Tarasoff v. Regents of the University of California* decision presented numerous challenges to psychotherapists. Whereas the psychiatric community initially believed that the obstacles placed by the Tarasoff duty were insurmountable, a duty to warn or protect is legally mandated or permitted in most jurisdictions, has been largely accepted as ethical by professional standards, and has become a part of regular psychotherapy practice.

The ethical and legal considerations for psychiatrists and psychotherapists in the treatment role when a Tarasoff duty is triggered must be carefully considered, as they may conflict with other considerations in rare scenarios. In such situations, psychotherapists must balance their duties to advance the well-being of their patients, protect potential victims, promote public safety, and avoid legal liability. Therapists have duties toward the patient and must protect the psychotherapist-patient relationship as much as realistically possible. Therapists also have duties toward potential victims of a patient's violence, originating in the special relationship the therapist has with potential victims of their patients to foresee violent behavior. There may be rare situations in which the psychotherapist believes that warning the potential victim would be likely to precipitate violence. In certain jurisdictions, such as California, it may be legally permissible to not warn the potential victim and protect the patient and potential victim via involuntary hospitalization of the patient and notifying the police. Although this action may not provide the psychotherapist full legal immunity from liability, it may be the most ethical, as it maximizes the welfare of the patient and protection of a vulnerable third party by mitigating against a foreseeable violent outcome.

The Tarasoff duty has shifted dramatically since its inception in 1974. In California, there remains confusion as to whether the statutory duty mandates warning the victim in every situation a duty is triggered, or simply allows for warning the potential victim, in addition to notifying the police for firearm prohibition purposes, to be a method of gaining statutory immunity from liability. Case law has now established that universities have a similar special relationship to protect students from self-harm or violence and face liability concerns that will likely affect the treatment of people with mental illness on college campuses (e.g., *Nguyen v. Massachusetts Institute of Technology* 2018; *Regents v. Superior Court of Los Angeles County* 2018). Additionally, the recent *Turner v. Rivera* (2021) appellate decision created further ambiguity about what psychotherapists should do to avoid legal liability when patients communicate serious threats of harm. The U.S. Court of Appeals for the Ninth Circuit affirmed the district court's judgment that the psychiatrist (Rivera) was liable for professional negligence in warning the patient's boss of the patient's threat. The Ninth Circuit Court reasoned that Rivera was liable in this case because she made the warning despite not actually believing or predicting that the patient posed a serious risk of inflicting grave bodily harm on the victim. If she had not warned the boss of the death threat, however, and the boss was later killed by the patient, it is likely that Rivera would have been found liable. This decision reinforces the double bind of liability concerns that have plagued psychotherapists since the original *Tarasoff* decision.

The continuing legal evolution of the Tarasoff duty necessitates a delicate balancing act between patient confidentiality and public safety, prompting complex risk assessment and prediction challenges and presenting practitioners with a perplexing dilemma of when to breach confidentiality in the face of potential harm. This dilemma is further complicated by case law and statutes that can be interpreted in ways to conclude liability for the psychotherapist in hindsight, no matter what action was taken when the patient communicated a threat (i.e., liability for warning and liability for not warning). Psychotherapists should understand the potential legal consequences in these *Tarasoff* situations so that they may be informed of liability risks when attempting to do what is ethically best in these difficult situations. Additionally, certain actions, depending on the jurisdiction, to protect the patient and potential victim that are legally permissible (e.g., involuntary hospitalization and notifying the police) may be chosen over actions that in particular situations may not be most protective of the patient and third party (e.g., warning the potential victim when it is foreseeable that doing so will lead to violence) but could offer full legal immunity from liability.

References

American Psychiatric Association: The Principles of Medical Ethics With Annotations Especially Applicable to Psychiatry. American Psychiatric Association, 2013. Available at: https://www.psychiatry.org/File%20Library/Practice/Ethics%20Documents/principles2013--final.pdf. Accessed August 13, 2024.

American Psychological Association: Ethical Principles of Psychologists and Code of Conduct. Washington, DC, American Psychological Association, 2017. Available at: https://www.apa.org/ethics/code. Accessed October 9, 2024.

Appelbaum PS: Tarasoff and the clinician: problems in fulfilling the duty to protect. Am J Psychiatry 142(4):425–429, 1985 3976915

Appelbaum PS: Law & psychiatry: "Depressed? Get out!": dealing with suicidal students on college campuses. Psychiatr Serv 57(7):914–916, 2006 16816275

Appelbaum PS: Responsibility for suicide or violence on campus. Psychiatr Serv 70(4):350–352, 2019 30841841

Aronson RH: The mental health provider privilege in the wake of Jaffe v. Redmond. Oklahoma Law Rev 54:591–612, 2001

Beauchamp TL, Childress JF: Principles of Biomedical Ethics, 7th Edition. New York, Oxford University Press, 2013

Beck JC: Violent patients and the Tarasoff duty in private psychiatric practice. J Psychiatry Law 13(3–4):361–376, 1985 11649765

Buckner F, Firestone M: "Where the public peril begins": 25 years after Tarasoff. J Leg Med 21(2):187–222, 2000 10911695

Carlsen v Koivumaki, 227 Cal App 4th 879 (2014)

Cohen RN: Tarasoff v. Regents of the University of California: the duty to warn—common law and statutory problems for California psychotherapists. Calif West Law Rev 14(1):153–182, 1978 11664959

Crocker EM: Judicial expansion of the Tarasoff doctrine: doctors' dilemma. J Psychiatry Law 13(1–2):83–99, 1985 11658739

Edwards G: Tarasoff, duty to warn laws, and suicide. Int Rev Law Econ 34:1–8, 2013

Edwards G: Doing their duty: an empirical analysis of the unintended effect of Tarasoff v. Regents on homicidal activity. J Law Econ 57(2):321–348, 2014

Givelber DJ, Bowers WJ, Blitch CL: Tarasoff, myth and reality: an empirical study of private law in action. Wis Law Rev 1984(2):443–497, 1984 11653756

Goodman TA: From Tarasoff to Hopper: the evolution of the therapist's duty to protect third parties. Behav Sci Law 3(2):195–225, 1985

Gutheil TG: Moral justification for Tarasoff-type warnings and breach of confidentiality: a clinician's perspective. Behav Sci Law 19(3):345–353, 2001 11443696

Jaffee v Redmond, 518 U.S. 1 (1996)

Johnson R, Persad G, Sisti D: The Tarasoff rule: the implications of interstate variation and gaps in professional training. Focus Am Psychiatr Publ 17(4):435–442, 2019 32015727

Lanterman-Petris-Short Act, Cal. Welf. & Inst. Code §§ 5000–5550 (1967)

Nguyen v Massachusetts Institute of Technology, 479 Mass 436, 96 NE3d 128 (2018)

People v Poddar, 518 Cal Rptr 910, 518 P2d 342 (1974)

Regents of the University of California v Superior Court of Los Angeles County, 240 Cal Rptr 3d, 29 Cal App 5th 890 (2018)

Runck B: Survey shows therapists misunderstand Tarasoff rule. Hosp Community Psychiatry 35(5):429–430, 1984 6724538

Simone S, Fulero SM: Tarasoff and the duty to protect. J Aggress Maltreat Trauma 11(1–2):145–168, 2005

Slovenko R: Article commentary: the therapist's duty to warn or protect third persons. J Psychiatry Law 16(1):139–209, 1988

Sones AC, Weinstock R, Darby WC, et al: Therapists need clarity on duty to warn of patients' violent threats. Daily Journal, February 19, 2021

Stone AA: The Tarasoff decisions: suing psychotherapists to safeguard society. Harv Law Rev 90(2):358–378, 1976 1028678

Tarasoff v Regents of the University of California, 118 Cal Rptr 129, 529 P2d 553 (1974)

Tarasoff v Regents of the University of California, 131 Cal Rptr 14, 551 P2d 334 (1976)

Turner v Rivera, No. 19–16497 (9th Cir. Feb. 2, 2021)

Venner S, Sivasubramaniam D, Luebbers S, et al: Cross-cultural reliability and rater bias in forensic risk assessment: a review of the literature. Psychol Crime Law 27(2):105–121, 2021

Weinstock R: Confidentiality and the new duty to protect: the therapist's dilemma. Hosp Community Psychiatry 39(6):607–609, 1988 3402920

Weinstock R: Dialectical principlism: an approach to finding the most ethical action. J Am Acad Psychiatry Law 43(1):10–20, 2015 25770274

Weinstock R, Weinstock D: Clinical flexibility and confidentiality: effects of reporting laws. Psychiatr Q 60(3):195–214, 1989 2641975

Weinstock R, Darby WC, Bonnici DM, et al: The ever-evolving duty to protect in California. J Am Acad Psychiatry Law 43(2):262, 2015 26071515

Wise TP: Where the public peril begins: a survey of psychotherapists to determine the effects of Tarasoff. Stanford Law Rev 31(1):165–190, 1978 11665029

13

Balancing Ethical Considerations for Assisted Outpatient Treatment

Michael R. MacIntyre, M.D.

Jeffrey W. Swanson, Ph.D.

Jon E. Sherin, M.D., Ph.D.

Marvin Swartz, M.D.

Assisted outpatient treatment (AOT), also known as involuntary outpatient commitment, requires certain severely mentally ill persons, by order of a court, to adhere to mental health treatment recommendations in the community. AOT was designed as a tool to assist patients whose capacity to consent to treatment and insight into their serious mental illness (SMI) fluctuate over time, resulting in stopping medications and disengaging from mental health services. Many severely and chronically mentally ill persons receive care only when involuntarily committed to a psychiatric facility. As legal standards for involuntary inpatient care have tightened and psychiatric hospital bed capacity has declined over time, many patients who experience a mental health crisis are hospitalized only for a short period of time—until they are stabilized. As soon as they no longer meet strict hospitalization criteria, they are discharged—often with little or no follow-up—and may stop taking their prescribed medication. Subsequently, a cycle ensues of rehospitalization once symptoms worsen, a process termed the *revolving door*.

AOT strives to solve this problem by providing a mechanism to ensure that certain people engage in outpatient mental health treatment with the support of comprehensive services and a multidisciplinary treatment team. Although most states have involuntary outpatient commitment laws, they vary widely in their application. In terms of implementation, infrastructure, and oversight, New York has developed one of the most comprehensive AOT programs in the country, with a focus on providing intensive, multidisciplinary case management, medication, and housing support as well as other court-mandated services to help ensure an individual's stability outside of a hospital setting (Swartz et al. 2009).

Several ethical considerations arise when mandating outpatient treatment for persons not at imminent risk of danger to themselves or others. Traditional medical ethical principles of autonomy, beneficence, nonmaleficence, and distributive justice must be promoted and balanced (Beauchamp and Childress 2013). Some believe that AOT unnecessarily limits autonomy and can be a coercive infringement on one's civil liberties. Conversely, health care providers adhere to the principle of beneficence when they advocate for AOT for their patients with severe psychiatric symptoms to improve functioning and decrease suffering. When people refuse necessary treatment owing to poor insight, AOT may prevent harm by limiting the need for inpatient hospitalizations or incarceration. Distributive justice concerns arise when examining the utilization of resources to provide AOT, because prioritizing involuntary treatment of patients might limit access to care for those voluntarily seeking help (Swanson et al. 2010). However, a pattern of repeated involuntary hospitalizations and criminal justice involvement is both harmful to the person with SMI and costly to society. Research suggests that appropriately funding AOT programs can prevent such outcomes and ultimately lead to greater access to care for both voluntary and involuntary patients (Swanson et al. 2010, 2013).

Multiple groups have competing interests regarding AOT, including the patients who receive treatment, their family members, treating clinicians, civil commitment courts, and society at large (members of the general public, persons voluntarily seeking treatment services, and the state responsible for funding treatment). Competent patients have a right to make their own medical decisions, including refusing care.

However, poor decisions made by those whose illness renders them incapable of properly weighing the risks and benefits of care can lead to harm to the individual and to society. The state has an obligation to patients unable to care for themselves, and also to protect society from potential harm. Reconciling these competing interests is not a simple task. In this chapter, we review the various ethical aspects of AOT that must be addressed for successful implementation. We review the benefits and costs of AOT and the competing interests of various stakeholders. By reviewing the latest research, we describe how to ethically address controversies that arise regarding involuntary outpatient commitment.

Benefits of Assisted Outpatient Treatment

Over the years, psychiatric care has largely transitioned from inpatient to outpatient settings. People with SMI who do not meet strict criteria for involuntary (or even voluntary) hospitalization may still require intensive community-based services to recover and optimally manage their illness. Those with SMI, and especially those with prominent psychotic symptoms such as seen in schizophrenia, frequently lack appropriate insight into their illness and lack the ability to engage in treatment in the outpatient setting without assistance. Although courts and most reasonable practitioners generally advocate for individuals to make treatment decisions when they fully understand the risks and benefits, untreated SMI may impair the ability to make truly informed decisions. In one study, more than half of patients with schizophrenia demonstrated impaired decision-making capacity regarding treatment decisions (Grisso et al. 1995).

AOT provides one mechanism for assisting those with SMI and impaired capacity to obtain necessary care in the outpatient setting. Given the complexities of AOT, a perfect randomized controlled trial may never clearly prove its benefits; however, a number of well-conducted, large-scale, quasi-experimental, and naturalistic studies provide sufficient evidence for the benefits of AOT (Swanson and Swartz 2014). Sustained outpatient commitment has been associated with fewer hospitalizations, shorter lengths of stay, less violence, and less criminal victimization (Swartz et al. 2001).

AOT has the potential to serve as an engagement tool, benefiting both patients and providers. Several interventions along a continuum allow a patient to appropriately engage in self-determination of their mental health treatment. For example, a patient with a high degree of insight may participate in shared decision-making with a provider, during which a physician uses their expertise to explain treatment options and a patient contributes their values and preferences before a final treatment plan is collaboratively created. Similarly, a patient may exert autonomy by completing a psychiatric advance directive. This allows the patient, while competent, to define the type of psychiatric care (such as medications, hospitalization, or electroconvulsive therapy) they wish to have in the future, if they were to lose competency and become incapacitated by a recurrence of severe symptoms of the psychiatric illness. This is a powerful tool: the U.S. Court of Appeals ruled that forcing treatment against the wishes of a clearly expressed psychiatric directive created by a patient while competent represented a violation of the Americans With Disabilities Act (*Hargrave v. Vermont* 2003). At the other end of the spectrum are tools such as conservatorship, in which an appointed individual is legally authorized to make decisions for those unable to provide for basic needs such as food, clothing, or shelter. Although conservatees lose autonomy to make many decisions, they potentially retain much more liberty living with assistance in an outpatient setting rather than requiring long-term psychiatric hospitalization.

AOT has similar potential to engage a patient in care appropriate to their needs and ultimately to increase autonomy. The goal should be to engage a patient in care for the length of time necessary to treat impairing symptoms, place them on a path to recovery, and restore sufficient autonomy so that AOT and involuntary hospitalization are no longer necessary. In fact, research has shown that successful implementation of AOT, even if it requires a degree of coercion, can lead to a decreased risk of being arrested, an outcome that would potentially involve a far more coercive criminal justice setting and prevent a person from receiving optimal treatment (Link et al. 2011).

One often-cited major study, the Oxford Community Treatment Order Evaluation Trial (OCTET), found no difference at 12 months in outcomes, including hospital readmissions and clinical functioning, during a randomized controlled trial of two types of mandated community treatment orders in the United Kingdom (Burns et al. 2013). The OCTET study was designed, however, to compare outcomes for hospitalized psychiatric patients who are discharged under two different programs of legally supervised outpatient treatment—a community treatment order versus conditional release (Swanson and Swartz 2014).

Experts have highlighted this study's lack of generalizability as complicating the answer to whether outpatient commitment is an effective legal tool compared with truly voluntary treatment.

Patient Perspectives

Given the potentially coercive nature of AOT and its infringement on individual rights, it is important to consider how we define positive outcomes and who benefits from AOT. Psychiatrists, patients, families, and society at large have different concepts of benefit and sometimes competing interests when it comes to involuntary treatment, yet most studies on AOT fail to consider the patient's perspective. Although AOT has benefits that a treating psychiatrist would consider positive— such as fewer hospitalizations, shorter lengths of stay, and less criminal victimization (Swartz et al. 2001)—these are based on average group effects and not guaranteed outcomes for any individual. A patient might not agree that the potential benefits are worth involuntary commitment to outpatient treatment. In one study, only 27% of patients mandated to outpatient treatment believed that the court-ordered intervention had benefited them personally after 1 year. In the subset of patients who experienced positive outcomes—avoiding rehospitalization or arrest and functioning well in the community after a year—the proportion who endorsed the personal benefit of outpatient commitment was higher, but still only 45%. These findings suggest that outpatient commitment cannot be ethically justified solely based on a retrospective perception of personal benefit in the eyes of affected individuals. Rather, other societal justifications must be brought to bear to undergird the ethical foundations of outpatient commitment. Still, given the potentially coercive nature of outpatient commitment, an ethical analysis of the benefits of this intervention requires attention to the patient's perspective (Swartz et al. 2003b).

Alan Stone has argued that the value of involuntary psychiatric treatment is confirmed when patients who initially object are ultimately grateful that clinicians overrode their refusals, an idea referred to as the *thank-you theory* (Stone 1975). Although this makes sense intuitively, it may not accurately reflect the nuances of involuntary outpatient commitment. As mentioned earlier, only a minority of outpatient-committed individuals retrospectively perceive that mandated treatment personally benefited them. However, and somewhat paradoxically, studies also suggest that a majority of those subjected to outpatient commitment believe that outpatient commitment is effective and fair in general (that is, when applied to other people). In one study of consumers with schizophrenia and other related psychotic disorders who were under mandated community treatment orders, 62% regarded the treatment mandate as generally effective, and 55% found the treatment mandate to be generally fair (Swartz et al. 2004). Although some people with psychosis see benefit from involuntary treatment, these studies still show that a large proportion of consumers are unhappy with AOT. In particular, single and noncohabitating patients, African Americans, and patients with substance abuse problems reported the highest levels of perceived coercion under outpatient commitment (Swartz et al. 2002).

Another study showed that AOT participants with longer periods of court-ordered treatment had a significantly better perceived quality of life at 1 year of follow-up (Swanson et al. 2003). At the same time, higher levels of perceived coercion were associated with longer periods of outpatient commitment—an adverse effect that moderated the positive impact on quality of life. The study did also suggest that the benefits of treatment under AOT outweighed the coercive side effects. Other research along these lines has shown that the strength of consumers' preferences for remaining in the community and avoiding hospitalization is substantially greater than the strength of preferences for avoiding court-ordered outpatient treatment (Swartz et al. 2003b).

Thank-you theory, despite its insights regarding involuntary treatment in general, is an oversimplified and insufficient ethical analysis. Switching from asking "Does the patient agree with the intervention once they are treated?" to "Does the patient accept the trade-offs of the intervention?" allows for a more nuanced analysis of the issues. The importance of *trade-offs* must regularly be considered during mental health treatment. For example, given the potentially unpleasant side-effect profile of psychiatric medications, a patient may never view taking medications such as lithium or an antipsychotic as desirable. They may never say "thank you" to psychiatrists who recommend the treatment. They may say they do not like being on a medication. However, a patient may develop sufficient insight to see that, although not ideal, taking a medication may be preferable to the consequences of no medication, such as recurrent hospitalizations or manic episodes. That is, although patients with SMI may never be happy that their mental health condition requires medication, they may still appreciate medication as a preferred alternative and worth the trade-offs. Some may also realize, then, that outpatient commitment is a legal tool that can ensure access to such beneficial treatment.

Rather than ask whether patients approve of AOT, it makes sense to consider whether patients prefer AOT to the likely alternatives. Although AOT may be restrictive and coercive, if it decreases hospitalizations, incarcerations, and conservatorships, it is likely many people would choose AOT over these alternatives. This was indeed the case in at least one study of stakeholder groups' opinions on AOT, including consumers with psychotic illness. Various mental health stakeholder groups were presented with vignettes explaining different treatment options and potential outcomes. Researchers found that those with psychoses prioritized avoiding involuntary rehospitalization more than any other outcome. Additionally, those with psychoses prioritized limiting interpersonal violence and maintaining interpersonal relationships, with a comparatively weak preference for avoiding outpatient commitment (Swartz et al. 2003a).

Cost

An infringement on civil liberties can be justified only if the resources are available to achieve the desired goal. For example, successful treatment of adults with SMI requires comprehensive treatment teams with psychiatrists, therapists, and case managers, as well as stable housing environments and access to both locked and unlocked treatment facilities. Research has shown that AOT can help improve outcomes, but only if paired with appropriate clinical treatment (Swanson and Swartz 2014; Swartz et al. 2001). Providing this care may require a large up-front public investment in the behavioral health care system.

To function appropriately, AOT must be thoughtfully implemented and receive appropriate funding. Legislation often seems destined to fail. Although at least 45 states have statutory authorization for involuntary outpatient treatment, only a minority actively implement such laws (Fitch and Swanson 2019; Meldrum et al. 2016). Some laws appear to be written in such a way as to preclude AOT from being widely adopted (Appelbaum 2003, 2005). In California, for example, AOT programs are subject to each individual county's approval and funding, leading to inconsistencies in implementation of AOT across the state. A patient with an AOT order issued in one county could move to the next county where the AOT order is not enforceable.

Initial costs to fully fund the treatment necessary for AOT may be substantial. These costs must come from somewhere, whether it is increased spending by the state or reappropriation of funds from other enterprises. Some have expressed concern that using mental health funding for involuntary outpatient treatment diverts access to care from those voluntarily and willingly seeking help. Alternatively, the costs of treatment nonadherence can be significant. Irregular medication use is one of the strongest predictors of hospital utilization and costs; hospital costs are four times higher for nonadherent patients than for those who take psychotropic medications regularly (Svarstad et al. 2001). The increase in services for those who refuse treatment also diverts resources from those voluntarily seeking treatment. Potentially, providing earlier care and limiting resource utilization may actually increase the availability of care to others.

Swanson and colleagues studied the cost-effectiveness of AOT programs in New York, the state with the most robust AOT system to date. The researchers analyzed 3 years of data and found that total net costs of care declined by 43% following the initiation of court-ordered treatment and an additional 13% in the second year (Swanson et al. 2013). Although spending on outpatient care increased, the increase was more than offset by a decrease in repeated hospitalizations and a decrease in costs related to criminal recidivism and days incarcerated. The researchers concluded that AOT can reduce overall service costs for those with SMI and even improve overall outpatient service costs for those voluntarily participating in intensive community-based services, provided the jurisdiction commits to a substantial investment of resources to adequately fund intensive outpatient services in connection with court-ordered treatment (Swanson et al. 2013). These findings were consistent with a similar study of involuntary outpatient commitment in North Carolina, where the same researchers found that if the state invested in intensive outpatient services, AOT resulted in lower overall costs for mental health care at 6 months of implementation and further savings for community-based services if court orders were extended beyond that period (Swartz et al. 2001).

Successfully Using Assisted Outpatient Treatment

As with any intervention, unique factors alter the ethical calculus for implementation of AOT. Several issues distinct to the individual patient, the availability of resources, and the structure of the community may affect an AOT program. Such nuances alter when AOT orders should be renewed or for how long they should be granted, which may be further complicated by how the community conceptualizes AOT. If AOT is used to force treatment on anyone who is mentally ill and has poor insight, a lack of defined goals and indeterminate length of coercion would be unjustifiable. When AOT is rather conceptualized as an engagement tool to help an individual build insight and regain capacity to make mental health decisions, the short-term infringement on civil rights may be more easily justified for resultant sustained, long-term improvements in autonomy and increased freedom. For example, a person refusing treatment for psychotic and delusional reasons lacks this decision-making capacity but, if treated successfully with AOT, may regain the ability to clearly express their wishes for care in a rational and informed manner. In such a case, rather than committing someone to a life of involuntary care, AOT can be conceptualized as having the goal of successfully enhancing an individual's autonomy by improving their health to the extent that they no longer require AOT.

The treatment setting in which involuntary commitment orders are applied also changes the ethics calculations. In New York State, 84% of AOT orders are to step down from inpatient hospitalization to outpatient care (Robbins et al. 2010). Applying AOT to someone who is acutely ill, with evidence of recent and likely repeated hospitalizations, implies different ethical considerations than for someone who is currently living sufficiently well in the community that they do not require inpatient hospitalization. AOT recipients in a hospital effectively do not experience an increase in restrictions (involuntary hospitalization is far more restrictive than AOT). Although the debate around AOT often focuses on people in a community setting who are facing restrictions on freedom, they are a distinct and small percentage of those receiving AOT orders.

The current stringent requirements for psychiatric hospitalization do not necessarily mean that people who are "not committable" have a high quality of life and are functioning well in the community. It is true that AOT for someone who is not at imminent risk of hospitalization or conservatorship may be overly paternalistic, but AOT to avoid the need for a conservatorship would appear to be more acceptable. The goal is to maximize therapeutic benefit while minimizing infringement on a patient's autonomy. That is, AOT is a tool to keep the patient engaged in an appropriate level of care rather than allowing their mental health to deteriorate until a highly restrictive environment is necessary. When AOT is initiated from an outpatient setting, some degree of certainty about its benefits is necessary to justify the infringement on civil liberties. To limit abuses, appropriate criteria for outpatient-initiated AOT must be clearly defined. Clinicians, policymakers, and researchers should work together to better understand what it means to live safely in a community, what patterns of behavior are suggestive of an individual's inability to continue to live safely, and when outpatient-initiated AOT evaluations should be initiated.

Racial Bias

When considering any treatment policy that may infringe on individual rights, care must be taken to ensure vulnerable groups are not unfairly disadvantaged. If AOT programs are to be ethically justified, they must be equitable as well as effective. Some critics have suggested that historically oppressed racial minority groups may disproportionately receive court mandates to outpatient treatment, raising the question whether AOT serves as a mechanism of social control rather than a pathway to recovery (New York Lawyers for the Public Interest 2005). Research has shown that Black patients are three to four times more likely than White patients to receive a diagnosis of a psychotic disorder, such as schizophrenia (Schwartz and Blankenship 2014). This discrepancy contributes to social stigma, increased psychiatric hospitalizations, increased use of psychotropic medications, relational and employment discrimination, and increased risk of suicide (Schwartz and Blankenship 2014). Furthermore, several research studies have concluded that clinicians overpredict the likelihood of future violence in Black men (Shadravan and Bath 2019). Although Black people make up a smaller percentage of the general population, a Black person in New York has an approximately five times greater chance of being placed in outpatient commitment than a White person (Swanson et al. 2009). Given the history of systemic racism and racial bias affecting treatment in medicine and mental health, it is essential to ensure racial equity in AOT programs.

Black people may be substantially overrepresented in AOT commitment orders, but that may not necessarily represent an unfair application of the policy (Swanson et al. 2009). The Institute of Medicine (IOM) recommends a framework that importantly distinguishes between "differences" and "disparities" in the interpretation of race-specific rates of health resource utilization (Institute of Medicine 2003). They recommend that "disparity" be specifically attributed to differences in health care quality attributable to systemic, legal, and regulatory factors that treat minorities differently or to discrimination, bias, and stereotyping within the health care system; differences attributable to variations in need, clinically appropriate decision-making, or patient preference are differences that should be factored out as important to study and understand, but not to be considered "disparities" (Institute of Medicine 2003; McGuire et al. 2006; Swanson et al. 2009).

The racial variations in AOT commitment orders from New York State show a difference, but not necessarily a disparity (Swanson et al. 2009). This distinction requires careful analysis of variations in need, clinical decision-making, and patient preference. Swanson et al. (2009) studied the association between race and New York State outpatient commitments to assess whether other factors may contribute to the notable differences. They found that the association was not statistically significant when accounting for other factors, including rates of involuntary hospitalization and involvement in the public-sector mental health care system, which itself is associated with poverty (Swanson et al. 2009). It is important to note that racial differences in these upstream determinants of "need" for AOT might themselves be the result of systemic discrimination. Thus, it is possible for AOT to be distributed fairly as a remedy for a problem that is unfairly distributed in the population. "Fairness" in this equation assumes that AOT is beneficial by providing access to effective treatment that is valuable to the individual, outweighing its costs and the adverse consequences of coercion.

Properly implemented AOT serves as an engagement tool and offers additional, state-funded resources to put those with SMI on a path to recovery. Members of racial minority groups often lack proper access to quality mental health care services and may not receive needed care (McGuire and Miranda 2008). When they do receive care, Black individuals it is likely to be in the public mental health system, and they are less likely to receive treatment for an SMI, factors contributing to a clinical presentation appropriate for AOT. AOT offers the potential to address these larger systemic issues and close the gaps in access to mental health care by using the authority of the legal system to ensure that care is provided to those who need it, regardless of race or personal resources. Given the benefits of AOT, the increased number of Black individuals receiving outpatient commitment orders suggests that AOT is being employed successfully to address and improve racial disparities in mental health care. Although AOT in New York State was applied equitably to Black and White individuals when accounting for the county of residence, socioeconomic factors, and degrees of illness (Swanson et al. 2009), racial justice must be a key outcome in future AOT research, policy development, and implementation.

How to Approach an Assisted Outpatient Treatment Case

Each case will have its own considerations, complexities, and nuances; nevertheless, we present the following example to illustrate the ethical issues that arise during outpatient commitment.

Case Example

An inpatient psychiatrist petitions the court in New York for involuntary outpatient commitment for her patient. The patient is a 26-year-old African American man with schizophrenia. He has been hospitalized several times, starting at age 19, for paranoid delusions and disorganized behavior. When symptomatic, he has limited insight into his mental illness. His hospital stays have been long and required court hearings and court-ordered medications. The patient improved when he received haloperidol decanoate during a hospitalization and was discharged. He did not show up for outpatient treatment or receive an injection after discharge. The patient was recently rehospitalized after hitting a police officer he thought was trying to harm him during a welfare check. The patient's mother explained that he has not been able to maintain employment since his illness was diagnosed. He often lives on the street, as he does not trust case managers who try to assist him with housing. His mother has struggled to assist him—she suffers from bipolar disorder, takes care of her two young children, and does not have disposable income.

Many ethical issues arise when considering this representative case. The psychiatrist acts by the principle of beneficence when recommending an intervention that will improve the health of her patient. Sustained outpatient commitment has been associated with shorter lengths of stay, less violence, and less criminal victimization (Swartz et al. 2001), which represent obvious benefits to this patient. Aside from the psychiatrist's duty to her patient, less violence and shorter lengths of stay (which make more resources available to others) provide a benefit to society.

Nonmaleficence must also be considered. The potential harms of forcing the patient into outpatient treatment include stigma and resentment toward the judicial system (which makes the order) and the mental health system (which requested it). The potential harm of lack of treatment or follow-up seems greater than any conceivable harm associated with a well-funded, comprehensive treatment program. The situation becomes more complicated if the AOT order is not supported with well-funded treatment services, including stable living opportunities. Additionally, the program needs oversight and design to ensure the patient's participation. If the program does not have the resources it needs to ensure the patient participates in the recommended mental health treatment plan, it may not be worth the infringements on autonomy.

In this case, the limitations on the patient's autonomy, and his right to refuse treatment services, likely serve as the most contentious aspect of the AOT order. A common argument holds that the patient refuses treatment because they are psychotic and paranoid, and that once they receive treatment, they will become rational and thankful that treatment was compelled. Empirical studies examining this thank-you theory of civil commitment have been mixed (Player 2015), but, as discussed earlier, although the patient may not be thankful for their care, they may prefer outpatient commitment to inpatient commitment. Indeed, in this scenario, the petitioning psychiatrist is using AOT as a tool to safely transition the patient from inpatient hospitalization to a less-restrictive outpatient environment. Without AOT and the promise of sustained care, the patient may not otherwise have a plan to ensure safe discharge and may remain in the hospital. Although AOT is still an infringement on his rights, it is less of an infringement than the alternative, which would be prolonged hospitalization. This argument can be extended when considering that the patient, although still in opposition to outpatient commitment, may prefer prolonged AOT to future inpatient hospitalizations.

A key issue to address is the protection of civil rights of those being committed. With no oversight, AOT could be abused or overapplied. In New York, to sign commitment orders based on the psychiatrist's petition, a court must find that AOT is the least restrictive alternative available for the person and must notify the patient, his nearest relative, and Mental Hygiene Legal Services (MHLS). The court must have a hearing no more than 3 days after receipt of the petition. The court requires that a written treatment plan benefits the specific patient, who must meet all of AOT's requirements, by clear and convincing evidence (New York M.H.Y. 9.60 2021). The patient has a right to appeal the ruling. The rigorous process is designed to protect the patient from capricious applications of AOT orders.

The patient also has the right to legal counsel through MHLS; however, the role of counsel remains controversial. Some believe that although counsel is necessary to guide the patient through the court process, they should work with the client to achieve the best outcome for that individual, even if it might result in undesired treatment. Conversely, some believe counsel should represent the stated interest of the client and fight outpatient commitment to the extent possible (if this is the goal of the patient). In one study, how legal counsel approached outpatient commitment varied greatly by jurisdiction (Swanson 2010). Whether regional differences in legal defense's approach to AOT result from economic pressures, social beliefs, or other factors remains unclear. However, policymakers should continue to consider the importance of due process in outpatient commitment laws.

Justice considerations are present in the case example. The patient is Black and thus more likely to be a recipient of outpatient commitment orders than a White patient, as discussed earlier. Scrutiny is required to ensure that he is not being unfairly diagnosed and that risk assessments are not overpredicting violence. In this example, the patient has a clear history of severe illness. He has perpetrated violent actions with a direct nexus to his disease. His mother acknowledges the difficulty in engaging him with care and his relative lack of access and support. In this case, using AOT as a mental health engagement tool offers a way to overcome socioeconomic bias and structural racism by providing necessary resources to a traditionally underserved person.

Some may argue that in a system with limited resources, providing services to people who actively refuse them is unfair to those voluntarily seeking care (Swanson et al. 2010). Whereas an AOT patient will receive comprehensive treatment, someone voluntarily seeking intensive services may be added to a growing waitlist. The voluntary patient, with no history of violence or recent hospitalizations attributable to treatment nonadherence, thus fails to qualify for AOT but could potentially decompensate and need to be hospitalized; the AOT patient who does not want treatment services receives them in the community and is able to avoid hospitalization. Ideally, reason and research suggest that, over time, successfully implemented AOT may increase the available resources to all mental health consumers. Even if aggressive AOT policies increased the wait times for voluntary Assertive Community Treatment teams for several years, in the long run, the highest utilizers would use fewer intensive resources.

For example, the dangerous patient in our example spends prolonged periods in the hospital. In the future, he may require state forensic hospital services. If his AOT treatment plan is successful, however, he will be hospitalized less often. By moving his care to the community, more inpatient beds will be available for longer periods of time for the acutely mentally ill who are not dangerous and are voluntarily seeking care. Rather than be turned away for "not meeting criteria" or being discharged prematurely for systems issues, those people will obtain the care they need and presumably use fewer resources in the future as well, resulting in more access for everyone.

Conclusion

Most mental health stakeholders agree that it is unacceptable to have more than 4 million severely mentally ill adults go without treatment each year, and that jails have become the largest treatment centers for people with SMI. AOT provides a legal tool with an individualized clinical purpose: to remediate a person's impaired decision-making as a pathway to treatment and better managed illness. Critics may see AOT as a hindrance to a patient's chance for self-determined recovery free from coercion and an obstacle to creating systemic reform in society. Some may find middle ground, believing AOT to be a reasonable solution to the greater problems of accessing mental health services.

We believe that AOT can be a useful tool when thoughtfully and ethically implemented. This case example is not meant to be an exhaustive discussion of all ethical issues that arise during the outpatient commitment process; rather, our goal is to show that even in a fairly simple AOT petition, numerous questions arise related to the traditional bioethics principles of autonomy, beneficence, nonmaleficence, and distributive justice. We hope to make the reader aware of what information should be considered and how to approach the difficult questions related to outpatient commitment.

Much about outpatient commitment remains unsettled and controversial. Increased longitudinal data may greatly strengthen the argument for AOT. Research is limited, with only short-term outcome data available. By observing outcomes in people with or without AOT orders for 10 years or more, researchers and policymakers will be able to determine whether AOT is an appropriate intervention. This research could determine whether mental health improves, in both individuals and the larger population, by using AOT to help break the pattern of revolving-door hospitalizations and incarcerations. It could show that long-term overall health costs decrease, allowing for more services to be provided to all. Current data and research focusing on 1- or 2-year outcomes limit the ability to draw conclusions on potential long-term benefits and leave debate about AOT lacking.

References

Appelbaum PS: Ambivalence codified: California's new outpatient commitment statute. Psychiatr Serv 54(1):26–28, 2003 12509662

Appelbaum PS: Assessing Kendra's Law: five years of outpatient commitment in New York. Psychiatr Serv 56(7):791–792, 2005 16024507

Beauchamp TL, Childress JF: Principles of Biomedical Ethics, 7th Edition. New York, Oxford University Press, 2013

Burns T, Rugkåsa J, Molodynski A, et al: Community treatment orders for patients with psychosis (OCTET): a randomised controlled trial. Lancet 381(9878):1627–1633, 2013 23537605

Fitch WL, Swanson JW: Civil Commitment and the Mental Health Care Continuum: Historical Trends and Principles for Law and Practice. Rockville, MD, Substance Abuse and Mental Health Services Administration, 2019. Available at: https://www.samhsa.gov/sites/default/files/civil-commitment-continuum-of-care.pdf. Accessed July 12, 2024.

Grisso T, Appelbaum PS, Mulvey EP, et al: The MacArthur Treatment Competence Study. II: Measures of abilities related to competence to consent to treatment. Law Hum Behav 19(2):127–148, 1995 11660291

Hargrave v Vermont, 340 F.3d 27 (2d Cir. 2003)

Institute of Medicine: Unequal Treatment: Confronting Racial and Ethnic Disparities in Health Care. Committee on Understanding and Eliminating Racial and Ethnic Disparities in Health Care. Edited by Smedley BD, Stith AY, Nelson AR. Washington, DC, National Academies Press, 2003

Link BG, Epperson MW, Perron BE, et al: Arrest outcomes associated with outpatient commitment in New York State. Psychiatr Serv 62(5):504–508, 2011 21532076

McGuire TG, Miranda J: New evidence regarding racial and ethnic disparities in mental health: policy implications. Health Aff (Millwood) 27(2):393–403, 2008 18332495

McGuire TG, Alegria M, Cook BL, et al: Implementing the Institute of Medicine definition of disparities: an application to mental health care. Health Serv Res 41(5):1979–2005, 2006 16987312

Meldrum ML, Kelly EL, Calderon R, et al: Implementation status of assisted outpatient treatment programs: a national survey. Psychiatr Serv 67(6):630–635, 2016 26828396

New York Consolidated Laws, Mental Hygiene Law, MHY § 9.60 Assisted Outpatient Treatment (2021)

New York Lawyers for the Public Interest (NYPLI): Implementation of "Kendra's Law" is severely biased. NYPLI, 2005. Available at https://www.nylpi.org/wp-content/uploads/2021/10/DLC-Report-on-Kendras-Law.pdf. Accessed October 9, 2024.

Player CT: Involuntary outpatient commitment: the limits of prevention. Stanford Law Pol Rev 26(159):159–238, 2015

Robbins PC, Keator KJ, Steadman HJ, et al: Assisted outpatient treatment in New York: regional differences in New York's assisted outpatient treatment program. Psychiatr Serv 61(10):970–975, 2010 20889633

Schwartz RC, Blankenship DM: Racial disparities in psychotic disorder diagnosis: a review of empirical literature. World J Psychiatry 4(4):133–140, 2014 25540728

Shadravan SM, Bath E: Invoking history and structural competency to minimize racial bias. J Am Acad Psychiatry Law 47(1):2–6, 2019 30852558

Stone AA: Mental Health and Law: A System in Transition. Rockville, MD, National Institute of Mental Health, Center for Studies of Crime and Delinquency, 1975

Svarsad BL, Shireman TI, Sweeney JK: Using drug claims data to assess the relationship of medication adherence with hospitalization and costs. Psychiatr Serv 52(6):805–811, 2001

Swanson J: What would Mary Douglas do? A commentary on Kahan et al., "Cultural cognition and public policy: the case of outpatient commitment laws." Law Hum Behav 34(3):176–185, 2010 19462224

Swanson JW, Swartz MS: Why the evidence for outpatient commitment is good enough. Psychiatr Serv 65(6):808–811, 2014 24881685

Swanson J, Swartz MS, Elbogen E, et al: Effects of involuntary outpatient commitment on subjective quality of life in persons with severe mental illness. Behav Sci Law 21(4):473–491, 2003

Swanson J, Swartz M, Van Dorn RA, et al: Racial disparities in involuntary outpatient commitment: are they real? Health Aff (Millwood) 28(3):816–826, 2009 19414892

Swanson JW, Van Dorn RA, Swartz MS, et al: Robbing Peter to pay Paul: did New York State's outpatient commitment program crowd out voluntary service recipients? Psychiatr Serv 61(10):988–995, 2010 20889636

Swanson JW, Van Dorn RA, Swartz MS, et al: The cost of assisted outpatient treatment: can it save states money? Am J Psychiatry 170(12):1423–1432, 2013 23896998

Swartz MS, Swanson JW, Hiday VA, et al: A randomized controlled trial of outpatient commitment in North Carolina. Psychiatr Serv 52(3):325–329, 2001 11239099

Swartz MS, Wagner HR, Swanson JW, et al: The perceived coerciveness of involuntary outpatient commitment: findings from an experimental study. J Am Acad Psychiatry Law 30(2):207–217, 2002 12108557

Swartz MS, Swanson JW, Monahan J: Endorsement of personal benefit of outpatient commitment among persons with severe mental illness. Psychol Public Policy Law 9(1–2):70–93, 2003a 16700137

Swartz MS, Swanson JW, Wagner HR, et al: Assessment of four stakeholder groups' preferences concerning outpatient commitment for persons with schizophrenia. Am J Psychiatry 160(6):1139–1146, 2003b 12777273

Swartz MS, Wagner HR, Swanson JW, et al: Consumers' perceptions of the
      fairness and effectiveness of mandated community treatment and related
      pressures. Psychiatr Serv 55(7):780–785, 2004 15232017
Swartz MS, Swanson JW, Steadman HJ, et al: New York State Assisted
      Outpatient Treatment Program Evaluation. June 30, 2009. Available at:
      https://static.prisonpolicy.org/scans/NYDPH-report.pdf. Accessed July
      13, 2024.

14

Ethical Issues in Forensic Psychiatry

Mental Health Firearm Prohibitions

Joseph R. Simpson, M.D., Ph.D.

Legal Regulation of Firearm Ownership on the Basis of Mental Health Factors

In the United States, the Second Amendment to the Constitution guarantees the right to "keep and bear arms" (U.S. Const. amend. II). Whether that right applies only to members of a state militia or to all citizens as individuals is a topic of great controversy. In 2008, the U.S. Supreme Court addressed the question (*District of Columbia et al. v. Heller* 2008). In a 5–4 decision, the Court ruled that the Second Amendment protects the *individual* right to possess firearms, unconnected to service in a militia. In 2010, the Supreme Court ruled that their decision in *Heller,* which covered only federal jurisdictions such as Washington, D.C., also applies to the states. Again in a 5–4 decision, the Court held that the Second Amendment is incorporated via the Fourteenth Amendment, meaning that the states must also follow the ruling in *Heller* (*McDonald v. City of Chicago* 2010).

In the *Heller* decision, it was noted in dicta that "nothing in our opinion should be taken to cast doubt on long-standing prohibitions on the possession of firearms by felons and the mentally ill" (*District of Columbia et al. v. Heller* 2008, p. 626). Since 1968, the federal government has barred individuals from owning firearms if they have been subject to certain types of legal proceedings as a result of a mental health condition.

Federal law specifies that people who have been "adjudicated as a mental defective" or "committed to a mental institution" are prohibited from possessing firearms (18 U.S.C. § 922 [g] [4] 2018). These two terms are explicated in the Code of Federal Regulations. "Adjudicated as a mental defective" is defined as

> a determination by a court, board, commission, or other lawful authority that a person, as a result of marked subnormal intelligence, or mental illness, incompetency, condition, or disease: (1) Is a danger to himself or to others; or (2) Lacks the mental capacity to contract or manage his own affairs. (27 C.F.R. § 478.11 2020)

(As the definition makes clear, the archaic term "defective" does not specifically refer to intellectual or cognitive capacity. Although there have been calls to update the language, the word remains in the current federal statute.)

"Committed to a mental institution" is defined as

> a formal commitment of a person to a mental institution by a court, board, commission, or other lawful authority. The term includes a commitment to a mental institution involuntarily. … [It] does not include a person in a mental institution for observation or a voluntary admission to a mental institution. (27 C.F.R. § 478.11 2020)

The exclusion of observation periods and voluntary inpatient treatment in the definition of "committed to a mental institution" is critical for the firearm rights of U.S. citizens. Congress decided in 1968 that having been involuntarily committed and receiving some type of due process review of that commitment—which is not present in an emergency detention for observation—constitutes a "bright line" for the purpose of determining who should be able to own a firearm. In other words, as far as federal law is concerned, there is no limit to the number of short-term emergency psychiatric detentions, or voluntary inpatient admissions, that a person can have; they will still be legally able to purchase and possess guns. But if either type of inpatient hospitalization evolves into an involuntary commitment, upheld by the review process provided for in that jurisdiction (such as in a probable-cause hearing, for example), the person loses the right to own guns.

This schema has not been modified in the past half-century, despite the paucity of evidence to suggest that the distinction between voluntary treatment and involuntary commitment is particularly useful to reduce firearm-related suicide or homicide or to protect the firearm rights of people who are not dangerous to themselves or others. At the time of writing, only one study (Swanson et al. 2020) appears to have directly examined this question, so further data are certainly needed.

In addition to the federal law, many states have their own prohibitions. Some remove firearm rights for varying periods of time in response to events or conditions not included in the federal law. For example, a state may prohibit firearm possession after voluntary psychiatric inpatient treatment of a specified duration, after an involuntary emergency detention, or even simply for having a mental health diagnosis (Norris et al. 2006; Simpson 2007). At the time of writing, there is no mechanism for one state to notify another about people it has prohibited from owning guns. This author is also not aware of any published legal case involving a person barred in one state, but who is not federally barred, being prohibited from possessing or purchasing a gun after changing their residency to another state.

The actions (and decisions not to act) of psychiatrists and other mental health professionals in the course of their work can have implications for their patients' firearm rights at several points. In some situations, the potential ramifications of a clinical decision on firearm rights raises ethical concerns for the practitioner. In addition, in some jurisdictions, practitioners are authorized or even required to report to a government agency patients thought to pose a danger, specifically for the purpose of preventing firearm ownership. This reporting is independent of other actions such as hospitalization or warning an identified victim (what is often referred to as a "Tarasoff warning," after *Tarasoff v. Regents of the University of California* [1976], the landmark California case which established a duty to protect when a patient makes a threat against an identifiable victim) (see Chapter 12, "The Tarasoff Duty to Protect").

The next two sections discuss the ethical questions that may confront clinicians in treatment situations and in jurisdictions that provide for reporting for the purpose of removal of firearms. The third section explores ethical questions that may arise in the context of proceedings to restore firearm rights, often referred to as an application for *relief from disabilities* (RFD). The final section provides resources that can help ethical practitioners improve their knowledge and understanding of the myriad and confusing issues at the points of interface between the mental health profession and legal schemes regulating firearm ownership. It must be pointed out that the legal landscape is evolving, and although ethical principles do not change (or change very slowly), all discussion of statutes, regulations, or case law herein should not be considered definitive.

Ethical Issues in Mental Health Firearm Prohibitions

Clinical Evaluations for Involuntary Detention

Psychiatry is a rarity among the medical specialties, in that therapeutic interventions such as hospitalization can, under the appropriate circumstances, be imposed on patients against their will and over their objection (Simpson and Carannante 2017). In many situations, the necessity of emergency detention for a period of observation is clear to those with training (if not always to the layperson) when the patient is adamant that they will not agree to voluntary hospitalization or lacks the capacity to consent due to their present mental condition. The same clarity also typically applies to the decision to initiate formal commitment proceedings later in the treatment course. For psychiatrists who work in some settings or otherwise evaluate patients in crisis, however (such as a psychiatric emergency service [PES], a mobile response unit, or a medical emergency department [ED]), the initial decision regarding whether to place someone on an emergency involuntary hold is not always so clear-cut.

A substantial body of literature has shown that many patients are pressured, induced, or even coerced into agreeing to be admitted to a psychiatric hospital voluntarily (Gilboy and Schmidt 1971; Lewis et al. 1984; Lidz et al. 1995; Monahan et al. 1995; Reed and Lewis 1990). There are several reasons for this, mostly involving a desire on the part of hospital staff to avoid paperwork, formal proceedings, testimony, and the like. In some cases, a desire—perhaps paternalistic—to help the patient avoid loss of gun rights because of an involuntary admission may be a factor. In a recent survey of more than 500 American psychiatrists and psychiatry trainees, some practitioners reported that they had used the threat of loss of gun rights as a negotiation technique to convince patients to sign in voluntarily (Newlon et al. 2020). Pressuring patients in this way quite obviously raises numerous ethical concerns; for the purposes of this chapter, we are concerned with the risk of potentially preserving firearm rights for a patient who is actually dangerous to self or others.

Although this author is not aware of any literature exploring the opposite situation (a patient being placed on involuntary status despite being potentially willing to agree to voluntary admission and possessing the capacity to do so, whether for the convenience of hospital staff, concern that the patient may change their mind and be more difficult to involuntarily detain after being allowed to enter voluntarily, or other reasons), my clinical experience, as well as common sense, suggests that this approach also can and does occur. Here another ethical concern arises: patients may lose gun rights unnecessarily if they were in reality willing to come into the hospital voluntarily but were nevertheless placed on an emergency hold. Note that this is primarily of concern only in those jurisdictions that take a more expansive approach to mental health firearm laws (prohibiting gun ownership for patients who have been detained on an emergency basis or for observation). In states where there is no prohibition unless federal criteria are met through a formal commitment, the likelihood that a patient will be committed unnecessarily and lose firearm rights without justification is presumably much lower. And of course, in the small minority of states that prohibit firearms for people who have been *voluntarily* hospitalized, the question shifts to whether to admit at all or to send the patient home. This is a choice between two very different courses of action (compared with the lesser difference between a voluntary or involuntary admission) and thus presumably less often one that is equivocal.

The forfeiture of firearm rights is one of the few long-lasting legal consequences of a psychiatric hospitalization. Other legal proceedings in which psychiatrists are involved have a more profound impact on a patient's rights, specifically the appointment of a guardian or conservator. People who are so affected by a mental condition that a substitute decision-maker is appointed, in addition to losing the power to make decisions about their mental health treatment and often where they will live, generally lose some or all of the other rights and privileges shared by the vast majority of American adults: the right to vote, to enter into contracts and marriages, to possess a driver's license, and, perhaps most consistently, to manage money. Of course, firearm rights are also lost in this circumstance, by the operation of the federal law discussed earlier, if the prohibition is not made explicit in the applicable state law. The lesser imposition on freedom of a short-term involuntary hospitalization or commitment generally has no impact on any of the rights just listed—with the exception of firearm rights. Although involuntary hospitalization can certainly have profound indirect effects on a person (for example, leading to loss of employment), as a legal matter, once they are released, their ability to engage in typical activities is not affected. Firearm ownership is the one exception.

Unfortunately, most psychiatrists are unaware of this fact, as demonstrated in two recent surveys (Nagle et al. 2021; Newlon et al. 2020). As it turns out, many psychiatrists are poorly equipped to consider the firearm-related ethical issues that arise when evaluating a patient who may pose a danger to themselves or others, whether encountered in an ED, office, or other circumstance. The psychiatrist has three possible choices: 1) leave the patient alone or release them from the encounter; 2) arrange for voluntary inpatient care, if appropriate; or 3) place the patient on a hold and admit them to an inpatient setting against their will (for the purposes of the subsequent analysis, only temporary holds, and not longer-term formal commitments, are considered here).

Not only is the temporary or emergency detention approximately five times more common in the United States than formal commitment (Swanson et al. 2020), but it can fairly be assumed that the decision to seek a hearing to extend a patient's involuntary treatment from short term to longer term is significantly less subject to ambiguity as a clinical matter. It is also a larger imposition on the rights of the patient; thus, one would hope, the decision to proceed is considered carefully by the hospital treatment team. The review process itself is an additional safeguard against unnecessary commitments (although not against premature discharges).

Careful decision-making does not necessarily obtain with short-term emergency holds of the 3- to 5-day variety and is not subject to independent review. When a patient presents to an ED in the middle of the night, intoxicated and dysphoric, having at some point said (or reportedly said) something about suicide, a busy on-call psychiatrist may find it easier to simply "write a hold" and move on to the next case, rather than spend time assessing the entire clinical picture or providing sufficient information to the patient that they decide to sign in to the hospital voluntarily.

So, what is the ethical issue that arises with the psychiatrist's decision, which is of a type made tens of thousands of times a year throughout this country? It is that it could have a hidden impact on the person in terms of future firearm rights, at least in the nearly half of states where an emergency detention leads to loss of those rights for some time (The Policy Surveillance Program 2016). Failure to consider this—perhaps believing that an emergency detention is really no big deal in the larger scheme of things—and using an emergency hold when another option is reasonable constitutes an ethical lapse, as it violates the principles of both nonmaleficence and autonomy.

A second ethical concern is the potential for a clinician's attitude toward firearms to influence the decision of whether to place a patient on an emergency hold. Theoretically, a psychiatrist who is fully aware of the consequences of a temporary hold for gun rights could be biased for or against detaining patients in close cases. If a psychiatrist believes that it is best to try to preserve gun rights when possible, they could develop a tendency toward initiating fewer holds, which could lead to a different form of maleficence than arbitrarily removing gun rights unnecessarily: harming the patient, who goes on to use their unconfiscated or newly purchased weapon for suicide or to harm others. Several empirical studies have demonstrated that access to firearms is correlated with increased risk of suicide (Anglemyer et al. 2014; Reisch et al. 2013; Swanson et al. 2015). Conversely, a psychiatrist who thinks that there are too many firearms in circulation, or just doesn't like guns, could use holds more frequently, harming some patients who are actually safe and could have been treated with a voluntary admission (for example) but who now lose gun rights, because of a bias (even if unconscious) against firearm ownership.

Another important question is whether to discuss the potential loss of firearm rights with the patient at the outset of the emergency evaluation. Not disclosing it could be considered a violation of autonomy, as the evaluator is withholding information that the patient may want as they decide whether to agree to a voluntary admission. Conversely, advising the patient of the link between an involuntary hold and loss of firearm rights could make the patient less candid in their answers to the evaluator's questions, thus reducing the quality of the assessment and increasing the risk of harm to the patient and others, should the wrong decision be made as a result of insufficient information.

In conclusion, where mental health firearm laws are concerned, ethical psychiatric practice includes: 1) understanding the relevant laws in one's jurisdiction and 2) recognizing any biases for or against individual firearm ownership (in general or for those who seek or receive mental health treatment) and striving to prevent any such biases from affecting clinical decisions regarding involuntary treatment. This is especially true when the psychiatrist is evaluating a patient for a possible temporary emergency detention; in such cases, the clinical picture is more likely to be ambiguous and to allow for more than one possible safe option for management.

Reporting Potentially Dangerous Patients for the Purpose of Firearm Removal

In August 2018, California governor Jerry Brown vetoed Assembly Bill (AB) 2888. The bill would have modified the state's Gun Violence Restraining Order (GVRO) law. At the time, California was one of a small number of states that had implemented a new approach designed to mitigate the risk of firearm violence (including suicide). GVRO laws are known as *extreme risk protection orders* in some jurisdictions, and sometimes colloquially referred to in the media and by advocacy groups as *red flag laws*.

At one point during the drafting of AB 2888 in the California legislature, it would have allowed "a mental health worker who has seen the person as a patient in the prior six months" to "file a petition requesting that the court issue an *ex parte* gun violence restraining order enjoining the subject of the petition from having in his or her custody or control, owning, purchasing, possessing, or receiving a firearm or ammunition" (AB 2888 2018). This provision was removed from the bill that was ultimately submitted to the governor. The final bill did include the addition of "an employer, a coworker, [or] an employee of a secondary or postsecondary school that the person has attended in the last six months" to the categories of people who could petition for a GVRO.

California's GVRO law, one of the first in the United States, was originally passed in 2014 and went into effect January 1, 2016. In its original form, it provided for immediate family members and law enforcement officers to file a GVRO petition. (A similar bill to add other categories, including mental health workers, had already been vetoed by Governor Brown in 2016 [AB 2607 2016]). In 2019, the legislature made a third attempt to broaden the categories. Governor Gavin Newsom signed AB 61 into law, which added employers, coworkers, and school employees, but not mental health workers (Cal. Penal Code § 18150 2019).

Most GVRO laws provide for the temporary removal of firearms after a hearing, for a period of weeks, which can be followed by a petition to remove the firearms for a longer period such as 1 year. The orders can be renewed if the subject remains dangerous. These laws have grown in popularity since 2014: at the time of writing, 19 states and the District of Columbia have some type of GVRO law (Giffords Law Center 2021). Only three jurisdictions currently allow mental health professionals to request the order: the District of Columbia, Hawaii, and Maryland (D.C. Code Ann. § 7–2510.01 et seq. 2021; Haw. Rev. Stat. Ann. § 134–61 et seq. 2019; Md. Code Ann., Pub. Safety § 5–601 et seq. 2018).

Some states also have other types of laws that provide for mental health professionals to report patients to state authorities when they are considered to be dangerous to themselves or others, specifically for the purpose of confiscating the individual's firearms and prohibiting them from obtaining more. These include New York's Secure Ammunition and Firearms Enforcement Act (SAFE Act), passed in 2013 (N.Y. Mental Hygiene Law § 9.46 2013), and an Illinois law requiring the reporting of individuals determined to pose a "clear and present danger" to self or others (405 Ill. Comp. Stat. 5/6–103.3 2015). In California, mental health professionals are required to report to law enforcement all patients who make a threat that triggers a so-called Tarasoff duty. This requirement was added to California law explicitly for the purpose of law enforcement reporting the patient to the state government, to terminate the patient's firearm rights for a 5-year period (Cal. Welfare and Institutions Code § 8105(c) 2014; Weinstock et al. 2015).

The ethical issues for psychiatrists in jurisdictions with a GVRO law that applies to mental health professionals, or a law allowing or requiring reporting of dangerous patients to the state for purposes of firearm restrictions, are similar to those discussed in the preceding section, with one additional complexity: instead of reporting an *action*, such as hospitalization, the psychiatrist here is reporting a *status* or *condition*, i.e., the status of being dangerous. If that condition rises to the level of necessitating involuntary hospitalization, the burden of reporting may be automatic; this is true throughout the United States for formal involuntary commitments and varies by jurisdiction for emergency detentions, as discussed in the previous section. But what about patients whose alleged dangerousness is not deemed sufficiently severe or imminent to require involuntary treatment? When do such patients merit a GVRO or other state report? If the psychiatrist is seeking a GVRO or reporting the patient, what is the reason that the patient is not eligible for involuntary hospitalization? We will leave aside the rare scenario in which a patient is making threats of harm toward self or others via phone, email, etc., but refuses to present to the treating psychiatrist's office or to an emergency department, and their whereabouts are unknown, so law enforcement cannot be sent to detain them. Generally, this would be a clear case where reporting would be indicated, if available in that jurisdiction, in the hopes of (at least) preventing a new gun purchase, potentially to be used for suicide or other violence.

Assuming that the patient is available for a face-to-face evaluation, any biases a psychiatrist has regarding firearms may find their way into the decision of whether to report. It is not difficult to imagine a psychiatrist with strong antigun views making reports or petitions whenever they encounter a patient who is prone to psychosis, has difficulty controlling anger, or has a substance abuse issue and the doctor knows or believes that the patient has access to firearms. If such a decision is not sufficiently particularized for the individual patient's clinical circumstances, it would violate the ethical principles of autonomy and nonmaleficence. Conversely, a psychiatrist who strongly favors gun rights could experience a distortion in clinical judgment and avoid reporting a patient who would be better served by having their access to firearms removed, at least temporarily.

As noted in the previous section, the best approach to ethical practice is to become aware of one's biases and strive to prevent them from influencing one's decisions regarding the reporting of potentially dangerous patients. Here as well, to practice ethically, it is essential that psychiatrists be aware of any reporting laws in their state.

Evaluations for Relief From Disabilities

Federal law provides for those who are prohibited from owning firearms to petition for restoration of firearm rights. This is commonly referred to as *relief from disabilities* or RFD. However, the federal statute does not provide for an RFD petition to be made directly to the federal government (e.g., to the FBI or Bureau of Alcohol, Tobacco, Firearms and Explosives [ATF]). Instead, federal law requires that prohibited individuals must use a state RFD process, if available. States can choose to (but are not required to) develop an RFD process. If they choose to, the program must be approved by ATF for its use to lead to the restoration of *federal* firearm rights. Many but not all states that have their own prohibitors also have RFD procedures in place for those bans. Patients must apply for relief from a federal prohibition in the state where the prohibiting commitment or adjudication occurred; they cannot simply move to another state and apply there. This is a complex area of law that can only be touched on in this chapter. The interested reader is referred to reviews of state laws (Norris et al. 2006; Simpson 2007) and of the RFD process generally (Gold and Vanderpool 2018a, 2018b).

State RFD processes vary widely by jurisdiction. Some state statutes require that an evaluation be performed; a subset specify that the evaluation include a risk assessment. The type of professional who may perform the evaluation is specified in some states but not others (Gold and Vanderpool 2018b). Depending on state law and local practice, requests may be made by law enforcement or other entities to treating primary care physicians or psychotherapists to provide a letter certifying that an applicant for RFD is safe (Pirelli et al. 2019). Of course, such requests are also made of forensic mental health practitioners, especially if the person seeking RFD has retained an attorney with experience in this area of the law.

Ethical considerations are especially salient in the RFD situation, since the person seeking it has already been prohibited from owning firearms by operation of state or federal law. This means that there is a presumption (which may be quite weak, depending on the length of time since the prohibition began) of high (or heightened) risk, and the burden of proof is on the petitioner rather than on the state. Yet the petitioner is unlikely to see it that way, and, especially if the prohibition stems from a long-ago event, they may be mystified that anyone would even think that there is any danger. For a treating provider, providing a negative report (or declining to give an opinion) could have a significant impact on the therapeutic relationship, even leading to termination of that relationship.

For the treating psychotherapist, the ethical principles of beneficence and autonomy (i.e., helping the patient obtain something they want, RFD) must be weighed against the principle of nonmaleficence— not providing assistance in obtaining RFD if they believe it is not in the patient's interests (i.e., when they consider the patient at risk of self-harm or violence).

In an independent forensic evaluation, of course, there is no therapeutic relationship. The forensic practitioner is obligated to recognize when they lack sufficient expertise to perform the requested evaluation and should decline it. This is a basic yet critical ethical principle that is codified in the ethics recommendations of the American Academy of Psychiatry and the Law (2005): "Expertise in the practice of forensic psychiatry should be claimed only in areas of actual knowledge, skills, training, and experience." In other words, an ethical expert will not take on an appointment if their knowledge is not sufficient to complete the job.

Certainly, if a treating clinician is not well versed in the process of performing a thorough RFD evaluation, the best course of action would be to decline to give an opinion and to suggest that the patient obtain an independent evaluation by a forensic evaluator with experience, if available. Even if the treating clinician does have a good understanding of the process, as mentioned above, the potential impact on the therapeutic alliance may preclude true objectivity, with referral to an independent evaluator often being the wisest option (if state law does not require that the RFD opinion be from a treating provider).

As discussed in the preceding two sections, it bears repeating that for RFD evaluations, any pro- or antigun biases need to be identified and disregarded if possible; no evaluation should be performed if the treating clinician or forensic expert realizes that they cannot set aside those biases to reach the most objective conclusion possible.

Resources for Improving Ethical Practice Relating to Mental Health Firearm Prohibitions

This chapter should make clear that fundamentally, the ethical issues raised by mental health firearm laws fall into two main categories. The first is the matter of having sufficient knowledge and understanding of both the law and the evidence base in this area to ethically render an opinion; the second is understanding one's own biases regarding the subject and striving to ensure that they do not influence one's professional decisions, whether that is a clinical decision that affects firearm rights (such as initiating emergency detention) or a decision about whether to provide an opinion in an RFD proceeding, and what that opinion will be.

Unfortunately, two surveys of psychiatrists have demonstrated that the state of knowledge of mental health firearms laws in our field is poor (Nagle et al. 2021; Newlon et al. 2020). This is a situation that needs to be addressed, ideally through required education in all forensic fellowships and psychiatric residency programs (Simpson 2021a, 2021b, 2021c, 2023). In the meantime, resources exist that allow for self-study for the interested practitioner. Three recent books, *Gun Violence and Mental Illness* (Gold and Simon 2016), *The Behavioral Science of Firearms* (Pirelli et al. 2019), and *Firearms and Clinical Practice* (Pirelli and DeMarco 2023), together can be expected to provide a solid framework for understanding the issues and include numerous references for further reading.

The second question, that of identifying and setting aside biases, may prove to be a more difficult challenge, at least for some. Increasing one's knowledge is greatly beneficial for reducing bias. It can reasonably be hoped that a good understanding of the ramifications of various types of involuntary treatment on firearm rights and an awareness of one's personal slant regarding firearms should be sufficient to resolve most ethical questions in treatment decisions, such as whether to hospitalize someone and whether this needs to be involuntary. For example, it would seem safe to assume that once educated, few practitioners would consciously choose to behave unethically by gratuitously placing on temporary hold a patient who doesn't require it solely to reduce the number of people with access to firearms in society or, conversely, by releasing patients who are dangerous from the PES or ED simply in the belief that the firearm restrictions that would follow are not appropriate or necessary.

For RFD proceedings, however, increased knowledge and a recognition of one's biases may not always completely solve the problem. Away from a crisis situation, it is possible that some may feel that it is best to "let sleeping dogs lie" and not do anything to further an RFD petition, regardless of the current clinical picture, because of a general aversion to the private ownership of firearms. By the same token, some with strong pro-gun beliefs might find it impossible to acknowledge ongoing, but perhaps subtle, risks a patient presents. For practitioners who meet either of these descriptions, the only ethical course would be to decline to perform any RFD-type evaluations.

Conclusion

In the United States, legal regulation of ownership of firearms is a very active, and frequently changing, area of law. This is especially true at the state level. Mental health professionals have an ethical obligation to understand laws restricting firearm ownership rights on the basis of mental health considerations. They should be aware of the ethical issues that arise when performing an evaluation for involuntary hospitalization; reporting potentially dangerous patients for the purpose of firearm removal; and determining whether and how to conduct an evaluation for relief from disability. Fortunately, a growing body of literature is available to help the practitioner understand this complex area at the interface between law and mental health.

References

18 U.S.C. § 922 (g) (4) (2018)

27 C.F.R. § 478.11 (2020)

405 Ill. Comp. Stat. 5/6–103.3 (2015)

AB 2607 (California). Firearm restraining orders. July 1, 2016. Available at: https://leginfo.legislature.ca.gov/faces/billNavClient.xhtml?bill_id =201520160AB2607. Accessed March 28, 2021.

AB 2888 (California). Firearm restraining orders. Veto. March 22, 2018. Available at: https://trackbill.com/bill/california-assembly bill-2888-gun-violence-restraining-orders/1560022/. Accessed March 28th, 2021.

American Academy of Psychiatry and the Law: Ethics Guidelines for the Practice of Forensic Psychiatry. Adopted May 2005. Bloomfield, CT, American Academy of Psychiatry and the Law, 2005. Available at: https://www.aapl.org/ethics-guidelines. Accessed March 1, 2021.

Anglemyer A, Horvath T, Rutherford G: The accessibility of firearms and risk for suicide and homicide victimization among household members: a systematic review and meta-analysis. Ann Intern Med 160(2):101–110, 2014 24592495

Cal. Penal Code § 18150 (2019)

Cal. Welfare and Institutions Code § 8105(c) (2014)

D.C. Code Ann. § 7–2510.01 et seq. (2021)

District of Columbia et al. v Heller, 554 U.S. 570 (2008)

Giffords Law Center: Extreme Risk Protection Orders. Available at: https://giffords.org/lawcenter/gun-laws/browse-state-gun-laws/?filter0=,307. Accessed March 28, 2021.

Gilboy JA, Schmidt JR: "Voluntary" hospitalization of the mentally ill. Northwest Univ Law Rev 66(4):429–453, 1971

Gold LH, Simon RI (eds): Gun Violence and Mental Illness. Arlington, VA, American Psychiatric Association Publishing, 2016

Gold LH, Vanderpool D: Legal regulation of restoration of firearms rights after mental health prohibition. J Am Acad Psychiatry Law 46(3):298–308, 2018a 30368462

Gold LH, Vanderpool D: Psychiatric evidence and due process in firearms rights restoration. J Am Acad Psychiatry Law 46(3):309–321, 2018b 30368463

Haw. Rev. Stat. Ann. § 134–61 et seq. (2019)

Lewis DA, Goetz E, Schoenfield M, et al: The negotiation of involuntary civil commitment. Law Soc Rev 18(4):629–649, 1984

Lidz CW, Hoge SK, Gardner W, et al: Perceived coercion in mental hospital admission: pressures and process. Arch Gen Psychiatry 52(12):1034–1039, 1995 7492255

McDonald v City of Chicago, 561 U.S. 742 (2010)

Md. Code Ann., Pub. Safety § 5–601 et seq. (2018)

Monahan J, Hoge SK, Lidz C, et al: Coercion and commitment: understanding involuntary mental hospital admission. Int J Law Psychiatry 18(3):249–263, 1995 7591396

Nagle ME, Joshi KG, Frierson RL, et al: Knowledge and attitudes of psychiatrists about the gun rights of persons with mental illness. J Am Acad Psychiatry Law 49(1):28–37, 2021 33234536

Newlon C, Ayres I, Barnett B: Your liberty or your gun? A survey of psychiatrist understanding of mental health prohibitors. J Law Med Ethics 48(4 Suppl):155–163, 2020 33404305

Norris DM, Price M, Gutheil T, et al: Firearm laws, patients, and the roles of psychiatrists. Am J Psychiatry 163(8):1392–1396, 2006 16877652

N.Y. Mental Hygiene Law § 9.46, 2013

Pirelli G, DeMarco S: Firearms and Clinical Practice: A Handbook for Medical and Mental Health Professionals. New York, Oxford University Press, 2023

Pirelli G, Wechsler H, Cramer RJ: The Behavioral Science of Firearms: A Mental Health Perspective on Guns, Suicide, and Violence. New York, Oxford University Press, 2019

The Policy Surveillance Program: Short-Term Emergency Commitment Laws. 2016. Available at: http://lawatlas.org/datasets/short-term-civil-commitment. Accessed March 27, 2021.

Reed SC, Lewis DA: The negotiation of voluntary admission in Chicago's state mental hospitals. J Psychiatry Law 18(1–2):137–163, 1990

Reisch T, Steffen T, Habenstein A, et al: Change in suicide rates in Switzerland before and after firearm restriction resulting from the 2003 "Army XXI" reform. Am J Psychiatry 170(9):977–984, 2013 23897090

Simpson JR: Bad risk? An overview of laws prohibiting possession of firearms by individuals with a history of treatment for mental illness. J Am Acad Psychiatry Law 35(3):330–338, 2007 17872555

Simpson JR: Education on gun laws needed. Psychiatric News 56(5):34, 2021a

Simpson JR: The need for systematic training on gun rights and mental illness for forensic psychiatrists. J Am Acad Psychiatry Law 49:38–41, 2021b

Simpson JR: Psychiatrists and firearm laws: a disturbing lack of knowledge. AAPL Newsl 46(2):16, 21, 2021c

Simpson JR: Education about mental health firearm laws should be required in psychiatry residency programs. J Am Acad Psychiatry Law 51:13–17, 2023

Simpson JR, Carannante V: Hospitalization: voluntary and involuntary, in Principles and Practice of Forensic Psychiatry, 3rd Edition. Edited by Rosner R, Scott CL. Boca Raton, FL, CRC Press, 2017, pp 125–130

Swanson JW, Bonnie RJ, Appelbaum PS: Getting serious about reducing suicide: more "how" and less "why." JAMA 314(21):2229–2230, 2015 26524461

Swanson JW, Tong G, Robertson AG, et al: Gun-related and other violent
    crime after involuntary commitment and short-term emergency holds. J
    Am Acad Psychiatry Law 48(4):454–467, 2020 33020171
Tarasoff v Regents of the University of California, 17 Cal. 3d 425 (1976)
U.S. Const. amend. II
Weinstock R, Darby WC, Bonnici DM, et al: The ever-evolving duty to protect
    in California. J Am Acad Psychiatry Law 43(2):262, 2015 26071515

15

Ethical Challenges When Interacting With Professional Organizations, Governmental Agencies, and Community Mental Health Programs

Matthew W. Grover, M.D.

Bridget McCoy, M.D.

Debra A. Pinals, M.D.

Psychiatrists, trained as physicians, serve in a number of different roles. Engaging in treatment of patients is a fundamental aspect of the work and the core of psychiatry training. At the same time, psychiatrists often work in other capacities. Additional roles include acting as medical or general administrators in public or private clinical systems, serving as members of organizational groups, participating in governmental affairs, and engaging in regulatory or oversight processes. Ethical challenges arise across each of these roles. Unique challenges occur at the interface of public mental health systems that are underresourced and strained. In the public mental health system, many complex patient populations are served, such as those who have had "forensic" challenges with criminal courts, who may have been found incompetent to stand trial or not guilty by reason of insanity; the psychiatrist is either conducting the evaluation or helping to transition them to settings that are the "least restrictive." Regulatory factors and external pressures related to funding and payment authorizations can lead to care decisions that might look different between settings. In all of these scenarios, the psychiatrist must balance competing priorities and advocate for the best path forward. In this chapter, we review several of these types of contexts to provide an overview of some of the ethical challenges and ways to think through them.

Ethics and Leadership in Governmental Systems

Governmental systems exist at many levels, including municipal, county, state, and federal. Within each of these levels, there are separate funding streams and tables of organization that delineate leadership lines of authority. Many agencies will hire psychiatric medical directors who serve both to advise and to provide direct patient care or consultation. These roles have the potential to provide strong advocacy for the best patient care but can butt up against system limitations, leaders who view outcomes and goals differently, or personality clashes within the leadership infrastructure that can be detrimental to patient care. In complex scenarios, it has been argued that ethical issues in health care should be based on moral reasoning that stands on four basic principles: respect for autonomy, beneficence, nonmaleficence, and distributive justice, in addition to consideration of the scope of their application (Gillon 1994). If one takes respect for other human beings as a core value, application of these four principles may also require an analysis of context and potential consequences of decisions made (Gracia 1995). Take the following examples:

1. A patient has been waiting in the emergency department for 100 days for placement in an inpatient setting. The county mental health medical director is asked by the hospital chief executive officer to discharge the patient from the emergency department because of staffing coverage challenges.
2. A clinical program must be cut because of budget constraints, requiring many patients to risk losing services.

In each of these scenarios, the psychiatric medical leader is placed in an ethical and personal dilemma. A balancing of ethical principles can be helpful.

In the first example, there is the tension between beneficence and nonmaleficence. The patient has been waiting for far too long in the emergency department, where routine treatment initiation is limited. At the same time, the patient needs to remain at a hospital level of care (not clinically appropriate for discharge), and for cost and logistics reasons, the medical director is receiving pressure to discharge them. Sometimes these dilemmas can be at the psychiatrist's own risk, as there may be administrative directives that could lead to job loss if not followed.

For a psychiatrist, there can be competing agencies—agency to the patient and to management of resources so that the greatest number can benefit from them. In this scenario, discharging a patient who is not clinically appropriate for discharge based on an administrative edict could put in peril the psychiatrist's licensure. It is important for the psychiatrist to carefully explain why the patient is not appropriate for discharge; a second opinion may help. An appropriate plan needs to be formed that would not put the patient at risk but would allow the most efficient use of resources.

The second scenario involves the reality of budget limitations. Within governmental structures or large organizations, power dynamics and the personal legacy goals of politicians and leaders can drive some of the changes that affect individuals on the ground. For example, budget cuts made to appear cost-conscious might result in the second scenario. With ethical principles in mind, a medical leader is required to carefully analyze each situation to determine the best way to advise others within leadership and to identify alternative care sites for patients to avoid abandonment. Determining the best approach can be difficult, and standing up for it might involve significant risks.

According to utilitarian principles, there is a need to provide the greatest good for the greatest number, even if it means an individual's needs might be compromised for the needs of the larger population. This is often the ethical principle on which a leader must rely—for example, when resource limitations are a driving force in a dilemma. In the second scenario, it would be important to examine why this particular program was chosen for closure. There should be an intentional review of implications related to diversity and equity. For example, is the program in a neighborhood of poverty? Why was it selected instead of a similar program situated in a more affluent area? There should also be a review based on justice. Is it fair to close this program and not a different program? It is through these analyses that an administrative medical leader can thoughtfully inform or advise the system in which they are working and help set agendas and priorities.

In institutions where there are competing priorities between clinical leaders and management, it has been proffered that education, consultation, and policy development can be cornerstones to assist with ethical challenges (Suter 2006). Because there can be conflicting values in sorting out approaches for particular cases, Heeley (1998) suggested that leaders must create organizational integrity-based ethics that help shape actions based on the mission, vision, and core values of the organization. Heeley (1998) noted further that leaders hold a dialectic of competing values between Hippocratic patient-centered prioritization and population-based health care, which requires cost savings and at times yields to competitive market forces. Heeley (1998) further advised that leaders model and maximize integrity by squarely addressing when values at stake are in conflict.

Ethics and Leadership in Professional Organizations

Professional organizations such as the American Psychiatric Association (APA) have a long and rich history. Today, medical professional organizations aim to protect the interests of patients, organization members, and the organization itself. These organizations serve many functions, from providing collegial networks to producing practice guidelines and medical education training activities, disseminating information, and improving skills. They also produce public positions to promote policy. To do all these things effectively, the organization must also be a thriving and vital machine that has a strong infrastructure to support external activities.

Increasingly, professional training programs have developed to help advance an advocacy agenda by educating trainees specifically about how advocacy works (Kennedy et al. 2018). Working to support these organizations, psychiatrists can be tasked with considering key policy issues. Take, for example, the APA's position statements opposing physician participation in interrogation (American Psychiatric Association 2019) or in support of gay marriage (American Psychiatric Association 2013). From the personal experience of one of the authors (D.P.), promoting these position statements required extensive writing and rewriting to craft a statement that would garner support, followed by intense debate and ultimate passage by the governance structure of the organization. Each statement has had profound impacts on the direction of a broad array of policymakers in major venues. In each, there were dilemmas that involved debates about what was known versus conjectured and what was within the limits of psychiatric expertise as opposed to a political societal desire to see change. Policy statements that go beyond medical knowledge and science create numerous ethical difficulties for a leading medical organization. Psychiatry has a long history of being subject to and participating in political misuse (van Voren 2016). From a justice standpoint, individual members of organizations working on policy issues must be mindful of the potential to misuse the power of the position psychiatry offers, given the potential for such misuse to lead to dire consequences.

Overall, work within organized medicine has the potential for great good when approached with an eye toward beneficence toward each member, each patient, and society at large. At the same time, the work involves constant vigilance, given the risk of maleficence in the guise of advancing sound principles from the house of medicine and psychiatry.

Ethical Challenges Working Within State Governmental Institutions

Over the last 60 years, state psychiatric hospitals have evolved from providing custodial care for psychiatric patients to serving increasing numbers of *forensic patients*—those involved in the criminal justice system. Deinstitutionalization, changes in civil commitment statutes, diminishing financial support, and advancements in psychiatric treatment are just some of the factors that have contributed to the changing landscape of state psychiatric hospitals.

Psychiatrists working on inpatient psychiatric units in state hospitals experience challenges related to the low availability of inpatient beds, limited community mental health resources to facilitate discharge, and the difficulty of providing patient care in environments where outside interests, including the state court systems, are potential areas for conflict. The goals of the treating psychiatrist working with a patient may contrast with those of medical and administrative directors, who need to increase accessibility to scarce inpatient bed resources. Ethically, a patient's well-being may benefit from additional services that cannot be arranged before discharge. Such services and supports may serve the ethical principles of both beneficence and nonmaleficence. If a patient's history suggests that such services increase the amount of time a patient spends in the community (that is, not in the hospital), such interventions may also serve the principle of patient autonomy. A utilitarian approach, however, may suggest that the principle of justice is better served by increasing the access to beds for more acutely ill individuals who would benefit from a higher level of care.

Competency Restoration Challenges in State Hospital, Correctional, and Community Settings

As state hospitals serve increasing numbers of forensic patients, the number of court determinations in a state directly impacts care and bed availability. It has been estimated that patients admitted for the purpose of restoring their competency to stand trial (CST-CR, where CR stands for *competency restoration*) make up the highest proportion of forensic populations in state hospitals (Wik et al. 2020). Hospitalization on its face serves the ethical principle of beneficence, but because restoration patients may not need a hospital level of care, it may actually reflect a misuse of the system. From the perspective of nonmaleficence, one could argue that hospitalization is better than awaiting trial in jail. From a justice perspective, however, one could argue that it is unjust to crowd state hospitals with patients who don't need that level of care.

Factors within a correctional facility that could impact a defendant's health and ultimate presentation when they arrive at the state hospital—including restrictive housing, mental health deterioration due to treatment nonadherence or lack of available treatment, and victimization—are contradictory to the ethical principles of beneficence and nonmaleficence. Because the individual's criminal case halts when a CST evaluation is ordered, the court may not be able to address bail considerations that allow for release with supports and mental health diversion options. System reforms have been suggested that might better support justice, utilitarian goals, and more beneficial outcomes for more individuals who might be negatively affected by current practices (Pinals and Callahan 2020).

Once a defendant is hospitalized for CST-CR assessment, treatment is primarily focused on assisting the defendant in understanding the court processes and effectively working with their attorney, a focus that requires a combination of psychiatric treatment and legal education. It has been argued that the role of treatment providers in restoring a defendant's CST is ethically and clinically reasonable. For example, Mossman (2005) described why competence restoration is "medically appropriate," citing the potential negative impact of leaving a defendant to languish untreated or even stigmatizing individuals with mental illness by not accommodating their needs so that they can proceed to trial as other criminal defendants do. Of course, these arguments were made before the dramatic increase in volume and the ultimate result of waitlists to access services, which shifts some of the balance in deciding which value should be prioritized (legal vs. medical interests of the defendant).

Although restoration treatment modalities (usually medications when indicated and counseling/education around legal processes) support the defendant's legal rights, and perhaps arguably their legal best interests, such models exclude other aspects of care that might be needed to address the defendant's overall treatment, including a defendant's connection to their outpatient treatment providers, the need for substance use disorder treatment, housing insecurity, or vocational supports (Pinals and Callahan 2020). Thus, the true value of fidelity to the patient in terms of promoting their overall well-being within a health care setting is limited to addressing the ways in which their mental health impairments affect their functional capacities as a criminal defendant. To make the ethical challenges even more complex, once a defendant's CST is restored, they are returned to jail while awaiting trial, which in some cases has been associated with negative outcomes, including noncompliance with psychiatric medications, decompensation, and the potential need for reevaluation of CST (Boutros et al. 2018). If charges are dismissed, a defendant could potentially be released without coordinated reentry back to the community (Pinals and Callahan 2020). These outcomes after CST-CR and the return to pretrial detention in a correctional setting raise a number of ethical challenges with regard to the principles of nonmaleficence, beneficence, autonomy, and justice as they relate to the defendant.

Given the lack of available inpatient beds, successful alternatives to hospital-based CST-CR have evolved in both correctional and community settings. Kapoor (2020) argued that the jail setting, which is inherently not therapeutic, places many constraints on positive clinical treatment practices. An arrangement that allows for ongoing CST-CR services while other needs are addressed optimizes defendant autonomy and allows providers to operate under principles of beneficence and nonmaleficence. However, such arrangements are more common for defendants who are adherent with medications, engaged in treatment, and charged with nonviolent crimes (Mikolajewski et al. 2017). Ultimately, a continuum of services would allow the greatest flexibility in balancing ethical principles as they relate to the defendant versus the same principles as applied to the needs and safety of the community.

For defendants ultimately found "unrestorable," state hospitals can pursue involuntary inpatient civil commitment for the individual, enabling them to work toward community transition without any interruption in their treatment plan. However, Levitt and colleagues (2010) found that patients determined to be unrestorable had longer hospital stays and more often required court-ordered treatment over a patient's objection versus patients admitted through civil commitment involuntarily from the community.

Care and Treatment of Insanity Acquittees

Patients previously found not guilty by reason of insanity (*insanity acquittees*) by the courts make up a second group of forensic patients hospitalized in state psychiatric hospital settings. With multiple modalities of treatment available in the state hospital setting, many insanity acquittees function well with clinical improvement for many years. From the perspective of the psychiatrist, the principles of beneficence, nonmaleficence, and autonomy may all be best served by discharging the patient into the community with outpatient follow-up, supportive housing, and additional supportive services (e.g., vocational training, financial supports). However, the patient may not be granted conditional release or discharge because of the administrative or judicial oversight of the patient's legal case, based on their status as an insanity acquittee and fears that they will reoffend. Hospital administrators, state oversight committees, judges, or juries may decide that the safety of the community is of primary concern, leaning on the concepts of beneficence, nonmaleficence, and justice as they relate to a prior victim and the community (Kapoor et al. 2020). Psychiatrists working with these supervised patients must learn to consider the ethical needs of their patients, balanced by public concerns about their risks, and the awareness of the possible opposing views of a variety of stakeholders.

Notably, the success of community placement for insanity acquittees does not necessarily correlate with their length of psychiatric hospitalization (Miraglia and Hall 2011). Other studies have suggested that factors including supportive housing play an important role in maintaining community success of an insanity acquittee (Novosad et al. 2016). Identification and management of risk factors, along with the implementation of appropriate supports before conditional release, promote community safety while advancing the principles of beneficence, nonmaleficence, and autonomy for the patient.

Working With State Hospital Patients in a Pandemic

The COVID-19 pandemic involved infection control challenges in state hospital settings (and other settings such as nursing homes and prisons), where patients with severe psychiatric disorders may have lacked capacity to make decisions about medical care as it relates to medical assessment, testing, wearing masks, social distancing, vaccination, and room restrictions. Political pressures, as well as non-data-driven policies focused on reduced spread of infectious disease, may have driven decision-making processes without consideration of the overall clinical needs of patients.

Other aspects of patient care, including community transitions, were affected by pandemic-related policies. Considerations such as alternative settings for patient visitors, outdoor areas with utilization of masks, social distancing, and COVID-19 testing relied on the principles of beneficence and nonmaleficence. Management of pandemic concerns for state hospitals required careful thought and balance between enhancing rehabilitation options, advancing access to the community, and implementing restrictions to prevent viral spread. The evolving understanding of the virus created the need to continually pivot, rebalancing ethical and clinical concerns to protect patients and others.

Ethical Challenges in Acute-Care and Community Settings

An ongoing conversation in psychiatry weighs the need for inpatient psychiatric services against maintenance of mental health in the community. The National Association of State Mental Health Program

Directors suggested that while the ask is often for "more beds," the answer is much more complicated, and the goal should be to develop a more comprehensive continuum of care that includes community and inpatient services (Pinals and Fuller 2017). However, as clinicians continue to operate in a less-than-ideal continuum of care in the community, ethical challenges arise in many areas, including decisions about allocation of resources, payment for services (in particular involuntary services), and how to address the needs of patients increasingly interacting with the criminal justice system.

Scarcity of Resources

Fewer acute inpatient psychiatric beds are available in the community now than there were 50–70 years ago (Pinals and Fuller 2017). Additionally, general demand for mental health services often outweighs the available community resources (Parks and Radke 2014), leaving the community clinician to make difficult decisions about allocation of resources. Green and Bloch (2006) discussed this "process of moral deliberation" on both micro and macro levels and suggested two approaches to the micro-allocation of resources: implicit rationing and a more systemized approach typically based in cost-effectiveness.

Implicit rationing assigns the clinician as the decision-maker, operating under the ethical concepts of beneficence and nonmaleficence to allocate resources in the best way to advance the well-being of patients (Green and Bloch 2006). Clinicians in the position of making difficult decisions in resource-poor systems may use this principle, which relies heavily on the idea of triage and determining what services are most needed by which patients. For example, when large numbers of patients are boarding in an emergency department of a hospital awaiting psychiatric admission, a clinician may decide to discharge a chronically ill patient who has been acutely stabilized, even though the patient would benefit from a longer stay. In this scenario, the clinician considers the principles of beneficence and nonmaleficence as they relate to both the patient being discharged and the individual awaiting hospitalization in the emergency department. Critics (Eddy 1992) have suggested that there is too much room for bias in this model and rather support a more explicit and objective cost-effectiveness approach with the goal of meeting the needs of all patients as efficiently as possible, rather than focusing on a few (Green and Bloch 2006).

As the number of state and longer-term placement beds decreases (Lamb and Weinberger 2005), those with serious mental illness struggling to stay in the community end up in acute psychiatric hospital settings, including emergency departments. Psychiatric staff, who have to consider extended waits in emergency departments, limited outpatient resources, and limited long-term facilities, set priorities and parameters around who will be admitted and how long they will stay (Lamb and Weinberger 2005). Consider the following case example:

Case Example

An acute inpatient psychiatrist is caring for a patient with schizoaffective disorder who presented to the hospital with psychosis, mania, and extreme agitation. After a prolonged acute inpatient stay of nearly 5 weeks, the patient was stabilized on medications that require close outpatient follow-up. The patient's most recent address (and therefore managed care insurance) is out of state, which limits the social worker's ability to connect them to outpatient psychiatric services without a 3-week delay. Additionally, the patient is currently homeless, and they do not have any income or current family supports. The patient's psychiatric symptoms have improved, they are engaged in treatment, and they express limited insight into their condition but a willingness to follow up in the community.

The patient requests to leave the hospital. The inpatient psychiatrist must weigh the patient's autonomy against beneficence and nonmaleficence. Because of the limitations in accessible resources, holding the patient in the hospital longer would take up a bed needed for someone boarding in the emergency department. Notably, the patient's acute symptoms have stabilized, and prolonging the hospitalization is unlikely to change their access to resources.

This example highlights some of the ethical challenges community psychiatrists face in a continuum of care that is lacking in resources. There is unlikely to be an ideal solution, leading individual clinicians to examine each scenario through the lens of clinical needs, legal obligations, and ethical principles, with no clear right or wrong answer. The clinician may find support through a multidisciplinary team, other clinicians in the system, hospital administration staff, or professional organizations to provide guidance in how to weigh a patient's autonomy versus beneficence and nonmaleficence and, when the need arises, to take a utilitarian approach and attempt to do the most good for the greatest number of people.

Crises will continue to be a part of psychiatric care, and alternatives to inpatient psychiatric services or outpatient clinic-based services do exist. As the need for more services continues to be recognized, the development and implementation of additional services may help allay some of the ethical dilemmas that clinicians face regarding scarce resources. Some examples include psychiatric urgent care centers, crisis stabilization centers, extended observation units, crisis residential services, and living-room/peer-run crisis centers (Pinals 2020; Substance Abuse and Mental Health Services Administration 2020). Additionally, expansion of programs such as assertive community treatment, court-ordered outpatient commitment, and telepsychiatry services could be implemented with the goal of reducing the burden on the system and decreasing ethical dilemmas related to scarcity of resources.

Payment for Involuntary Psychiatric Care and Unintended Financial Consequences

One aspect of involuntary treatment that has not garnered much attention is surprise medical billing (Morris and Kleinman 2020). Patients may receive bills for medical services that they did not wish to receive, and they may receive bills for services that they attempted to refuse. Even if the patient is not charged out-of-pocket expenses, they may receive many other charges for deductibles, copayments, and coinsurance (Morris and Kleinman 2020).

The irony in this financial situation, and the dilemma it presents, is that all too often, patients being involuntarily psychiatrically hospitalized are already struggling with a number of psychosocial stressors, including limited finances. The financial impact of admission creates a justice and equity issue, as those of means are less negatively impacted. Additionally, the issue of billing patients after an involuntary intervention may demand greater consideration from the psychiatric world (Morris and Kleinman 2020). Taken together, the various burdens of hospitalization, curtailment of liberty, and potential financial impact can take their toll on patients. Clinicians would do well to have a frank conversation with patients about their mental health and their concerns about the hospitalization itself, any involvement in court hearings, and even their finances, to support beneficence and aid the patient in their recovery and overall well-being.

Caring for the Patient With Criminal Justice Involvement

People with serious mental illness are overrepresented in the criminal justice system (Parisi et al. 2022). The sequential intercept model was developed to help communities identify gaps in services for those with mental illness or substance use disorders involved with the criminal justice system, to divert them to treatment (Munetz and Griffin 2006; Substance Abuse and Mental Health Services Administration 2024). It was previously assumed that untreated symptoms of mental illness drove at least some criminal behavior, and that connection to mental health services would therefore reduce recidivism (Parisi et al. 2022). Although connection to mental health services has been shown to reduce symptoms, it has not been shown to have an impact on criminal justice involvement, leading to a call to expand services to address both mental illness and criminogenic risk factors (Parisi et al. 2022). The community clinician may best serve the patient and community by becoming familiar with models of risk, need, and responsivity principles, which have been shown to reduce criminal recidivism (Skeem et al. 2011), and incorporating them into individual and clinic practice. By expanding the context of treatment to criminogenic needs of patients involved in the criminal justice system, clinicians may be able to connect with patients on aspects of their life and care that are meaningful, identifying sources of increased stress and potential barriers to treatment.

Arresting Patients Versus Continuing to Treat Difficult Patients

The practice of psychiatric care includes working with individuals who are behaviorally challenged, and some may be assaultive. An ethical dilemma facing clinicians is how to make the decision about continuing to treat assaultive patients versus supporting their arrest or moving them to alternative treatment placements. Clinicians must take into account factors such as severity of violence, motivation for violence, diagnoses, and active symptoms when determining the most appropriate course of action available (Rachlin 1994). Overreliance on arrest creates other dilemmas, such as patients leaving health care settings and instead going to jails, where medical and psychiatric care may be inadequate. Clinicians are always balancing utilitarian and individual goals while considering the safety of staff on the unit, other patients, and the therapeutic milieu. Decisions about a patient's care and arrest should not be made based on others' comfort, but the balance of safety on an inpatient psychiatric unit is a delicate one, and patients and staff must feel safe enough to provide and participate in an effective therapeutic environment. At the same time, inadequate treatment provision is not a justification for criminalization of patients. Rigorous efforts must be made to ensure all treatment modalities have been exhausted in the course of treatment. If the ultimate goal is to provide patient care, arrests of patients should be an extremely rare outcome, if it happens at all.

Conclusion

Government systems, including state hospitals, offer unique opportunities for psychiatrists to have a role in patient care, policy development, and solutions to challenges at the interface of psychiatry and the criminal justice system. Psychiatrists working in state hospitals and acute-care settings may balance the principles of medical ethics differently than hospital, state agency, or even advocacy organizational leadership. Conflicts arise across settings, including challenges related to the limited community resources that create further challenges. Psychiatrists should be aware of potential areas of conflict and carefully balance ethical principles in a variety of organizational, advocacy, and patient-care contexts from the state hospital to the community.

References

American Psychiatric Association: APA Official Actions: Position Statement on Issues Related to Homosexuality. Arlington, VA, American Psychiatric Association, 2013. Available at: https://www.psychiatry.org/File%20Library/About-APA/Organization-Documents-Policies/Policies/Position-2013-Homosexuality.pdf. Accessed December 2, 2024.

American Psychiatric Association: APA Official Actions: Position Statement on Psychiatric Participation in Interrogation of Detainees. Arlington, VA, American Psychiatric Association, 2019. Available at: https://www.psychiatry.org/File%20Library/About-APA/Organization-Documents-Policies/Policies/Position-Psychiatric-Participation-in-Interrogation-of-Detainees.pdf. Accessed December 2, 2024.

Boutros A, Kang SS, Boutros NN: A cyclical path to recovery: calling into question the wisdom of incarceration after restoration. Int J Law Psychiatry 57:100–105, 2018 29548496

Eddy DM: Cost-effectiveness analysis: is it up to the task? JAMA 267(24):3342–3348, 1992 1597918

Gillon R: Medical ethics: four principles plus attention to scope. BMJ 309(6948):184–188, 1994 8044100

Gracia D: Hard times, hard choices: founding bioethics today. Bioethics 9(3–4):192–206, 1995 11653036

Green SA, Bloch S: Resource allocation, in An Anthology of Psychiatric Ethics. New York, Oxford University Press, 2006, pp 385–389

Heeley GF: Leading with integrity: how to balance conflicting values. Health Prog 79(5):60–62, 1998 10187522

Kapoor R: A continuum of competency restoration services need not include jail. J Am Acad Psychiatry Law 48(1):52–55, 2020 32047078

Kapoor R, Wasser TD, Funaro MC, et al: Hospital treatment of persons found not guilty by reason of insanity. Behav Sci Law 38(5):426–440, 2020 32897589

Kennedy KG, Vance MC; Council on Advocacy and Government Relations: APA Resource Document: Advocacy Teaching in Psychiatry Residency Training Programs. Arlington, VA, American Psychiatric Association, 2018. Available at: https://www.psychiatry.org/getattachment/aa7b03d1 -9296-4b85-9915-72281e416cb9/Resource-Document-2018-Advocacy -Teaching-in-Psychiatry-Residency-Training.pdf. Accessed December 2, 2024.

Lamb HR, Weinberger LE: The shift of psychiatric inpatient care from hospitals to jails and prisons. J Am Acad Psychiatry Law 33(4):529–534, 2005 16394231

Levitt GA, Vora I, Tyler K, et al: Civil commitment outcomes of incompetent defendants. J Am Acad Psychiatry Law 38(3):349–358, 2010 20852220

Mikolajewski AJ, Manguno-Mire GM, Coffman KL, et al: Patient characteristics and outcomes related to successful outpatient competency restoration. Behav Sci Law 35(3):225–238, 2017 28429375

Miraglia R, Hall D: The effect of length of hospitalization on re-arrest among insanity plea acquittees. J Am Acad Psychiatry Law 39(4):524–534, 2011 22159980

Morris NP, Kleinman RA: Involuntary commitments: billing patients for forced psychiatric care. Am J Psychiatry 177(12):1115–1116, 2020 33256438

Mossman D: Is Prosecution "Medically Appropriate"? University of Cincinnati College of Law Faculty Articles and Other Publications, Paper 20, 2005. Available at: https://scholarship.law.uc.edu/fac_pubs/20/. Accessed December 2, 2024.

Munetz MR, Griffin PA: Use of the sequential intercept model as an approach to decriminalization of people with serious mental illness. Psychiatr Serv 57(4):544–549, 2006 16603751

Novosad D, Banfe S, Britton J, et al: Conditional release placements of insanity acquittees in Oregon: 2012–2014. Behav Sci Law 34(2–3):366–377, 2016 26969885

Parisi A, Wilson AB, Villodas M, et al: A systematic review of interventions targeting criminogenic risk factors among persons with serious mental illness. Psychiatr Serv 73(8):897–909, 2022 34911352

Parks J, Radke AQ (eds): The Vital Role of State Psychiatric Hospitals. Alexandria, VA, National Association of State Mental Health Program Directors, 2014. Available at: https://www.nasmhpd.org/sites/default/files/The%20Vital%20Role%20of%20State%20Psychiatric%20Hospitals Technical%20Report_July_2014.pdf. Accessed December 2, 2024.

Pinals DA: Crisis Services: Meeting Needs, Saving Lives. Arlington, VA, National Association of State Mental Health Program Directors, 2020. Available at: https://www.nasmhpd.org/sites/default/files/2020paper1 .pdf. Accessed December 2, 2024.

Pinals DA, Callahan L: Evaluation and restoration of competence to stand trial: intercepting the forensic system using the sequential intercept model. Psychiatr Serv 71(7):698–705, 2020 32237983

Pinals DA, Fuller DA: Beyond Beds: The Vital Role of a Full Continuum of Psychiatric Care. Arlington, VA, National Association of State Mental Health Program Directors and Treatment Advocacy Center, 2017. Available at: https://nasmhpd.org/sites/default/files/TAC.Paper_ .1Beyond_Beds.pdf. Accessed December 2, 2024.

Rachlin S: The prosecution of violent psychiatric inpatients: one respectable intervention. Bull Am Acad Psychiatry Law 22(2):239–247, 1994 7949412

Skeem JL, Manchak S, Peterson JK: Correctional policy for offenders with mental illness: creating a new paradigm for recidivism reduction. Law Hum Behav 35(2):110–126, 2011 20390443

Substance Abuse and Mental Health Services Administration: National Guidelines for Behavioral Health Crisis Care: A Best Practice Toolkit. Rockville, MD, Substance Abuse and Mental Health Services Administration, 2020. Available at: https://www.samhsa.gov/sites /default/files/national-guidelines-for-behavioral-health-crisis-care -02242020.pdf. Accessed December 2, 2024.

Substance Abuse and Mental Health Services Administration: The Sequential Intercept Model. May 24, 2024. Available at: https://www.samhsa.gov/ criminal-juvenile-justice/sim-overview. Accessed December 2, 2024.

Suter RE: Organizational ethics. Emerg Med Clin North Am 24(3):579–603, 2006 16877131

van Voren R: Ending political abuse of psychiatry: where we are at and what needs to be done. BJPsych Bull 40(1):30–33, 2016 26958357

Wik A, Hollen V, Fisher WH: Forensic patients in state psychiatric hospitals: 1999–2016. CNS Spectr 25(2):196–206, 2020 31221229

16

Ethical Challenges Regarding Informed Consent, Reporting Laws, and Confidentiality Violations

Katrina Hui, M.D., M.S.
Steven K. Hoge, M.D.
Carl Erik Fisher, M.D.

In clinical practice, physicians hold both an ethical and a legal fiduciary duty to act in the best interests of the patient. Patients are recognized as beneficiaries of knowledge and skill from their physicians. Inherent in the relationship is an imbalance of power, based on the specialized knowledge and authority of the physician. Physicians often exercise varying degrees of paternalism, with the goal of beneficence to the patient. Unfortunately, tensions arise when decisions threaten to undermine patient autonomy. These conflicts become apparent in several exceptional contexts posing challenges or threats to this background norm, including those related to informed consent, reporting laws, and confidentiality.

Over the course of medical training and practice, physicians develop a deep concern for patients' interests and maintenance of the doctor-patient relationship. Clinicians strive to act in their patients' interests, often even when it imposes societal costs. For example, ordering confirmatory tests may not be supported by guidelines but will allay worry for some patients. In general, the added costs are believed to be offset by value gained in promoting patient trust in the therapeutic enterprise. Clinical ethics have been generated by the profession through practice, embodied in the principles of ethics, and enforced by professional organizations, state medical boards, credentialing, and privileging.

In this chapter, we address questions that arise regarding confidentiality, informed consent, and the regulation of psychiatric practice and medicine more broadly—topics that at times present challenges regarding professional responsibility and the doctor-patient relationship. We also discuss exceptions to these principles and a selection of complex and contemporary cases, with special attention toward pragmatic issues directly relevant to psychiatry.

Forensic Psychiatrists as Consultants

The demands of acting as a consultant in treatment settings differ significantly from those that fall on forensic clinicians in legal settings. Forensic psychiatrists working in legal settings—retained by attorneys, courts, or forensic institutions—are concerned with the accuracy of their opinions. Often the rules governing practice have been well established in law and determined by a calculus driven by the needs of fairly administering justice. In traditional forensic settings, experts are not operating as care providers and do not form treatment relationships with the people they assess, and thus are not governed by ordinary clinical ethics driven by fiduciary responsibilities. Forensic clinicians are usually directed by nonphysicians (e.g., lawyers and judges) regarding the limits of their discretionary behavior, and the principles applied are not rooted in fiduciary duties or the demands of sustaining treatment relationships.

By contrast, in clinical settings, forensic clinicians, as experts in the legal regulation of psychiatric practice, bring their experience to the task of reconciling external rules with clinical ethics and provide guidance on how to maintain therapeutic focus and sustain treatment relationships. Treating clinicians face challenges in responding to competing legal demands that threaten their fundamental ethics principles. To further complicate matters, in institutional settings, attorneys and risk managers are important actors in providing information and direction to clinicians. Consulting forensic psychiatrists can play an important role in providing guidance to clinicians about how to "do the right thing" in these circumstances.

Confidentiality in Clinical Settings

The ethical responsibility to protect the confidentiality of patients' medical information dates back many centuries to the Hippocratic Oath. Confidentiality stems from the value placed on patient autonomy and privacy interests. In psychiatry in particular, confidentiality has been considered to have important utilitarian value and to be essential to clinical practice. Absent strong professional commitment to privacy, patients would not seek treatment or disclose sensitive information essential to assessment and care.

The Health Insurance Portability and Accountability Act (HIPAA) of 1996 authorized the creation of federal regulations regarding confidentiality (termed "medical privacy") and the protection of health information. The resulting Privacy Rule went into effect in 2003. A detailed review of the HIPAA regulations is beyond the scope of this chapter, but a few points deserve discussion, as they underscore the importance of professional ethics in managing patient confidentiality. The HIPAA regulations set a floor for the protection of privacy. Professional standards as applied by clinicians may determine that a higher level of protection is necessary. Moreover, states may require higher standards in the enforcement of professional norms. The numerous provisions of HIPAA that apply to disclosure of private information to third parties are permissive in nature; they do not mandate disclosure. Therefore, clinicians have the discretion to apply professional judgment to protect the specified information. In institutional settings, clinicians and their consultants should be prepared to interact with hospital attorneys, risk managers, privacy officers, and record keepers on decisions to disclose and the scope of disclosure. These individuals are not bound by professional medical ethics and may place less weight on the protection of confidentiality, particularly when there is a risk of liability. HIPAA applies to clinicians or health care organizations that engage in defined electronic transmission of health-related information, generally related to insurance and billing transactions rather than broader applications around disclosure of protected health information. Thus, many clinicians are not required to comply with the HIPAA Privacy Rule.

Exceptions

The ethical obligation to protect patient privacy is not absolute and may be outweighed by other superseding values. Here, we briefly review various discretionary and mandatory exceptions to confidentiality, many of which involve secondary duties to society or others.

Discretionary Exceptions

Some clinical situations may compel a clinician to disclose confidential information without patient authorization. Emergencies, patient incompetence, and the initiation of involuntary commitment are common examples, which involve professional judgments made regarding patients' needs in a specific clinical situation based on individualized assessments. In general, such exceptions are not controversial, because the clinician is acting in the patient's best interests.

More problematic disclosures relate to clinicians' duties to protect third parties from patients' violent acts, as they may introduce a *duty to protect* or *duty to warn* other individuals, introducing an explicitly new duty to balance against the usual primary duty to act in the best interests of the patient. The case of *Tarasoff* (1974, 1976), which is discussed in Chapter 12, and related rulings established a legal duty for clinicians to protect third parties.

Most states have case law or statutes that have established a clinician's duty to third parties. These laws vary regarding what triggers this secondary duty and how the duty can be discharged. States also differ in how they define the scope of protection. For example, some states impose liability for property damage as well as personal violence. Other states may extend liability to the consequences of reckless driving or having unprotected sex (e.g., for patients with HIV). Other states have remained silent on the issue of clinicians' duties to protect third parties. In those instances, experts recommend that the duty be implemented in some form regardless.

Forensic psychiatrists are often called on to provide consultations in clinical settings when concerns arise around these complicated discretionary exceptions. Nonforensic clinicians have some level of awareness of a duty to third parties but are accustomed by training and practice to place their patients' interests first. Consequently, they often are uncomfortable responding to the unfamiliar demand of protecting third parties, for fear of undermining their relationship with the patient. In some cases, the clinician may ask the consultant to warn the third party, thereby resolving the ethical tension quickly by ensuring that the legal duty has been fulfilled outside the therapeutic relationship.

Consultants also play an important role in helping clinicians to reconcile the legal duty to protect third parties with the traditional ethical duty to act in patients' interests. Patients who threaten, commit violent acts, or behave recklessly are likely to suffer as a result of criminal justice involvement, other legal actions, and various social impairments. Legal responsibilities may incentivize clinicians to pay attention to reducing these behaviors; however, they also have beneficial effects on patients' social adaptation and functioning. To sustain the treatment relationship, it is important for clinicians to act from within the therapeutic alliance to the greatest extent possible.

Mandatory Disclosures

Numerous legally mandated reporting obligations require breaching doctor-patient confidentiality. Many of these reporting requirements have a public health purpose around societal protections. For example, states require physicians to report various communicable diseases, including sexually transmitted diseases, so that outbreaks can be curtailed by contact tracing. In addition, states require that suspected child abuse be reported, and many states have enacted similar laws to cover vulnerable groups such as those with disabilities or the elderly. These statutes vary as to the categories of mandated reporters and the circumstances in which reporting is required.

Mandatory reporting laws extend to circumstances that are arguably discriminatory toward individuals with mental disorders. For instance, most states report mental health data to the National Instant Criminal Background System, which must be checked before purchase of a firearm. Individuals are prohibited from possessing a firearm if they have been convicted of a serious crime, committed domestic violence, or fall into another specified category, often related to mental illness. Under federal law, individuals who have been involuntarily committed, adjudicated as incompetent, or found to be impaired in criminal proceedings are prohibited from gun ownership. (Issues surrounding firearms are covered in more detail in Chapter 14, "Ethical Issues in Forensic Psychiatry: Mental Health Firearm Prohibitions".) States may expand the restrictions beyond those specified, including to those who have been the subject of emergency commitment (without adjudication), outpatient commitment, or voluntary psychiatric hospitalization. Unlike the situations discussed in the previous section, these reporting requirements are not based on individualized assessment or clinical judgment. For example, in cases where there is concern for a child's well-being, the clinician is not responsible for determining whether child abuse has occurred or assessing whether there is ongoing risk. They are instead mandated to involve Child Protective Services, who perform their own investigation. On the one hand, the clinician is not placed in the position of making a judgment that may be contrary to the patient's preferences and interests. On the other hand, the result inevitably is that there will be some degree of unnecessary reporting that has no social utility and may still affect the therapeutic relationship by involving an external government agency. However, the extent to which these reporting requirements influence individuals with psychiatric problems to avoid treatment is not known.

Criminal Justice and the Legal Process

Forensic psychiatrists may also be consulted on a range of issues related to criminal justice and the legal process that arise in clinical practice. In this section, we briefly review the importance of protection of confidentiality in the contexts of subpoenas and reporting past crimes.

Legal Process

Clinicians and mental health systems may receive subpoenas to appear in court regarding their patients or to produce their records, or both. These documents are generated by litigants and do not necessarily mean that the records can be disclosed or introduced into evidence at a civil or criminal trial. In many instances, mental health information will be protected by testimonial privilege. In brief, privilege protects privacy by barring access to covered information in legal proceedings. The privilege is held by the patient, so barring incompetence or other special circumstances, the patient's lawyer will need to exercise an objection and contest the request. Ultimately, the determination of whether the requested testimony or record production is privileged will be decided by the court. Upon receipt of a subpoena, the clinician should notify their personal or facility attorney.

Reporting Past Crimes

Clinicians are not under a legal obligation to report past crimes committed by their patients. The federal and state courts have rejected such an obligation, termed *misprision.* (note that some mental health systems and hospitals may have contrary policies). Repeated criminal behavior, however, may lead to concerns about future harmful behavior and, as discussed above, may lead to assessment and interventions related to the duty to protect third parties.

The Role of Governmental Regulation

Certain other exceptions to confidentiality arise from different justifications. Here, we discuss another exemplary exception to the usually expected confidentiality and primary duty to the patient, one that involves a particular type of governmental incursion into the doctor-patient relationship motivated by considerations of law enforcement and police power. Then, we briefly discuss other related examples that introduce similar complications to the primary duty to the patient.

Prescription Monitoring—The Case of Opioids

The U.S. opioid overdose crisis was at a new record high in 2019—nearly 72,000 deaths—and overdose deaths further surged by another 20% during the COVID-19 pandemic (Goodnough 2021). The dominant image of the victim of the overdose crisis has generally been white and middle-class, which has powerfully influenced public sentiment and spurred political action to curb the use of prescription opioids, to a degree not seen in the long-running crises of overdose and harm in other communities, particularly communities of color (Netherland and Hansen 2016). There are two caveats about the overdose crisis worth making from the outset. First, the overdose epidemic is not limited to opioids, as a surge in both methamphetamine and benzodiazepine use is contributing to substance-related harms and deaths (Jones et al. 2020; Lembke et al. 2018). Second, after crackdowns on prescription opioid use, there has been a rising involvement of fentanyl and fentanyl analogs in street opioids. Nevertheless, it is clear that overprescription of opioids has played an important role in the overdose crisis, especially from its inception in the 1990s and early 2000s, when concerted marketing efforts from companies such as Purdue Pharma helped to encourage more liberal prescriptions of opioids and obscure the dangers of addiction (Keefe 2021). In response to these complicated and overlapping contributors to the overdose crisis, state and federal governments have instituted an array of initiatives, including some that impinge on the doctor-patient relationship.

Among "supply reduction" initiatives—which include efforts to limit illegal sales and diversion, disrupt supply chains, and other law enforcement methods—Prescription Drug Monitoring Programs (PDMPs) have become one of the most popular state-level initiatives to restrain opioid prescribing. PDMPs are statewide databases that track the prescription and dispensation of controlled substances and provide information to physicians and pharmacists about patient prescription histories.

PDMPs, in keeping with their state-by-state regulation, take a variety of forms. When PDMP use is optional, utilization rates by providers are very low, often less than 25% (Dave et al. 2021). In contrast, when states institute universal registration and mandatory-access provisions, requiring all providers to register and query the PDMP before issuing and dispensing prescriptions for controlled substances, emerging evidence indicates that rates of opioid-related harms decrease. However, findings are not homogeneous, and there are also worrying signs that although rigorous PDMPs might reduce prescription opioid deaths and other harms, they unduly increase deaths and harms related to synthetic opioids such as fentanyl (Delcher et al. 2020). One systematic review has concluded that "evidence that PDMP implementation either increases or decreases nonfatal or fatal overdoses is largely insufficient" (Fink et al. 2018, p. 8).

PDMPs are hotly debated, and a complete discussion of their costs, benefits, and alternatives is beyond the scope of this chapter. Instead, we focus on a select review of certain themes illustrating the tensions inherent in governmental incursion into the doctor-patient relationship, particularly in regard to confidentiality. Unlike the duties to warn or protect discussed above, which involve balancing a duty to the patient against a duty to third parties, PDMPs introduce a more generalized duty to participate in the state's policing of substance use.

The earliest PDMP-like system dates back to 1914, when New York State established a system to track opioid prescriptions that required prescribing physicians to submit duplicate prescription forms to a centralized state database (Holmgren et al. 2020). This development was contemporaneous with the Harrison Narcotics Tax Act of 1914, which marked the beginning of a period of strong social opprobrium toward and harsh regulation of opioids and other substances (Fisher 2022). California enacted a similar "triplicate prescription program" in 1939, administered by their Bureau of Narcotic Enforcement—of note, an arm of law enforcement, not medical practice or regulation.

It was only during a time of rapid development in drug policy in the 1960s and 1970s that the legality of PDMPs was tested in court. In *Whalen v. Roe* (1977), a group of New York patients and physicians challenged the legality of the state's PDMP, which registered the names and addresses of everyone who was prescribed Schedule II substances. The case rose to the level of the Supreme Court, which ruled that the PDMP did not violate a "right to privacy" as protected by the Fourteenth Amendment, in part because the PDMP was a law enforcement tool (i.e., one enacted for the purpose of preventing diversion) and not an instrument of public health (Holmgren et al. 2020).

This history illustrates the tensions inherent in PDMPs regarding the doctor-patient relationship and confidentiality. Although PDMPs, like most supply-side interventions, are politically popular, they lack definitive evidence for their benefits as public health measures and come with certain costs. Patients who are no longer able to access medications or willing to discuss pain relief with their physicians are likely to take matters into their own hands by obtaining illicit substances with unpredictable potency and adulterants (Mueller et al. 2021). This concern is only one facet of a farther-reaching potential consequence: restrictive policies meant to govern prescribing may exacerbate stigma, fear, and mistrust, thus damaging doctor-patient communication and driving more dangerous outcomes beyond opioid prescriptions.

Both as originally conceived and in practice, PDMPs are law enforcement mechanisms. To the extent that opioid prescribing needs to be reduced, the question still remains whether PDMPs are the appropriate curb on overprescription. By their nature, they move the locus of control of prescribing patterns away from the medical profession and toward nonmedical regulation. The effect of PDMPs on curbing prescriptions seems to introduce coercion and intimidation from the state into the doctor-patient encounter rather than bringing providers into line with best practices. Indeed, studies of clinicians providing care to patients with chronic pain found that they were fearful of losing their licenses for perceived inappropriate prescribing and felt that their primary responsibility had shifted from providing treatment to policing patients (Webster et al. 2019). Despite this reality (and the 1977 ruling of the Supreme Court), in political rhetoric, PDMPs are commonly positioned as a public health tool rather than a law enforcement mechanism, and several jurisdictions have moved PDMPs from narcotics enforcement to public health departments in their state administrations. Nevertheless, local and state police continue to use PDMPs to surveil both prescribers and patients (Holmgren et al. 2020).

Other Cases

The tensions, costs, and benefits of governmental incursion into the practice of medicine and the doctor-patient relationship can be applied in various degrees to other situations. One contemporary example for brief consideration relates to COVID-19 regulations. In various jurisdictions, health officials have swiftly enacted policies regarding contact tracing and quarantine, and (especially in the case of rapidly evolving digital applications for contact tracing) the data protection and health privacy implications appear to be rapidly outpacing existing laws and regulation (Bhattacharya and Ramos 2021). These cases invoke themes similar to those regarding PDMPs: the patient's right to privacy, balancing individual versus collective health, and the relative priority accorded to police power versus public health purposes of governmental regulation of medical practice.

Informed Consent

The basis for informed consent in the United States dates back to 1947 under the Nuremberg Code, which emphasized the process as an ethical imperative, in response to the widespread and inhumane experimentation led by physician researchers on prisoners in Nazi concentration camps. The significance of informed consent gained more public awareness and acceptance after the now infamous Tuskegee syphilis experiments. That research, spearheaded by the U.S. Public Health Service and the Centers for Disease Control, took place over 40 years. At no point were African American subjects with syphilis informed about their diagnosis or offered penicillin, which became adopted as the standard treatment for the illness early in the study. These two cases called into question the moral decision-making of physicians. Informed consent consequently has been developed in response to historically questionable practices of researchers and clinicians and has now been adopted as an important standard by professional and regulatory bodies. It is a requirement of research studies involving human subjects (Code of Federal Regulations 2018) and furthermore has become an essential part of the provision of care within clinical settings.

Informed consent emphasizes the importance of a collaborative decision made between physician and patient (Berg et al. 2001). At its core, informed consent places a priority on choice and the well-being of patients or subjects, although these two at times conflict and can create tensions in the therapeutic relationship. Informed consent has also been heavily influenced by interests protected under the law, including the right to bodily integrity and individual autonomy. These interests have translated to the legal duties to disclose information and also to obtain consent before administering treatment. Nonetheless, there is significant variability based on jurisdiction about the specifics of these legal duties.

Broadly speaking, informed consent requires voluntariness of choice, understanding of and access to relevant information, and the mental competence to make the decision at issue (Appelbaum and Gutheil 2007). In medicolegal spheres, informed consent was originally conceived to avoid claims of battery against a patient (see *Schloendorff v. New York Hospital* 1914). However, its application has evolved over time to place a greater emphasis on patient autonomy and choice. It is now deemed negligence if physicians fail to discuss the relevant risks, benefits, and alternatives of a proposed treatment. Arguably the most well-known case that shaped these legal obligations was *Salgo v. Leland Stanford Etc. Bd. Trustees* (1957), which coined the term "informed consent." Salgo, the patient, underwent a translumbar aortography and suffered hemiplegia, a rare but established complication about which Salgo alleged he had not been advised. The California Court of Appeals ruled that "a physician violates his duty to his patient and subjects himself to liability if he withholds any facts which are necessary to form the basis of an intelligent consent by the patient to the proposed treatment." Interestingly, the court also described exceptions should a physician believe that disclosure itself would cause harm.

In practice, the specifics of what information (in terms of the risks, benefits, and alternatives to a proposed intervention) needs to be disclosed in the process of informed consent have been debated. Previously, clinicians used a "reasonable practitioner" standard, that is, what would be deemed customary or acceptable to discuss by others in the profession. However, this standard has come under criticism for overprioritizing clinicians and neglecting patient-specific considerations. Consequently, the majority of jurisdictions now employ a "reasonable patient" standard, that is, what material risks and benefits about a proposed treatment the patient would want to know before making a decision.

Informed consent also requires that patients can engage in the consent process. Legally, patients are presumed competent unless determined otherwise. To demonstrate competence, a patient must be able to understand information relevant to the decision, appreciate their situation and its consequences, manipulate the relevant information rationally, and express a stable, voluntary choice (Appelbaum and Gutheil 2007). It is important to note that competence is decision specific; incompetence about a particular type of treatment does not imply incompetence about other treatments.

Exceptions

As with confidentiality, the prioritization of patient choice in decision-making is not absolute. Here we discuss a couple of exceptions to informed consent based on concerns around nonmaleficence, and then we review notable examples of government incursion on physician "free speech" in an attempt to regulate the consent process and show how those statutes compromised physicians' primary duty to the patient.

There are several common exceptions to the duty to obtain informed consent that have generally been deemed morally permissible based on competing values. More straightforward exceptions include emergency situations in which the patient is not physically or mentally capable of providing informed consent (Kambam 2017). In those situations, autonomy is overridden by the need to preserve health: the process of obtaining consent may also lead to detrimental effects, and physicians pursue treatment in the patient's best interests based on implied consent to a lifesaving procedure that most reasonable patients would accept. Other important exceptions include situations in which a patient is unable to make treatment decisions and consent is obtained instead from a substitute decision-maker. Patients themselves may opt out of a discussion required for consent, waive the right to receive information, and defer the responsibility of decision-making to the physician, an action known as a *therapeutic waiver of consent*. Involuntary treatment is another exception to patient autonomy and informed consent, which are overridden by interests such as the risk of harm to the patient or third parties.

Other Exceptions

Several contemporary cases demonstrate a tension between the limits of informed consent and government regulations to protect third-party interests. These examples bring to light controversial limits placed on informed consent, particularly those due to the possible harms involved in the process of the provision of information. We offer a brief discussion of these examples here.

Therapeutic privilege is perhaps the most widely known and controversial exception to informed consent. Therapeutic privilege refers to the privilege of physicians to withhold information because disclosure would have harmful effects on the patient by causing psychological distress and damaging decision-making capacity (Kambam 2017). In such a case, the purported promotion of health and nonmaleficence supersedes the patient's right to information. Many types of information are potentially distressing to patients, for instance, disclosures about life-threatening diagnoses or bad outcomes. In the past, many clinicians would often cite therapeutic privilege as their motivation behind withholding information from patients. In fact, it was common practice for clinicians to withhold poor prognoses or likelihood of death for fear of causing unnecessary distress, further worsening patient well-being, and impeding judgment. In reality, it remains unclear what type of information would impede decision-making altogether. In *Canterbury v. Spence* (1972), the courts reported that therapeutic privilege is applicable only where "risk-disclosure poses such a threat of detriment to the patient as to become unfeasible or contraindicted from a medical point of view" and also clarified that anticipated disagreement with patient decisions was insufficient. Interpretation of therapeutic privilege continues to be poorly defined, and although clinicians have attempted to broaden the scope of therapeutic privilege, in very few cases has therapeutic privilege been upheld in courts when legally challenged.

Relatedly, there is a growing body of evidence that informed consent itself can play a role in patient outcomes. The process of providing consent can pose certain harms, including both psychological and physical distress, by priming patients to expect certain negative outcomes. More widely known is the *placebo effect*, the phenomenon whereby individuals' positive expectations of an intervention lead to improvement or positive effects independent of the mechanism of the intervention itself, but there is growing attention to the corollary phenomenon of the *nocebo effect*. In the nocebo effect, negative expectations lead to negative effects independent of an intervention. Similar to therapeutic privilege, this phenomenon presents conflicting duties to the patient around nonmaleficence and autonomy. Research about the nocebo effect remains in its infancy, and standards about how the nocebo effect may inform medical discussions and therapeutic privilege have not yet been established. In clinical practice, physicians already use their discretion to withhold certain information about less common or more benign risks to avoid the nocebo effect.

Physician Gag Laws

Several recent top-down governmental policies in certain states regulate the doctor-patient relationship and place limits on clinician disclosure of information. These cases have caused widespread debate owing to perceptions of the policies being motivated by political and financial interests rather than public health and scientific evidence. Many of the policies have had limited supporting medical evidence, thereby posing significant physical and psychological risks to patients. Although some of these regulations have been repealed, they illustrate the harms of government restrictions on clinician disclosure of information, which is often an important component of acting as fiduciary to patients. For example, in Pennsylvania, Act 13, signed in 2012, included a "medical gag rule" that allowed physicians access to a full list of chemicals used in natural gas drilling if these chemicals were deemed important for diagnosis or treatment. However, the law required clinicians to sign a confidentiality agreement to obtain the data. In doing so, it prohibited them from sharing information with patients and other physicians, limiting the dissemination of knowledge about potentially hazardous chemicals used in the fracking process that caused environmental contamination. Furthermore, the confidentiality agreements also placed restrictions on medical documentation about the chemicals as causative agents, based on the argument that they were industry trade secrets. This state law was heavily influenced by special interests of the oil and gas industry and marked an unusual departure for policymakers to protect these particular industry interests over those of its state citizens and regulate physician free speech. Act 13 was challenged by environmental activists and a physician and was repealed in 2014 by the Pennsylvania Supreme Court.

Conclusion

Physicians hold a fiduciary duty to their patients to act in their best interests and promote patient autonomy by protecting confidentiality and providing informed consent. Although these professional responsibilities have been codified in standards of practice and by regulatory bodies, they are not absolute. Challenges to upholding these funda-mental duties based on competing interests and government regula-tion create dilemmas in professional practice and may, at times, call for special expertise from forensic psychiatrists around navigating these ethically complex situations.

References

Appelbaum PS, Gutheil TG: Clinical Handbook of Psychiatry and the Law. Philadelphia, PA, Lippincott Williams and Wilkins, 2007

Berg JW, Appelbaum PS, Lidz CW, et al: Informed Consent: Legal Theory and Clinical Practice. New York, Oxford University Press, 2001

Bhattacharya D, Ramos L: COVID-19: privacy and confidentiality issues with contact tracing apps, in Proceedings of the 54th Hawaii International Conference on System Sciences, 2021, pp 2009–2018

Canterbury v Spence, 464 F.2d 772 (D.C. Cir. 1972)

Dave D, Deza M, Horn B: Prescription drug monitoring programs, opioid abuse, and crime. South Econ J 87(3):808–848, 2021

Delcher C, Pauly N, Moyo P: Advances in prescription drug monitoring program research: a literature synthesis (June 2018 to December 2019). Curr Opin Psychiatry 33(4):326–333, 2020 32250984

Fink DS, Schleimer JP, Sarvet A, et al: Association between prescription drug monitoring programs and nonfatal and fatal drug overdoses: a systematic review. Ann Intern Med 168(11):783–790, 2018 29801093

Fisher CE: The Urge: Our History of Addiction. New York, Penguin Press, 2022

Goodnough A: Overdose deaths have surged during the pandemic, CDC data shows. The New York Times, April 14, 2021. Available at: https://www.nytimes.com/2021/04/14/health/overdose-deaths-fentanyl-opiods-coronaviurs-pandemic.html. Accessed April 14, 2021.

Holmgren AJ, Botelho A, Brandt AM: A history of prescription drug monitoring programs in the United States: political appeal and public health efficacy. Am J Public Health 110(8):1191–1197, 2020 32552023

Jones CM, Olsen EO, O'Donnell J, et al: Resurgent methamphetamine use at treatment admission in the United States, 2008–2017. Am J Public Health 110(4):509–516, 2020 32078347

Kambam PR: Informed consent and competence, in Principles and Practice of Forensic Psychiatry. Boca Raton, CRC Press, 2017, pp 145–154

Keefe PR: Empire of Pain. New York, Doubleday, 2021

Lembke A, Papac J, Humphreys K: Our other prescription drug problem. N Engl J Med 378(8):693–695, 2018 29466163

Mueller SR, Glanz JM, Nguyen AP, et al: Restrictive opioid prescribing policies and evolving risk environments: a qualitative study of the perspectives of patients who experienced an accidental opioid overdose. Int J Drug Policy 92:103077, 2021 33423916

Netherland J, Hansen HB: The war on drugs that wasn't: wasted whiteness, "dirty doctors," and race in media coverage of prescription opioid misuse. Cult Med Psychiatry 40(4):664–686, 2016 27272904

Code of Federal Regulations. Part 46 -- Protection of Human Subjects. Title 45 (2018)

Salgo v Leland Stanford Etc. Bd. Trustees, 154 Cal.App.2d 560, 317 P.2d 170 (Cal. Ct. App. 1957)

Schloendorff v New York Hospital, 211 N.Y. 125, 105 N.E. 92 (N.Y. 1914)

Tarasoff v Regents of the University of California, 118 Cal Rptr 129, 529 P2d 553 (1974)

Tarasoff v Regents of the University of California, 551 Cal Rptr 14, 551 P2d 334 (1976)

Webster F, Rice K, Katz J, et al: An ethnography of chronic pain management in primary care: the social organization of physicians' work in the midst of the opioid crisis. PLoS One 14(5):e0215148, 2019 31042733

Whalen v Roe, 429 U.S. 589 (1977)

17

Termination of Pregnancy, Ethics, and Decisional Capacity[1]

Susan Hatters Friedman, M.D.

Jacqueline Landess, M.D., J.D.

Nina Ross, M.D.

Aimee Kaempf, M.D.

The decision to have an abortion can be fraught and time-sensitive. A woman's decisional capacity to consent to abortion may be called into question, particularly when she has a psychiatric diagnosis or an intellectual disability. In many states, minors seeking abortions without parental notification may require assessment for capacity. When psychiatrists are called on to assess decisional capacity, they must be aware of their personal feelings about abortion and not allow those opinions to influence their assessment of the woman's capacity for this medical procedure. Psychiatrists must also be knowledgeable about their state laws and about non–research-based beliefs that are promoted regarding the mental health risks of abortion.

[1] The authors gratefully acknowledge the insights of Professor Jessie Hill.

Of late, the landscape has shifted rapidly regarding availability and legality of abortions in America. Before *Roe v. Wade,* a woman's ability to access an abortion was limited. State laws varied, but in many states a woman could obtain an abortion only under certain circumstances, such as if the pregnancy severely impaired her mental or physical health, if the pregnancy was the result of rape or incest, or if the child would be born with severe mental or physical problems (Friedman et al. 2022; Morgan 1979). In *Roe v. Wade* (1973), the U.S. Supreme Court held that prohibiting abortion violated a woman's constitutional right to privacy. Nonetheless, despite the legality of abortion after *Roe v. Wade,* a woman who wished to have an abortion potentially faced many logistical challenges, such as accessing an abortion provider, obtaining an abortion in a timely manner, and navigating logistical and legal requirements. Those challenges could be further exacerbated by psychiatric illness. *Roe v. Wade* was overturned in 2022 with the Supreme Court's ruling in *Dobbs v. Jackson Women's Mental Health Organization* (2022), which limited legal pregnancy terminations and affected psychiatric patients and psychiatrists' practices (Friedman 2023; Friedman et al. 2022).

Steps to Obtaining an Abortion

A woman first needs to be aware that she is pregnant. The average woman is aware of her pregnancy at about 5½ weeks (Branum and Ahrens 2017). About a quarter (23%) of women learn of their pregnancy late, meaning after 7 weeks (Branum and Ahrens 2017). Factors associated with late pregnancy awareness include being younger, having fewer years of education, having lower socioeconomic status, being unmarried, and having an unintended pregnancy (Branum and Ahrens 2017). Women with serious mental illness are more likely to have unplanned and unwanted pregnancies relative to women without serious mental illness (Miller 1997), increasing their odds of late detection of pregnancy.

A woman must then navigate her jurisdiction's legal requirements for abortion, including timeliness. States vary in the timing allowed. Many states prohibit abortions after 22 weeks since the last menstrual period, except when the health or life of the woman is in danger (Guttmacher Institute 2021b), and other states are moving to block abortion entirely. Thus, there is a limited amount of decision-making time between knowledge of pregnancy and abortion. Many states also require abortion counseling; some mandate in-person counseling (Guttmacher Institute 2021b). Many states require that women wait for a period of time between counseling and the actual procedure; this time period ranges from 24 hours to 3 days (Guttmacher Institute 2021b). Access to abortion care therefore may require multiple trips to a provider's office. In addition, accessing a provider to perform the abortion may be an obstacle, especially in rural areas (Guttmacher Institute 2019; Jones et al. 2019). Women with severe mental illness are likely to have less-strong support networks (Miller 1997), which may impair their ability to attend multiple physician appointments in a short period of time.

There are also financial barriers to having an abortion. Several states have restrictions regarding when state funds can be used for an abortion (Guttmacher Institute 2021b). The Hyde Amendment, passed in 1977, prohibits federal Medicaid funding for abortion in the United States unless the abortion endangers the woman's life or was the product of rape or incest (Hyde Amendment Codification Act 2013). Some states have their own policies that require Medicaid to pay for all medically necessary abortions (Guttmacher Institute 2021a). In practice, however, barriers to proving these circumstances (in a timely fashion and given travel necessities) limit coverage for qualifying abortions (Kacanek et al. 2010). Even if an abortion is legally allowed, a woman may face additional challenges. Navigating insurance coverage may present a further barrier for a woman who wishes to obtain an abortion; private insurance companies in many states also limit coverage for abortions (Guttmacher Institute 2021b).

Patients with psychiatric illness may have illness exacerbations during pregnancy, creating further barriers to obtaining an abortion. Psychiatric illness exacerbations have varying and often unpredictable rates of resolution. A woman who has been psychiatrically hospitalized or incarcerated may face additional barriers to obtaining an abortion, including institutional regulations regarding such services as well as unclear practices for assessing a woman's capacity to consent to an abortion. Capacity to consent to an abortion should be evaluated as would capacity to consent to any other medical procedure. However, providers may perceive that capacity to consent to an abortion requires a higher threshold of capacity, possibly because of discomfort with the topic of abortion itself.

Of note, there has been much interest in potential psychiatric sequelae of abortions. Research has established that abortion does not worsen mental health and that mental health prior to an abortion is the most reliable predictor of mental health after an abortion (Steinberg et al. 2016). Nonetheless, at the time of this writing, 22 states require that a woman seeking an abortion receive counseling about psychological sequela of an abortion, and 8 of those states mandate inclusion of information about negative emotional responses to abortions (Guttmacher Institute 2021b). *Roe v. Wade* (1973) itself noted that unwanted pregnancy or motherhood could itself cause significant psychological harm. Abortion has not been demonstrated to negatively impact mental health outcomes; research positing that abortion negatively impacts mental health has had serious methodological flaws, including omission of conflicting data and conflation of association with causation. For example, a study that posited that abortion causes mental health problems failed to evaluate pre-abortion rates of mental health problems (Robinson et al. 2012) and thus did not address a major confounding factor, that is, pre-abortion mental health, nor did it establish a temporal relationship between the abortion and mental health sequelae (Robinson et al. 2012). In fact, the development of methodologically flawed papers in this area is so pronounced that the American Psychological Association has called for caution when interpreting studies in this field (American Psychological Association 2008). These methodological flaws include comparisons to inappropriate control groups, inadequate controlling for confounding variables, poor definition and assessment of outcomes being measured, and interpretation problems such as interpreting correlation as causation (American Psychological Association 2008). Studies that are more rigorously designed, with careful attention to best statistical practice, have demonstrated that abortion does not worsen mental health outcomes (Biggs et al. 2015, 2016, 2017; Foster et al. 2015; Steinberg et al. 2016). Rather, women who were denied a wanted abortion often had worsened mental health outcomes compared with women who were able to obtain a wanted abortion (Biggs et al. 2015, 2016, 2017; Foster et al. 2015; Steinberg et al. 2016). Despite this strong evidence base, physicians in some states are legally required to counsel their patients that abortion causes adverse mental health problems (Guttmacher Institute 2021b). Physicians in those states therefore face an ethical dilemma: choosing between the state's legal requirements and accurately communicating evidence-based information to their patients. Physicians should consider providing the context for the information that they are required to provide, and thus may mitigate some impact of the inaccuracies.

Informed Consent

Informed consent is the process whereby communication between a clinician and a patient helps a patient to make knowledgeable decisions about medical care. Informed consent is an ethical and legal obligation stemming from an individual's right to determine what happens to their own body. As Justice Benjamin Cardozo noted: "Every human being of adult years and sound mind has a right to determine what shall be done with his own body" (*Schloendorff v. Society of New York Hospitals* 1914). Without a patient's informed consent, a physician is not authorized to provide nonemergent treatment. Informed consent consists of three basic components: 1) competency of the patient to make decisions, 2) disclosure to the patient of relevant information, and 3) lack of coercion (or voluntariness) in decision-making (American Medical Association 2016). Standards for what information must be disclosed by providers to meet informed consent requirements differ by state but generally include the following (American Medical Association 2016):

1. The diagnosis or medical condition;
2. The nature and purpose of the proposed intervention;
3. The risks and benefits of the proposed intervention; and
4. The risks and benefits of other treatment options, including forgoing treatment.

Adequate and appropriate information is usually based on a reasonable physician or reasonable patient standard and includes such details as the nature, risk, and benefits of a procedure along with available alternatives. State laws might further define the scope of reasonable disclosure; for instance, in Wisconsin, physicians are not required to disclose "extremely remote possibilities [of medical treatment] that might falsely or detrimentally alarm the patient" (Medical Practices 2020).

Medical Decision-Making Capacity

Medical decision-making capacity, an essential element of informed consent, refers to a patient's ability to make informed decisions about treatment. Four key skills are involved: 1) the ability to communicate choices, 2) the ability to understand relevant information, 3) the ability to appreciate the situation and its consequences, and 4) the ability to rationally manipulate information (Appelbaum and Grisso 1988). Medical decision-making capacity may fluctuate over time, depending on a patient's mental state, and is task specific, with higher-stakes decisions requiring more stringent criteria for competency (Appelbaum and Grisso 1988). The ethics principle of autonomy dictates that patients should be involved in health care decisions to the greatest extent possible, in accordance with decision-making capacity (American Medical Association 2016). Adults are presumed to have medical decision-making capacity unless determined otherwise (American Medical Association 2016).

Informed Consent and Abortion

In the United States, approximately 50% of all pregnancies are unintended, and 18%–21% of pregnancies end in abortion (Jones and Jerman 2017). The informed-consent process is especially important when a woman is considering whether to terminate a pregnancy, because such decisions are time-sensitive, irreversible, and life-changing (American College of Obstetricians and Gynecologists 2021; Ross et. al 2022b). Capacity to consent to an abortion should be evaluated similarly to capacity to consent to any serious, irreversible medical procedure (Friedman et al. 2022). The decision-making process may be complicated by the presence of conflicting views among involved parties, sociopolitical controversies, and powerful emotions elicited among patients and health care providers (American College of Obstetricians and Gynecologists 2021). Even when a woman is certain of the decision to receive an abortion, she may experience emotional, spiritual, or moral ambivalence that should be explored, normalized, and validated (Perrucci 2012). Ambivalence surrounding important life choices is common and does not signify an underlying mental disorder or preclude women from having medical decision-making capacity (Brody et al. 2016).

The American College of Obstetricians and Gynecologists (ACOG) recommends a shared decision-making model of informed consent that emphasizes a patient-centered discussion of treatment options within the framework of the patient's own values and preferences. Pre-abortion counseling entails a comprehensive, accurate, and understandable explanation of all available pregnancy termination options, including the risks and benefits of each. When reviewing alternatives to abortion, such as continuing pregnancy and adoption, clinicians should take an impartial, nondirective approach. Efforts by the clinician to influence or persuade a woman in her decision undermine professional integrity and violate ethical obligations of respect for patient autonomy, beneficence, and nonmaleficence (American College of Obstetricians and Gynecologists 2021).

In the United States, nearly all states allow health care providers to refuse abortion services on the grounds of conscientious objection

(Guttmacher Institute 2021b). Conscientious objection is based on the physician's right to protect their own moral integrity and may conflict with other professional and ethical duties, including those related to the informed-consent process. Clinicians who conscientiously refuse to provide abortion services are obligated to provide prior notice of their objection to potential patients and to impart unbiased, scientifically accurate, and professionally accepted information regarding reproductive health choices so that patients may make informed decisions about care. Providers refusing abortions on moral or religious grounds have a duty to refer patients considering pregnancy termination in a timely manner to providers who do offer such services (American College of Obstetricians and Gynecologists 2007).

In some U.S. jurisdictions, policies designed to restrict abortion access confound the informed-consent process by mandating that abortion providers present women with government-authored materials regarding fetal development and possible physical and psychological repercussions of abortion, some of which may be medically inaccurate or misleading (Daniels et al. 2016; Vandewalker 2012).

Informed-Consent Laws

Abortion "informed-consent" laws are controversial. Many require the physician to disclose specific and detailed information that may be related only peripherally or not at all to the information needed for adequate informed consent. In *Planned Parenthood of Southeastern PA v. Casey* (1992), the court upheld the constitutionality of an abortion informed-consent law in Pennsylvania. The court found that the state had an "important and legitimate interest in potential life" that was established "from the outset of the pregnancy" such that "states are free to enact laws to provide a reasonable framework for a woman to make a decision that has such profound and lasting meaning." The court found that abortion informed-consent laws did not violate physician-patient privacy and stated that information provided to the woman should be truthful, realistic, nonjudgmental, and scientifically accurate.

Many states require women to receive counseling before an abortion, including requiring physicians to provide certain information to the patient before the procedure, often in the form of state-produced written materials (Guttmacher Institute 2021b). Typically, state health departments develop these "informed-consent" brochures. It is not clear whether knowledgeable medical professionals are always consulted in the development of these materials, and Daniels et al. (2016) found that up to one-third of statements in state-sponsored informed-consent materials were medically inaccurate.

The type of information provided to the patient is not typical of that provided for other medical procedures; for instance, women may be given graphic accounts of the abortion surgical techniques and in-depth descriptions of fetal development throughout all stages of pregnancy, even if the woman is seeking a first-trimester termination. Other examples of "informed-consent" provisions include the following:

1. Women may be told that there is a potential association between abortions and breast cancer, even though the National Cancer Institute and other experts have issued categorical statements to the contrary (National Cancer Institute 2010).
2. Some states inform women that abortions lead to an increased risk of infertility. This information is misleading, because the conditions in question (for example, uterine infection) are quite rare and, even when they do occur, do not always lead to infertility (Hakim-Elahi et al. 1990).
3. Women may be told that they could experience a range of psychological consequences following an abortion, despite evidence that the best predictor of a woman's mental health following an abortion is the state of her mental health before the procedure (Steinberg et al. 2016).
4. Some states mandate ultrasounds before an abortion and require the provider to offer the woman an opportunity to view the fetal image or hear the fetal heartbeat (Gold and Nash 2007). For instance, a Kentucky law required the physician to describe fetal anatomy to the patient before the abortion and required the patient to listen to the fetal heartbeat. This law was appealed by the American Civil Liberties Union (ACLU) and progressed to the U.S. Supreme Court. The high court declined to hear the appeal, leaving the law in place (SCOTUSblog 2021).
5. Some states require physicians to inform a woman seeking a medically induced abortion that the abortion may be reversed, even though the American Medical Association and others have stated that there is no medical evidence to support this claim.

Importantly, two-thirds of women seeking abortions live in a state where physicians are required to give women these state-authored informational "informed-consent" packets (Daniels et al. 2016).

Critics contend that abortion "informed-consent" laws undermine patient autonomy and privacy and are thinly veiled attempts to restrict or discourage abortions through shame, fear, and other tactics (Gold and Nash 2007; Vandewalker 2012). Defenders of these laws contend that women are unaware of the psychological consequences of abortion and should thus be fully informed before proceeding; this thinking extends to the Supreme Court: Justice Anthony Kennedy commented, "While we find no reliable data to measure the phenomenon, it seems unexceptionable to conclude some women come to regret their choice to abort the infant life they once created and sustained. Severe depression and loss of esteem can follow" (*Gonzales v. Carhart* 2007).

Abortion and Mental Illness/Intellectual Disability

Historically, women with psychiatric illness or intellectual disability have been denied reproductive rights, including access to abortion (American College of Obstetricians and Gynecologists 2017). Women with mental disorders have several risk factors for pregnancy complications and unintended or unwanted pregnancies, including higher rates of contraception non-adherence, sexual victimization, risky sexual encounters, substance use, and medical comorbidities; thus pregnancy termination is a relevant consideration in this group.

The presence of a mental disorder does not equate to incapacity, and pro forma assessment of decision-making capacity for women requesting abortion is not necessary. Nonetheless, when a woman with psychiatric illness or intellectual disability seeks an abortion, medical decision-making capacity can be called into question. Capacity assessment involves a detailed discussion with the patient regarding the pregnancy and available options using clear, understandable language with an emphasis on determining whether she appreciates her current situation and the consequences of termination versus carrying the pregnancy to term (Zalpuri et al. 2015). Given that women with mental disorders may be susceptible to coercion by partners or others, it is important to ascertain that whatever the woman's choice, it is voluntary and free of any undue influence (Zalpuri et al. 2015).

If a woman is found to lack decisional capacity regarding pregnancy care, clinicians should determine whether capacity can be restored and, if so, work to treat the cause of incapacitation so that the patient may participate in the informed-consent process to the greatest degree possible

(Zalpuri et al. 2015). In situations where capacity cannot be restored, a suitable surrogate must be identified (American Medical Association 2016). Surrogate decision-making typically follows a substituted judgment standard, whereby decisions are made based on the patient's previously expressed preferences and values, if known (American College of Obstetricians and Gynecologists 2021). A best-interest standard may be applied in situations where a woman's wishes are unknown or a patient has never had the capacity to make informed health care decisions (American College of Obstetricians and Gynecologists 2021). Even patients who lack full medical decision-making capacity should be included in the process wherever possible to bolster substituted judgment and maximize autonomy. Some jurisdictions limit the power of surrogate decision-makers with regard to pregnancy termination, and additional legal or administrative procedures may be needed (Zalpuri et al. 2015). Strategizing and anticipating reproductive needs with women while they have medical decision-making capacity can help to avoid future ethical dilemmas and guide treatment decisions, should psychiatric decompensation occur (Acera Pozzi et al. 2014).

Guardianship and Abortion

Guardianship is founded on the concept of *parens patriae*, which allows a state to intervene on behalf of a citizen who needs protection, lacks decision-making capacity, and cannot care for themselves owing to psychiatric, intellectual, cognitive, or other impairment. A judge or commissioner in a probate court determines whether guardianship should be granted on an emergency, temporary, or permanent basis. The ward may be under a limited (also known as a partial) guardianship (for instance, needing a guardian only to make financial decisions) or a full guardianship. Interestingly, limited or partial guardianships are ordered much less frequently than are full guardianships (Teaster et al. 2007). Often, a guardian may be a family member or friend, but approximately one-quarter of guardians are professional guardians with no prior knowledge of the individual (Teaster et al. 2007).

In making a judicial determination regarding guardianship, judges often rely on clinical evaluations of capacity. Definitions and procedural requirements of incapacity and the standards clinicians must follow when evaluating capacity vary considerably by state; a 2007 survey (Moye et al. 2007) noted that 30 states required clinical evaluation of capacity, 15 states left it to the discretion of the judge, and 5 states provided no guidance in the matter.

Once guardianship is granted, the guardian should follow established statutory standards (when they exist) in making decisions for the ward. Of note, multiple states provide no decision-making standard for the guardian to use when making medical decisions (Cohen et al. 2015). Other states follow a *substituted judgment* or a *best interests* standard, the first standard asking what the ward would have decided if competent, and the second asking what is best for the ward, using an "objective" standard. However, the ward's communicated preferences should be taken into account even under the best-interests model (French 2005; McCaman 2013).

States may also enumerate specific medical decisions the ward may make independently or only with guardianship approval. Most state laws do not comment on a ward's evaluative capacity to consent to an abortion. This presents a potential dilemma, particularly in cases where the woman's communicated desires do not align with the guardian's.

A Florida case, *Lefebvre v. N. Broward Hospital District* (1990), illustrates this dilemma. Ms. Lefebvre was treated for bipolar disorder and psychosis for years with lithium. She stopped taking lithium when she discovered she was pregnant and rapidly decompensated to the point of requiring involuntary admission to the psychiatric hospital. She also was not given lithium during her hospital admission because of an opinion that lithium would severely damage the fetus. A hospital psychiatrist filed a petition with the court stating it would be in Lefebvre's and the fetus's best interests to terminate the pregnancy, as she would continue to be dangerous without lithium. The petition was also supported by Lefebvre's father, who was appointed as a "guardian advocate" by the court. At least one staff member testified that Lefebvre communicated a desire to continue with the pregnancy. Ultimately, the trial court authorized North Broward Hospital to seek an abortion.

The appellate court reversed the trial court's decision because the court had not followed proper statutory procedure. Under Florida law, this included appointing an attorney to act on the incapacitated person's behalf; obtaining independent medical, psychological, and social evaluations of the person; holding a judicial meeting with the incapacitated person allowing the person "to express his or her personal views or desires"; and finding by clear and convincing evidence that the person lacked capacity to consent to an abortion. A guardian would then be appointed on the incapacitated person's behalf, and the guardian must obtain court approval for the abortion (Fla. Stat. Ann. 2020a, 2020b). Florida's scheme is time-intensive but implements procedural safeguards that ensure a woman's preference is heard by the court. Furthermore, a guardian is specifically appointed for the purpose of determining whether an abortion is in the woman's best interest. (Of note, these guardianship laws do not extend to the fetus.) In *In re Guardianship of J.D.S.* (2004), the wife of a Florida state attorney attempted to seek fetal guardianship of a severely intellectually disabled woman's fetus, under the presumption that the woman might obtain a guardian and seek an abortion. The court held that fetal guardianship was not proper or allowed under the existing statutes.

In summary, abortions for women who are under or needing guardianship are minimally addressed in the existing literature. It appears that most states do not explicitly address capacity to consent to abortions in their guardianship laws, so it is not clear how this dilemma is approached when the question arises. Given the state-to-state variability in guardianship clinical evaluations and standards of incapacity, women under guardianship may still retain the ability, to some degree, to assist their guardian in making certain medical or reproductive decisions. The woman's preference should be taken into consideration when using either a substituted-judgment or best-interests standard, and statutory guidance should be followed when it is available.

Minors, Informed Consent for Abortion, and Judicial Bypass

Many states have parental involvement laws requiring that pregnant teenagers younger than 18 notify at least one parent (or the parent provide consent) for the minor to obtain an abortion (Hawkins 2018). However, in America, once a woman has had her eighteenth birthday, she is considered an adult and able to make her own health care decisions. These laws stem from the dual ideas that these adolescent females need protection and the teens' parents' rights require protection. Similar to adult women who obtain abortions, adolescents do not appear to have increased difficulties with self-esteem or depression either in the short term or up to 5 years postabortion (Warren et al. 2010). Stotland (2011) noted a lack of evidence that parental consent improved outcomes and suggested that it may even lead to violence or exclusion from the family.

In 1979, the U.S. Supreme Court ruled in *Bellotti v. Baird* (1979) that a Massachusetts law that required minors to seek or obtain parental consent before an abortion was unconstitutional. The court emphasized that minors must have an alternative to parental consent to abortion, such as seeking judicial authorization, noting that minors should be allowed to prove they are mature and possess adequate decision-making capabilities to pursue an abortion rather than relying solely on an "absolute third-party veto." The justices sought to balance the parental interest in raising their (pregnant) minor with the rights of the minor. *Judicial bypass for abortion* is the mechanism through which pregnant minors can obtain an abortion without parental consent by petitioning the court. This procedure exists in the majority of states (Hawkins 2018). Hawkins (2018) noted that many states use a standard of "clear and convincing evidence," with the burden of proof being on the minor. To grant a judicial bypass of parental consent for abortion, the court must generally determine either that the young woman is "sufficiently mature and well enough informed to intelligently decide whether to have an abortion" or that notifying her parents is not in her best interest, usually owing to maltreatment (Friedman et al. 2015, p. 401).

To obtain a judicial bypass, the pregnant adolescent must research her options, decide not to alert her parents to her pregnancy, and likely skip school to meet her attorney and file her case. Further hurdles are obtaining medical proof of pregnancy and proof of having completed pre-abortion counseling and a mental health evaluation before the court date. For the pregnant minor to navigate the barriers judicial bypass presents, she must be proactive (Friedman et al. 2015). In a study of 55 Jane Doe anonymous judicial bypass assessments completed at a metropolitan Ohio juvenile court psychiatric clinic (Friedman et al. 2015), the majority of the pregnant adolescents pursuing judicial bypass were 16 and older. Most held part-time jobs and were in long-term relationships with the involved male. Although this group of pregnant adolescents had not discussed the decision to have an abortion with their parents, most had discussed the abortion and options with a trusted adult. Despite the politically charged nature of this assessment, 95% were eventually granted a judicial bypass. Friedman et al. (2015) noted that "this may represent a selection bias for those pregnant minors who were persistent, proactive, assertive, and informed about the judicial bypass option, have better nonparental supports, and who are better able to overcome the barriers of this challenging process" (p. 40).

Age 16 is often considered the age of consent for sexual activity, so the distinction between the age of 16 for sexual activity and an average age above 16 among those seeking a judicial bypass for abortion may be seen as a logical conflict. Further, 16-year-olds are allowed to obtain a driver's license, are able to be charged in adult court, and can serve adult sentences. Finally, minors are allowed to obtain treatment for sexually transmitted infections without parental consent and are allowed to access contraception without parental involvement in Title X–funded programs, which are both medical issues related to reproduction. As Friedman et al. (2015) noted, "thus society has accepted the premise that adolescents, even before the age of 18, can make decisions on their own of great importance and are already being held responsible for these decisions" (p. 403).

Steinberg et al. (2009) have researched adolescent decision-making and found that mid-aged adolescents possess the capacity to make medical decisions similar to that of adults when there are not time constraints or increased stress and when there are adequate supports. Of note, in the Jane Doe study mentioned earlier, adolescents had discussed the pregnancy with the involved male or a trusted adult, such as a counselor or a friend's parents. They had various reasons for not discussing their pregnancy and abortion plans with their own parents, such as fears of violence or of being kicked out of the house.

A Chicago study (Kavanagh et al. 2012) indicated that among pregnant minors presenting for abortion, most had discussed their options with an adult, be it their parents or another adult. Two Arkansas studies (Altindag and Joyce 2017; Joyce 2010) noted that approximately 1 in 10 adolescent abortions occurred through the judicial bypass procedure. Of note, those seeking judicial bypass in Arkansas were likely to be 17 years old, to be Hispanic and non-residents of Arkansas (crossing state lines), and to have fewer previous pregnancies than those who had abortions with parental involvement (Altindag and Joyce 2017).

A study examining the well-organized Illinois Judicial Bypass Coordination Project's data from 2017 and 2018 found that most minors using this mechanism were 17 years old. They sought the bypass for various concerns, which included being forced to continue pregnancy, fears of being kicked out of the house, a poor relationship with their parents, and fears of abuse (Ralph et al. 2021). In Illinois, they traveled an average of 24 miles to the courthouse (range of 1–270 miles). On average, almost a week (6.4 days) elapsed between the bypass request and the hearing. A wait time of a week and the need to travel may be critical in this abortion timeline, especially in a population likely to discover pregnancy later. (And this study was in a state that has a well-organized network.)

Twenty teens who had sought a judicial bypass for abortion in Texas (Coleman-Minahan et al. 2019) were interviewed about their experiences. These young women described difficulty getting away from school and obtaining transportation. They also "described the bypass process as 'intimidating' and 'scary' and described judges and guardians-ad-litem who shamed them, 'preached' at them, and discredited evidence of their maturity" (p. 20). Coleman-Minahan and colleagues noted, "We found the bypass process functions as a form of punishment and allows state actors to humiliate adolescents for their personal decisions. The bypass process was implemented to protect adolescents from alleged negative emotional consequences of abortion, yet our results suggest the bypass process itself causes emotional harm through unpredictability and humiliation" (p. 20).

Psychiatrists have provided opinions about abortions since before *Roe v. Wade,* given the pre–*Roe v. Wade* restrictions on abortions except in limited circumstances, such as a pregnancy posing a serious risk to maternal mental health (Friedman et al. 2022). Ironically, if a teenager is found not to be competent to provide informed consent in cases of abortion and does not obtain parental consent for the abortion, she will be expected to make decisions about prenatal care, delivery, and parenthood in only a few months' time.

The question the evaluating psychiatrist should ask in completing a judicial bypass evaluation is whether the minor should be considered "mature" and "informed." An assessment of the pregnant teenager's capacity to provide informed consent should be made. In doing such an assessment, one should be aware that in general there are fewer psychiatric and medical risks from abortion compared with vaginal delivery or C-section. As with other assessments of informed consent, does the teen have sufficient capacity, understand her options, demonstrate appropriate reasoning ability, and make the decision voluntarily and knowingly? Specifically, is the decision to have an abortion considered rational and well informed? Is it consistent with the adolescent's personal values? And finally, is there any coercion or inappropriate influence from others in making this decision? (Friedman et al. 2015).

Post-*Dobbs* Considerations

In the current American legal landscape, several additional issues bear consideration in the ethical practice of psychiatry. One must consider that the current illegality of abortion in some states can itself negatively impact mental health, and that there are significant consequences of being forced to carry an unwanted pregnancy (Ross et al. 2022a). This will disproportionately impact already marginalized populations, including psychiatric patients (Friedman et al. 2022). Further, as psychiatric patients are at elevated risk of unintentional pregnancies, psychiatrists should feel comfortable counseling their patients about emergency contraception options in advance of need, to encourage appropriate use (Makino et al. 2022). With abortion statutes now varying across states and continuing to shift, psychiatrists should be aware of the laws in their own jurisdictions. In states in which abortion has become criminalized, additional laws may be passed in which physicians are required to report their pregnant women patients; ethical considerations apply (Friedman et al. 2022), and psychiatrists should discuss the issue with their malpractice insurers (Landess et al. 2023).

Conclusion

Abortion-related choices are among the most profound and complex decisions encountered in medicine. Although the presence of serious mental illness, intellectual disability, or young age (adolescence) should not be a presumption of incapacity, some women with these conditions may have their decision-making capacity questioned. In some cases, capacity may fluctuate over time or be permanently impaired. Women should share in reproductive planning and care to the greatest extent possible without being pressured or coerced by others. Many poorly designed studies exist that make an association between abortion and damaged mental health. However, the best predictor of mental health after an abortion is mental health before the abortion.

American women face many barriers to obtaining an abortion, including medical misinformation promulgated by some so-called informed-consent statutes. In some situations, ethical and legal obligations conflict, and psychiatrists should be familiar with federal, state, and local requirements. Coordination of care between obstetrical and mental health teams can help ensure that patients are not deprived of medical decision-making rights while also protecting incapacitated individuals from making choices they may later regret. Psychiatrists completing evaluations of decisional capacity for abortion must be cautious not to let personal opinions about abortion bias their evaluations of capacity to consent to this medical procedure.

References

Acera Pozzi R, Yee LM, Brown K, et al: Pregnancy in the severely mentally ill patient as an opportunity for global coordination of care. Am J Obstet Gynecol 210(1):32–37, 2014 23911382

Altindag O, Joyce T: Judicial bypass for minors seeking abortions in Arkansas versus other states. Am J Public Health 107(8):1266–1271, 2017 28640684

American College of Obstetricians and Gynecologists: ACOG Committee Opinion No. 385: the limits of conscientious refusal in reproductive medicine. Obstet Gynecol 110(5):1203–1208, 2007 17978145

American College of Obstetricians and Gynecologists: ACOG Committee Opinion No. 695: sterilization of women: ethical issues and considerations. Obstet Gynecol 129(4):e109–e116, 2017 28333823

American College of Obstetricians and Gynecologists: ACOG Committee Opinion No. 819: informed consent and shared decision making in obstetrics and gynecology. Obstet Gynecol 137:e34–e41, 2021 33481530

American Medical Association: Opinions on Consent, Communication & Decision Making. AMA Code of Medical Ethics, 2016. Available at: https://www.ama-assn.org/sites/default/files/media-browser/code-of-medical-ethics-chapter-2.pdf. Accessed February 19, 2021.

American Psychological Association, Task Force on Mental Health and Abortion: Report of the APA Task Force on Mental Health and Abortion. 2008. Available at: http://www.apa.org/pi/wpo/mental-health-abortion-report.pdf. Accessed July 16, 2024.

Appelbaum PS, Grisso T: Assessing patients' capacities to consent to treatment. N Engl J Med 319(25):1635–1638, 1988 3200278

Bellotti v. Baird, 443 U.S. 622 (1979)

Biggs MA, Neuhaus JM, Foster DG: Mental health diagnoses 3 years after receiving or being denied an abortion in the United States. Am J Public Health 105(12):2557–2563, 2015 26469674

Biggs MA, Rowland B, McCulloch CE, et al: Does abortion increase women's risk for post-traumatic stress? Findings from a prospective longitudinal cohort study. BMJ Open 6(2):e009698, 2016 26832431

Biggs MA, Upadhyay UD, McCulloch CE, et al: Women's mental health and well-being 5 years after receiving or being denied an abortion: a prospective, longitudinal cohort study. JAMA Psychiatry 74(2):169–178, 2017 27973641

Branum AM, Ahrens KA: Trends in timing of pregnancy awareness among US women. Matern Child Health J 21(4):715–726, 2017 27449777

Brody BD, Chaudhry SK, Penzner JB, et al: A woman with major depression with psychotic features requesting a termination of pregnancy. Am J Psychiatry 173(1):12–15, 2016 26725341

Cohen AB, Wright MS, Cooney L Jr, et al: Guardianship and end-of-life decision making. JAMA Intern Med 175(10):1687–1691, 2015 26258634

Coleman-Minahan K, Stevenson AJ, et al: Young women's experiences obtaining judicial bypass for abortion in Texas. J Adolesc Health 64(1):20–25, 2019 30197199

Daniels CR, Ferguson J, Howard G, et al: Informed or misinformed consent? Abortion policy in the United States. J Health Polit Policy Law 41(2):181–209, 2016 26732319

Dobbs v Jackson Women's Health Organization 597 U.S. 215 (2022)

Fla. Stat. Ann. § 744.3215(4)(e) (2020a)

Fla. Stat. Ann. § 744.3725 (2020b)

Foster DG, Steinberg JR, Roberts SC, et al: A comparison of depression and anxiety symptom trajectories between women who had an abortion and women denied one. Psychol Med 45(10):2073–2082, 2015 25628123

French CM: Protecting the "right" to choose of women who are incompetent: ethical, doctrinal, and practical arguments against fetal representation. Case West Reserve Law Rev 56(2):511, 2005

Friedman SH: Searching for the whole truth: considering culture and gender in forensic psychiatric practice. J Am Acad Psychiatry Law 51(1):23–34, 2023 36732028

Friedman SH, Hendrix T, Haberman J, et al: Judicial bypass of parental consent for abortion: characteristics of pregnant minor "Jane Doe's." J Nerv Ment Dis 203(6):401–405, 2015 26034870

Friedman SH, Landess J, Ross N, et al: Evolving abortion law and forensic psychiatry. J Am Acad Psychiatry Law 50(4):494–501, 2022 36535784

Gold RB, Nash E: State abortion counseling policies and the fundamental principles of informed consent. Guttmacher Policy Rev 10(4):6–13, 2007

Gonzales v Carhart, 550 U.S. 124 (2007)

Guttmacher Institute: Abortion Incidence and Service Availability in the United States, 2017. 2019. Available at: https://www.guttmacher.org/report/abortion-incidence-service-availability-us-2017. Accessed July 16, 2024.

Guttmacher Institute: Medicaid coverage of abortion. 2021a. Available at: https://www.guttmacher.org/evidence-you-can-use/medicaid-coverage-abortion. Accessed July 16, 2024.

Guttmacher Institute: An overview of abortion laws. 2021b. Available at: https://www.guttmacher.org/state-policy/explore/overview-abortion-laws. Accessed July 16, 2024.

Hakim-Elahi E, Tovell HM, Burnhill MS: Complications of first-trimester abortion: a report of 170,000 cases. Obstet Gynecol 76(1):129–135, 1990 2359559

Hawkins H: Clearly unconvincing: how heightened evidentiary standards in judicial bypass hearings create an undue burden under whole woman's health. Am Univ Law Rev 67(6):1911–1945, 2018

Hyde Amendment Codification Act, U.S.C. § S.142 (2013)

In re Guardianship of J.D.S., 864 So. 2d 534 (2004)

Jones RK, Jerman J: Population group abortion rates and lifetime incidence of abortion: United States, 2008–2014. Am J Public Health 107(12):1904–1909, 2017 29048970

Jones RK, Witwer E, Jerman J: Abortion Incidence and Service Availability in the United States, 2017. Guttmacher Institute, 2019. Available at: https://www.guttmacher.org/report/abortion-incidence-service-availability-us-2017. https://doi.org/10.1363/2019.30760. Accessed January 13, 2025.

Joyce T: Parental consent for abortion and the judicial bypass option in Arkansas: effects and correlates. Perspect Sex Reprod Health 42(3):168–175, 2010 20887286

Kacanek D, Dennis A, Miller K, et al: Medicaid funding for abortion: providers' experiences with cases involving rape, incest and life endangerment. Perspect Sex Reprod Health 42(2):79–86, 2010 20618746

Kavanagh EK, Hasselbacher LA, Betham B, et al: Abortion-seeking minors' views on the Illinois parental notification law: a qualitative study. Perspect Sex Reprod Health 44(3):159–166, 2012 22958660

Landess J, Friedman SH, Kaempf A, et al: Abortion and the psychiatrist: practicing in post-Dobbs America. Psychiatr Times 40(1):16–17, 2023

Lefebvre v N. Broward Hospital District, 566 So. 2d 568 (1990)

Makino K, Friedman SH, Amin J, et al: Emergency contraception in psychiatric care. Curr Psychiatr 21(11):34–45, 2022

McCaman E: Limitations on choice: abortion for women with diminished capacity. Hastings Women's Law Journal 24(1):155–176, 2013

Medical Practices, Wis. Stat. § 448.30 (2020)

Miller LJ: Sexuality, reproduction, and family planning in women with schizophrenia. Schizophr Bull 23(4):623–635, 1997 9365999

Morgan RG: Roe v Wade and the lesson of the pre-Roe case law. Mich Law Rev 77(7):1724–1748, 1979 10245969

Moye J, Butz SW, Marson DC, et al: A conceptual model and assessment template for capacity evaluation in adult guardianship. Gerontologist 47(5):591–603, 2007 17989401

National Cancer Institute: Abortion, Miscarriage, and Breast Cancer Risk: 2003 Workshop. 2010. Available at: https://www.cancer.gov/types/breast/abortion-miscarriage-risk#summary-report. Accessed July 16, 2024.

Perrucci A: Decision Assessment and Counseling in Abortion Care: Philosophy and Practice. Lanham, MD, Roman and Littlefield, 2012

Planned Parenthood of Southeastern PA v Casey, 505 U.S. 833 (1992)

Ralph LJ, Chaiten L, Werth E, et al: Reasons for and logistical burdens of judicial bypass for abortion in Illinois. J Adolesc Health 68(1):71–78, 2021 33041202

Robinson GE, Stotland NL, Nadelson CC: Abortion and mental health: guidelines for proper scientific conduct ignored. Br J Psychiatry 200(1):78–80, 2012 22215872

Roe v Wade, 410 U.S. 113 (1973)

Ross N, Landess J, Kaempf A, et al: Pregnancy termination: what psychiatrists need to know. Curr Psychiatr 21(8):8–9, 2022a

Ross NE, Webster TG, Tastenhoye CA, et al: Reproductive decision-making capacity in women of childbearing age with psychiatric illness: a systematic review. J Acad Consult Liaison Psychiatry 63(1):61–70, 2022b 34461294

Schloendorff v. Society of New York Hospital, 105 N.E. 92 (N.Y. 1914)

SCOTUSblog: EMW Women's Surgical Center v Meier, Petition for Certiorari. December 9, 2019. Available at: https://www.scotusblog.com/case-files/cases/emw-womens-surgical-center-v-meier/. Accessed July 16, 2024.

Steinberg L, Cauffman E, Woolard J, et al: Are adolescents less mature than adults? Minors' access to abortion, the juvenile death penalty, and the alleged APA "flip-flop." Am Psychol 64(7):583–594, 2009 19824745

Steinberg JR, Tschann JM, Furgerson D, et al: Psychosocial factors and pre-abortion psychological health: the significance of stigma. Soc Sci Med 150:67–75, 2016 26735332

Stotland NL: Induced abortion and adolescent mental health. Curr Opin Obstet Gynecol 23(5):340–343, 2011 21836505

Teaster P, Wood E, Lawrence S, et al: Wards of the state: a national study of public guardianship. Stetson Law Rev 37:193–241, 2007

Vandewalker I: Abortion and informed Consent: how biased counseling laws mandate violations of medical ethics. Mich J Gend Law 19(1):1, 2012

Warren JT, Harvey SM, Henderson JT: Do depression and low self-esteem follow abortion among adolescents? Evidence from a national study. Perspect Sex Reprod Health 42(4):230–235, 2010 21126298

Zalpuri I, Byatt N, Gramann SB, et al: Decisional capacity in pregnancy: a complex case of pregnancy termination. Psychosomatics 56(3):292–297, 2015 25591494

18

Clinical Requests for Hastened Death in Individuals With Mental Illness

An Examination of Advance Directives and Physician Assistance in Dying

Michael F. Zito, M.D.

The ethical delivery of end-of-life care involves special considerations for individuals with mental illness, especially surrounding requests for hastened death. The clinician must contextualize such requests with relevant ethical, legal, and clinical factors, such as the relationship of the request to the individual's psychopathology. This chapter provides some grounding that can be used to think about these requests as they occur or as they are discussed in potential policy or law. First, predocumented treatment refusals are examined as they relate to care given after a suicide attempt, using the well-known case of Kerrie Wooltorton as an anchoring point. Then, issues related to physician-assisted death (PAD; also termed physician assistance in dying) are discussed. This second section summarizes the arguments for and against the act of providing these services when the individual's suffering stems from mental illness alone. These controversial topics are relevant to modern clinical practice and illustrate a framework for ethical decision-making that can be applied broadly. They also represent an area of practice that is actively evolving. The reader ought to be aware of the current state of policy and law in the relevant jurisdiction and the ethical standards being used. This is especially important because laws surrounding physician-assisted death are changing rapidly.

Advance Directives and Suicide

Informed decision-making is at the foundation of our health care system. To receive any given treatment, an individual must make an informed decision after consultation with their provider. Conversely, a competent adult may refuse any treatment, even if such a refusal is certain to result in death. This ability to refuse life-sustaining treatment is legally protected by decades of judicial consensus in the United States (Kim 2010).

Typically, a treatment decision is made contemporaneously—that is, at the time the clinical situation is occurring. In the past several decades, however, individuals have been able to document treatment-related preferences before the clinical situation, using documents known as *advance directives.* Advance directives are legal in all 50 states and the District of Columbia and are common in clinical practice (Olick 2012). They serve as a record of an individual's wishes that can inform treatment after the individual has fallen acutely ill and lost decision-making capacity. Most often, they serve to appoint a surrogate decision-maker, as in a spouse or a family member, but they also may describe various treatment preferences. Commonly, but not necessarily, they denote preferences against life-sustaining treatments such as mechanical ventilation and cardiopulmonary resuscitation.

The widespread use of advance directives represents societal progress when it comes to individual autonomy. They protect the treatment preferences of vulnerable individuals at their sickest moments. There are certain scenarios, however, in which the execution of an advance directive is clinically, ethically, or legally unclear. One such situation involves the treatment of an individual who presents with an advance directive limiting life-sustaining care after a suicide attempt. This situation is worthy of discussion per se, but it also illustrates, generally, several of the crucial factors surrounding end-of-life decision-making in individuals with mental illness.

Kerrie Wooltorton

The case of Kerrie Wooltorton illustrates well the complexities of this topic (David et al. 2010; Dresser 2010; McLean 2009; Muzaffar 2011). Wooltorton was a young woman who presented to the hospital in 2007 after ingesting ethylene glycol. She gave her providers a letter declining medical treatment other than comfort care. In the letter, she cited the risks of untreated ingestion, including death. After much investigation and deliberation, the decision was made to withhold lifesaving treatment, and Wooltorton died the next day. An inquest performed in 2009 supported the hospital's decision, stating that it would have been unlawful for the hospital to impose such treatments against her will. The outcome of this case has been the subject of controversy and propelled the subject of advance directives into public discourse (McLean 2009).

The Wooltorton case raises the following simple question: Should a clinician follow the wishes outlined in an advance directive after a suicide attempt? The response to this question is not simple and can be divided into two parts. First, one must think about the factors related to the document itself and its writing. Second, one must assess the case as a treatment refusal, per se, which is a complex clinical task involving many factors.

Considering the Document

Advance directives rest on a solid legal foundation, which can be found in past Supreme Court decisions as well as state and federal law (Olick 2012). An advance directive implies that the decisions documented therein were made by an individual with *decision-making capacity* (DMC) at the time of the document's signing (Muzaffar 2011; Olick 2012). Further, they take effect only after the individual loses capacity. Additionally, a later decision by a competent individual trumps what they had previously written in the directive.

An essential question at the signing of an advance directive is, then, does the patient have DMC? In the United States, one is determined to have capacity when one can demonstrate specific mental abilities;

capacity does not have to do with the outcome of the decision one makes. Said a different way, one is allowed to make an unfortunate, imprudent, or unpopular decision as long as one can demonstrate the proper decisional capabilities. A decision's being unusual or unfortunate, however, may cue the practitioner to evaluate more carefully for deficits in capacity. To meet criteria for DMC, one must adequately (1) *communicate* a choice, (2) *understand* the facts relevant to that choice, (3) *appreciate* the facts as they specifically apply to oneself, and (4) *reason* about the decision (Appelbaum and Grisso 1988). Capacity is presumed until an individual is determined to lack it, and it is typically determined by an attending physician with or without special consultation. Individuals with mental illness generally perform well on capacity assessments. A systematic metareview from 2020 found that up to 60%–70% of hospitalized individuals with severe mental illness have DMC (Calcedo-Barba et al. 2020). Note that an assessment of DMC is specific to the decision at hand. Decisions with graver consequences require a higher level of capacity than ones with clear benefits and few risks (Kim 2010). For example, consenting to a risky neurosurgical procedure will require a level of capacity that is greater than, for example, that required to accept antibiotic therapy for pneumonia. Also note that depression (among other mental illnesses) can, in severe forms, distort and impair one's ability to demonstrate the capabilities necessary for DMC (Kim 2010; Sullivan and Youngner 1994).

With this background in mind, how can one, in an effective and ethical manner, evaluate an advance directive after a suicide attempt? Nowland and colleagues (2019) surveyed this complex scenario by performing a systematic review and thematic analysis of extant literature on advance directives and suicidal behavior. The evidence they found was mostly in the form of case reports and analyses, but several important issues were identified.

For many authors surveyed in the Nowland review, the idea that the advance directive could itself be a component of suicidal behavior, written to increase the likelihood of death by suicide, was important in considering the document's validity or lack thereof (David et al. 2010; Kapur et al. 2010; Muzaffar 2011). That is, the writing of the advance directive could be considered a part of the disorder itself. This perspective was particularly important to authors from the field of psychiatry, a field that, for the most part, views suicidal behavior as pathological and treatable. To support the claim that the documents lacked validity, authors pointed to known clinical characteristics of suicidal behavior—that it is often impulsive, transient, and regretted after the fact (Kapur et al. 2010; Volpe and Levi 2012). These characteristics are not typically associated with autonomy in competent individuals. Competency, rather, is associated with long-standing, durable, and authentic beliefs, as opposed to transient ideation (Callaghan and Ryan 2011). As such, many authors suggested that perhaps any advance directive in play after a suicide attempt should have to undergo scrutiny (David et al. 2010; Kapur et al. 2010; Muzaffar 2011).

Many authors have examined the idea of *intent* behind an advance directive vis-à-vis suicide. Dresser (2010) pointed out that an advance directive associated with a suicide attempt may have been written with the intent to lead to death. This, to the author, placed the document in a different moral standing than a similar document written by a patient with a terminal physical condition. In the latter scenario, the document may be written with other intentions—to ease suffering or to facilitate a more dignified death. Both intent and causation, Dresser claimed, are important and have been hallmarks in decisions such as the U.S. Supreme Court decision in 1997 in *Vacco v. Quill* (Dresser 2010). Volpe (Volpe and Levi 2012), however, was less convinced of the importance of intent and causation. Volpe argued that the validity of wishes for treatment withdrawal should hold for intentional and unintentional injuries alike, and that the distinction may be arbitrary.

A recurring idea in this literature is that an advance directive may stem from thoughts and behavior that are bereft of durability, authenticity, and appreciation for their specific consequences. If we accept the chance that this is the case, how can we as practitioners do well by our patients to recognize this and act accordingly? Muzaffar (2011), though referring to advance decisions in the British legal system, offered some guidance. The most relevant, but perhaps most difficult, question to answer is,Was the patient competent at the time of making the advance decision? Unless the treating clinician is the same individual who assisted the patient with the document, this question will be difficult to answer. However, that does not mean that one cannot make an educated guess by using basic psychiatric skills, namely, careful history-taking and gathering of collateral sources of information. Moreover, forensic psychiatrists have training, expertise, and experience assessing a past mental state by performing evaluations, reviewing records, and interviewing collateral sources. In the hospital, this may involve a thorough interview with the patient centered around the decisions in question (if possible). It may also involve family meetings, contact with outside providers (particularly the individual who assisted with the directive), and a careful review of treatment history. And of course, reasonable efforts should be made to ensure that the patient was reasonably informed of medical facts and was not under undue influence at the time of signing (Muzaffar 2011).

An additional suggestion by Muzaffar (2011) captures the themes of *durability* and *consistency,* which in turn relate to individual autonomy and DMC. One may ask whether there has been evidence of decisions that indicate ambivalence or inconsistency—such as Wooltorton's presentation to the hospital after her suicide attempt, for example—which may have been driven by an ambivalence about death (David et al. 2010). McLean (2009), while affirming that ambivalence is an important behavioral characteristic to observe, noted that it, in isolation, does not indicate incapacity. A competent person does have the right to change their mind about preferences. That is not to say that it may not be useful in characterizing and contextualizing behaviors that stem from a diagnosable mental illness.

Another point worth mentioning, in reference to evaluating advance directives, is that human beings are particularly poor at predicting the future (Maclean 2006; Muzaffar 2011), which complicates the notion that predocumented wishes for a future situation will remain accurate. Some even go so far as to question whether an individual's present self (and its preferences) does not bear enough resemblance to their future self for advance directives to be useful (Maclean 2006). To remedy this inherent weakness in the documents, Muzaffar (2011) argued that advance directives ought to undergo frequent review. Even sporadic reviews may prompt important discussions about the patient's decisions, including the motivations driving them and the context. Finally, are there other abnormal features hinting that the document may be part of suicidal behavior? One might take note, for example, of unusual efforts to broaden the preferences or their scope or to enhance their power, such as by seeking a Physician Order for Life-Sustaining Treatment (Olick 2012), in an otherwise healthy person.

Many authors agree that, no matter the outcome, evaluating advance directives after a suicide attempt is clinically complex and requires more time than may be available (Chalfin et al. 2001), and the evaluation may occur in the absence of informative hospital policies (Callaghan and Ryan 2011). In the systematic review discussed earlier, Nowland found that physicians needed intensive validation checks to evaluate advance directives, as well as consensus across different parties in the clinical situation (e.g., family, consultants, hospital authorities) (David et al. 2010; Muzaffar 2011). These circumstances preclude a swift, simple clinical decision.

Considering a Treatment Refusal That Follows a Suicide Attempt

How can one think, generally, about contemporaneous treatment refusals following a suicide attempt? The four pillars of bioethical decision-making are useful here and deserve a brief review (Beauchamp and Childress 2001). First, *beneficence* describes the favoring of decisions that confer a biomedical *benefit* to the patient. Second, *nonmaleficence* supports choices that *avoid harm* done to the individual. Third, *autonomy* captures the importance of an individual's *rightful agency* in determining the care they receive and the acts done to their body. And finally, *justice* guides decision-makers to consider *equitable* delivery of benefits to all persons and groups in society. The clear majority of clinical decisions involve situations in which these pillars align. Disagreements between these concepts are a reason to pause and deepen one's ethical evaluation of the situation at hand.

The case of Kerrie Wooltorton, though prominently featuring a pre-written letter, is actually a case of contemporaneous treatment refusal, as she was conscious and interactive on presentation. She was found to have DMC, and her treatment refusal was honored. Authors who support this decision found the autonomy-related factors particularly compelling. Wooltorton communicated her choice in plain, written English and wrote a statement that listed the apparent medical facts related to her treatment refusal and her acceptance of the results of her refusal. Some authors found the letter sufficient to indicate her DMC (McLean 2009). Thus, in this case, the duty to honor autonomy was felt to be stronger than the duty to provide the lifesaving benefits of treatment. From a certain perspective, nonmaleficence was honored as well, if unwanted bodily acts (treatment) could be considered psychologically harmful.

Some authors, however, do not see the justification for putting autonomy front and center in the Wooltorton case. David et al. (2010), for example, raised doubt that the patient met criteria for DMC. Specifically, they focused on the ability to "use or weigh" information, which is written into law in the British Mental Capacity Act of 2005. The American analog of this ability is the *appreciation* criterion (Appelbaum and Grisso 1988). David argued that her severe (although treatable) personality disorder may have led to distorted thinking that specifically impacted her ability to use and weigh the relevant information. For example, she may not have been able to use the information to "appreciate that she has an illness that affects her mood and thinking" and manipulate this information in accordance with her personal values (David et al. 2010). This line of argument would characterize Wooltorton as a vulnerable patient, and thus the duty to maximize beneficence and nonmaleficence becomes more compelling.

Autonomy and beneficence are not the only concepts relevant here. In a case such as this, justice guides us to allocate treatments to all patients in accordance with their wishes. Just as with autonomy, justice in this specific sense applies only to individuals with DMC (Sontheimer 2008). Justice also guides us to avoid discriminatory treatment of certain groups. In this case, an individual with severe mental illness must not be deprived of the benefits of life-sustaining treatment when their treatment refusal results from that illness. Alternatively, one could argue that individuals with mental illness ought not to be unjustly deprived of the right to refuse treatment. That is, every effort must be made to confirm the DMC of such individuals to ensure that justice is maximized.

Certain clinical factors may be of importance to ethical analyses, such as *quality-of-life factors* and *shared decision-making*. For example, future poor quality of life could place limits on the benefits resulting from life-sustaining treatment (Chalfin et al. 2001), and input from family or loved ones may help to further characterize and contextualize suicidal behavior in relationship to the individual's wishes.

Physician Assistance in Dying for Psychiatric Conditions

In the previous section, we considered scenarios in which death is likely to occur imminently. Here, our focus shifts to points in time that are further from imminent death. Specifically, we discuss the practice of *physician assistance in dying* (PAD) and, when relevant, euthanasia. Note that the two practices together are often referred to as *euthanasia and assisted suicide* (EAS; other acronyms are also used in the literature). This chapter uses *psychiatric EAS* to describe cases in which EAS is provided when mental illness is the sole reason for the request—that is, in contrast to EAS for terminal physical conditions with requirements that death be foreseeable (e.g., a terminal disease being defined as an incurable and irreversible disease that has been medically confirmed and will, according to reasonable medical judgment, result in death within 6 months).

In the United States, state laws have legalized PAD in a growing number of jurisdictions, stemming from the landmark law passed in

Oregon in 1997 (Oregon Death With Dignity Act 2023). At the time of this publication, the American Medical Association maintains its opinion that "physician-assisted suicide is fundamentally incompatible with the physician's role as a healer," although it acknowledges a thoughtful moral basis for nonsanctioned beliefs, such as those related to relieving suffering at the end of life (American Medical Association 1997).

In the U.S. laws, PAD is permitted only in cases of terminal disease (expected to lead to death within 6 months) and involves the prescription of life-ending drugs as the result of an explicit request from a patient with decisional capacity, who takes the substance on their own. In some of these statutes, DMC is determined by two independent physicians, who may or may not be psychiatrists (Darby 2018). Certain state statutes require the involvement of mental health professionals to assess an individual's DMC in various circumstances. California requires a mental health assessment if there is any indication of a mental disorder (California End of Life Option Act 2022). The District of Columbia, Maine, New Mexico, Oregon, and Washington require a mental health assessment if there are concerns that an underlying psychiatric disorder is impairing a person's judgment regarding the request (D.C. Death With Dignity Act 2017; Maine Death With Dignity Act 2019; New Mexico End-of-Life Options Act 2021; Oregon Death With Dignity Act 2023; Washington Death With Dignity Act 2023). Colorado, New Jersey, and Vermont statutes require individuals to be referred for a psychiatric assessment when there is a concern regarding DMC (Colorado End-of-Life Options Act 2017; New Jersey Medical Aid in Dying for the Terminally Ill Act 2019; Vermont Patient Choice at End of Life 2023). Hawaii mandates a mental health capacity assessment "to determine if the patient is capable," that is, has the mental capacity to make an informed decision, "and does not appear to be suffering from undertreatment or nontreatment of depression or other conditions which may interfere with the patient's ability to make an informed decision" (Hawaii Our Care, Our Choice Act 2018). In addition to these statutes, several health systems have instituted guidelines that psychiatric evaluations be mandatory in this process or under certain conditions.

Whether PAD will be offered for indications other than terminal conditions (e.g., purported "irremediable" mental suffering) is the subject of current debate and represents an evolving area of the law. In 1994, a ruling by the Dutch Supreme Court supported the legalization of PAD and euthanasia in the Netherlands in cases in which the patient's suffering is due solely to a mental disorder. Currently, such practices are also legal in Belgium, Luxembourg, and Switzerland (Grassi et al. 2022; Kim and Lemmens 2016). Canadian legislatures are considering allowing PAD for people with mental illness as the sole reason for the request, but this is excluded until 2027 (Government of Canada 2024). An emerging literature (made up of mostly case series and surveys) has described trends related to psychiatric EAS in those countries and has found a small but increasing prevalence of these requests. For example, according to one registry in the Netherlands, the percentage of cases of EAS for psychiatric indications increased from 0% in 2009 to 1.07% in 2019 (Calati et al. 2021). This increasing prevalence, among other factors, has led to much recent discussion in the field of bioethics. This section highlights important arguments on the subject as well as the issues at stake if the practice is ultimately legalized in the United States.

The American Psychiatric Association (APA) has taken a clear stance on this practice, stating that "a psychiatrist should not prescribe or administer any intervention to a non–terminally ill person for the purpose of causing death" (American Psychiatric Association 2016). Many of the principal arguments against this practice stem from the opinion that such an act would violate *professional integrity*. That is, the practice deviates from the core set of ethical behaviors that define a physician. For Miller, permissibility of PAD hinges on what we consider the core behaviors of a physician. In his line of reasoning, medical EAS may actually be permissible, as "helping patients achieve a peaceful and dignified death" is integral to a physician's identity (Miller and Brody 1995, p. 11). He distinguishes psychiatric EAS from this role, however, because this practice does not occur close to the time of natural or unpreventable death. For Miller and others, self-determination and relief of suffering are important considerations but are not paramount, and they do not trump considerations of professional identity (Miller 2015).

What, then, are the principal arguments in favor of the permissibility of psychiatric EAS? As of 2023, numerous review articles had been published on the arguments for and against psychiatric EAS (Grassi et al. 2022; Nicolini et al. 2020; van Veen et al. 2020). One of the central arguments in favor of this practice is based on the *parity* of mental and physical suffering (Schuklenk and van de Vathorst 2015). This argument holds that if individuals are allowed to access EAS for unbearable suffering due to a physical condition such as cancer, they should not be excluded if their suffering is from a mental disorder. A major problem with this argument is that although suffering from mental illness may be comparable to subjective experiences of suffering in persons with a terminal physical disease, there is a lack of consensus that a mental illness could ever be categorized as terminal (where death is reasonably and imminently foreseeable). Moreover, prioritizing suffering as the most important justification for EAS may ignore other factors of importance, such as upholding professional integrity (Miller 2015). Further, many authors argue against this type of parity—that there are important differences between physical and mental illness that impact the ethics of assisted death (Kelly and McLoughlin 2002).

One of the most important differences between mental and physical illness is the ease with which a state of irremediable suffering, or a treatment-resistant illness, can be identified (van Veen et al. 2020). In the setting of cancer, for example, practitioners can usually identify when additional treatment will not significantly alter the course of disease. With mental illness, this same task is distinctly challenging. For example, it is difficult to assess whether past psychiatric treatments were effective. For medication trials, daily compliance with the medication at an adequate dose and sufficient time would need to be confirmed. Assessing compliance, effort, and engagement with psychotherapy, such as work done outside of therapy sessions in cognitive-behavioral therapy, may present similar challenges in determining whether the person did not or could not benefit from therapy to alter the course of their mental illness. There is also no consensus on how many types of treatment must have failed for a mental illness to be truly irremediable (Kim and Lemmens 2016; van Veen et al. 2020). Some PAD laws consider only treatment options that are acceptable to the particular patient when determining whether the mental illness is resistant to treatment (Appelbaum 2016).

A study by Kim et al. (2016) analyzed 66 Dutch cases for psychiatric EAS from 2011 to 2014 and found that 56% of patients had previously declined some form of recommended treatment for reasons such as lack of motivation, concerns about side effects or risks, doubts about treatment efficacy, or a combination of factors. In the same study, personality disorders were comorbid in 52% of the patients requesting psychiatric EAS, 56% of cases were complicated by prominent loneliness and social isolation, and 20% of patients had never been psychiatrically hospitalized.

Consider major depressive disorder as an example. There is no universally accepted definition of treatment-resistant depression (TRD). In fact, definitions of TRD are quite variable. Some definitions are broad enough to account for 12%–20% of depression cases, and some definitions even consider failure of a single antidepressant trial as evidence of treatment resistance (Mrazek et al. 2014). Further, many clinical factors complicate the idea that TRD may cause irremediable suffering. A label of TRD may not include vital information such as whether the individual has undergone trials of multiple medication classes (e.g., monoamine oxidase inhibitors), electroconvulsive therapy, transcranial magnetic stimulation, adequate trials of evidence-based psychotherapies, or novel and emerging treatments. It may not indicate that personality disorders have been properly ruled out or targeted with treatment. It also does not necessarily account for factors such as social isolation or loneliness, which may respond to basic psychosocial support and other interventions. It would also indicate nothing about comorbidities such as chronic pain or substance use disorders, which are treatable and may exacerbate distress. Aside from the determination of its diagnostic criteria, there are additional challenges in understanding just how futile treatment would be for individuals with TRD. For example, many authors point out the realistic prospect of emerging treatments for depression, such as neurostimulatory interventions (e.g., deep brain stimulation) or novel psychedelic therapies (e.g., psilocybin). Last, one cannot discount the possibility of spontaneous recovery, even if rare, or the human capacity for creativity and resilience.

With a limited evidence base on TRD, confirming that there is "no reasonable alternative" may involve a considerable amount of subjectivity. Many authors consider this problematic. Vandenberghe (2018), for example, argued for a maximal objectivity of this criterion, and that it can only be met for individuals with long-term access to high-quality, affordable mental health care. For many, the verification that requests for EAS are a true "last resort" is crucial to their ethical permissibility (Miller 2015). Similarly, for many authors, irremediability is difficult to substantiate in patients who have refused certain treatment in the past (van Veen et al. 2020). Subjective variability in determining irremediability is less of a problem for other authors, mostly nonclinicians, who argue that personal judgment, under the guidance of a physician, is sufficient (Nicolini et al. 2020; Schuklenk and van de Vathorst 2015).

A different way of articulating these concerns about irremediability is to say that entry criteria for psychiatric EAS might yield too many *false positives*. That is, our present ability to identify intractable illness lacks proper resolution, and many individuals not actually meeting criteria would receive the service. The retrospective data from the Netherlands add weight to the concern that non–intractably ill individuals may receive EAS (Kim et al. 2016). For example, in 12% of cases, the psychiatrist thought the criteria were not met, but the death occurred anyway (Kim et al. 2016). It is worth mentioning that epidemiologic data have been published since that study, including psychiatric EAS requests that did not end in death. These data provide additional context for the situation in the Netherlands and underscore the rarity of the practice: 68% of requests were rejected during the observation period, and 20% of requests were withdrawn, such that nearly 90% of requests did not end in completion of EAS (van Veen et al. 2022).

Decision-making capacity is a precondition to the honoring of an individual's personal judgment, and it is indeed crucial to the discussion of psychiatric EAS. Those in favor of psychiatric EAS reasonably point to the observation that mental illness, even when severe, does not preclude the presence of capacity. This observation is grounded in studies that have observed high levels of capacity in psychiatric inpatients (Calcedo-Barba et al. 2020). Berghmans and colleagues explained that a person's wish for death, when arising from a "rational evaluation of one's former, present and future situation, and…not the result of compelling influences connected to the patient's mental illness," may be permissible (Berghmans et al. 2013, p. 437). Many proponents have spoken about the threshold of capacity for psychiatric EAS, namely, that it should be in line with other clinical decisions to minimize violations of autonomy (Nicolini et al. 2020). In regard to capacity and the "rational" quality of requests for psychiatric EAS, Schuklenk and van de Vathorst (2015) discussed the fact that depression both influences one's worldview in a negative way and causes the state of suffering. They implied that these two processes may be separable or independent. As such, one may have a negative view of their prospects, but that view may very well be an accurate assessment of disease's impact on their life.

Opponents of psychiatric EAS point to factors related to DMC in their arguments against the practice. A decision as gravely consequential as assisted death is believed by many to demand a high threshold of capacity (den Hartogh 2015), which runs contrary to the idea that the threshold be similar to that of other clinical decisions. Despite the significant prevalence of DMC in psychiatric populations, mental disorders such as depression and psychosis can interfere with capacity, and this possibility needs to be carefully evaluated and likely replicated by multiple examiners. A 2013 systematic review of medical ethical and empirical literature found that depression was most likely to alter the domain of *appreciation* (Hindmarch et al. 2013). Appreciation is often challenging to discern from *understanding* and involves an individualized deliberation on how the consequences apply specifically to the individual's situation (Kim 2010). Additionally, Elliott (1997) argued that the concepts of accountability and minimal self-concern are inherent to capacity. That is, it is not enough to understand and manipulate information, but one must also demonstrate on some level that one cares about the risk and has accounted for it in an individual way. Depression has been argued to affect cognition in multiple ways that are relevant to capacity, such as distorting the calculation of pleasure and pain in one's life (Sullivan and Youngner 1994) and distorting the ability to objectively evaluate one's future (Owen et al. 2018). Alarmingly, a 2016 retrospective review of psychiatric EAS capacity assessments in the Netherlands found inconsistent documentation practices, and only a minority of assessments mentioned capacity-specific abilities (Doernberg et al. 2016).

Several authors have brought up concerns about the impact that psychiatric EAS would have on the physician-patient relationship, and on society at large. Appelbaum, for example, asked, "will psychiatrists conclude from the legalization of assisted death that it is acceptable to give up on treating some patients?" (Appelbaum 2016). This question has important implications from the perspective of countertransference and the types of options offered to patients in treatment. Other authors have pointed to the possibility that a patient may be ambivalent but see access to psychiatric EAS as a "permission" of sorts to end one's life (Miller 2015). Several authors have asked whether psychiatric EAS would lead to a common hopelessness among individuals suffering from depression, or whether there would be less motivation to improve psychiatric services (Nicolini et al. 2020; van Veen et al. 2020). Miller wondered, gravely, about the greater meaning of psychiatric EAS: "Do we want to live in a society in which physicians help patients with depression end their lives?" (Miller 2015). And importantly, Sinyor and Schaffer (2020) pointed out the immense risks in making permanent policy changes based on a dearth of scientific data, where the societal effects (especially those on suicide rates) are unknown. When surveyed, only a minority (36.9%) of a U.S. general population sample supported PAD for nonterminal conditions in the context of inadequate resources, and that support was even less when participants were specifically asked about mental illness (Berens et al. 2022).

It should be clearly noted that the purpose of this section is to survey the foremost arguments that are exchanged in this ongoing, evolving ethical discussion. This author's recommendation, in line with the stated APA position as well as U.S. law, is that no psychiatrist ought to supply the means for an individual to end their life for a nonterminal condition, which would include PAD for individuals with mental illness as the sole reason for the request. Psychiatrists may play an important role in capacity assessments for legal PAD for those with terminal disease by assessing whether treatable depressive or other psychiatric symptoms impede a person's decision-making capacity for PAD; this role would serve as an important safeguard to promote beneficence and nonmaleficence principles, as well as autonomy, by honoring and prioritizing a person's durable and authentic beliefs rather than impulsive acts or transient desires that are the product of mental illness and inconsistent with a person's long-standing values.

Conclusion

Clinical requests for hastened death can take different forms. In this chapter, two types of requests are discussed: treatment refusals documented in advance directives and explicit requests for physician assistance in dying. An ethical response to these requests must be balanced, thorough, compassionate, and grounded in the law. The best tools available to psychiatrists confronting these requests are the basic tenets of ethical clinical practice. Foundationally, the ethical principles of Beauchamp and Childress (2001) provide a framework to help clinicians think about the factors at stake and clarify when ethical pillars are in conflict. Basic psychiatric skills are also of utmost utility. Good psychiatric interviewing, family involvement, knowledge of evidence-based treatments, and a thoughtful and flexible differential diagnosis will all help to resolve ethical dilemmas that emerge in end-of-life care.

References

American Medical Association: Code of Medical Ethics. Chicago, IL, American Medical Association, 1997

American Psychiatric Association: Position Statement on Medical Euthanasia. 2016. Available at: https://www.psychiatry.org/File%20Library/About-APA/Organization-Documents-Policies/Policies/Position-2016-Medical-Euthanasia.pdf. Accessed July 17, 2024.

Appelbaum PS: Physician-assisted death for patients with mental disorders: reasons for concern. JAMA Psychiatry 73(4):325–326, 2016 26864504

Appelbaum PS, Grisso T: Assessing patients' capacities to consent to treatment. N Engl J Med 319(25):1635–1638, 1988 3200278

Beauchamp TL, Childress JF: Principles of Biomedical Ethics, 5th Edition. New York, Oxford University Press, 2001

Berens N, Wasserman D, Wakim P, et al: Resource limitation and "forced irremediability" in physician-assisted deaths for nonterminal mental and physical conditions: a survey of the US public. J Acad Consult Liaison Psychiatry 63(4):302–313, 2022 35026471

Berghmans R, Widdershoven G, Widdershoven-Heerding I: Physician-assisted suicide in psychiatry and loss of hope. Int J Law Psychiatry 36(5–6):436–443, 2013 23830024

Calati R, Olié E, Dassa D, et al: Euthanasia and assisted suicide in psychiatric patients: a systematic review of the literature. J Psychiatric Res 135:153–173, 2021 33486164

Calcedo-Barba A, Fructuoso A, Martinez-Raga J, et al: A meta-review of literature reviews assessing the capacity of patients with severe mental disorders to make decisions about their healthcare. BMC Psychiatry 20(1):339, 2020 32605645

California End of Life Option Act, Ca. Health and Safety Code § 443.1 (2022)

Callaghan S, Ryan CJ: Refusing medical treatment after attempted suicide: rethinking capacity and coercive treatment in light of the Kerrie Wooltorton case. J Law Med 18(4):811–819, 2011 21774276

Chalfin DB, Crippen D, Franklin C, et al: "Round-table" ethical debate: is a suicide note an authoritative "living will"? Crit Care 5(3):115–124, 2001 11353927

Colorado End-of-Life Options Act, Colo. Rev. Stat. § 25–48–101–123 (2017)

Darby WC: Physician aid in dying: the role of the psychiatrist. Presented at the 49th Annual Meeting of the American Academy of Psychiatry and the Law, Austin, TX, October 25–28, 2018

David AS, Hotopf M, Moran P, et al: Mentally disordered or lacking capacity? Lessons for management of serious deliberate self harm. BMJ 341(7773):c4489, 2010 20823014

D.C. Death With Dignity Act, D.C. Code § 7–661.06 (2017)

den Hartogh G: Why extra caution is needed in the case of depressed patients. J Med Ethics 41(8):588–589, 2015 26112612

Doernberg SN, Peteet JR, Kim SYH: Capacity evaluations of psychiatric patients requesting assisted death in the Netherlands. Psychosomatics 57(6):556–565, 2016 27590345

Dresser R: Suicide attempts and treatment refusals. Hastings Cent Rep 40(3):10–11, 2010 20549864

Elliott C: Caring about risks: are severely depressed patients competent to consent to research? Arch Gen Psychiatry 54(2):113–116, 1997 9040277

Government of Canada: Medical assistance in dying: overview. March 14, 2024. Available at: https://www.canada.ca/en/health-canada/services/health-services-benefits/medical-assistance-dying.html. Accessed July 17, 2024.

Grassi L, Folesani F, Marella M, et al: Debating euthanasia and physician-assisted death in people with psychiatric disorders. Curr Psychiatry Rep 24(6):325–335, 2022 35678920

Hawaii Our Care, Our Choice Act, Haw. Stat. § 2739 (2018)

Hindmarch T, Hotopf M, Owen GS: Depression and decision-making capacity for treatment or research: a systematic review. BMC Med Ethics 14(1):54, 2013 24330745

Kapur N, Clements C, Bateman N, et al: Advance directives and suicidal behaviour. BMJ 341(7773):c4557, 2010 20823015

Kelly BD, McLoughlin DM: Euthanasia, assisted suicide and psychiatry: a Pandora's box. Br J Psychiatry 181:278–279, 2002 12356652

Kim SYH: Evaluation of Capacity to Consent to Treatment and Research. New York, Oxford University Press, 2010

Kim SYH, Lemmens T: Should assisted dying for psychiatric disorders be legalized in Canada? CMAJ 188(14):E337–E339, 2016 27328688

Kim SYH, De Vries RG, Peteet JR: Euthanasia and assisted suicide of patients with psychiatric disorders in the Netherlands 2011 to 2014. JAMA Psychiatry 73(4):362–368, 2016 26864709

Maclean AR: Advance directives, future selves and decision-making. Med Law Rev 14(3):291–320, 2006 16901976

Maine Death With Dignity Act, Me. Stat. § 2140 (2019)

McLean SAM: Live and let die. BMJ 339:b4112, 2009 19812136

Miller FG: Treatment-resistant depression and physician-assisted death. J Med Ethics 41(11):885–886, 2015 26401050

Miller FG, Brody H: Professional integrity and physician-assisted death. Hastings Cent Rep 25(3):8–17, 1995 7649748

Mrazek DA, Hornberger JC, Altar CA, et al: A review of the clinical, economic, and societal burden of treatment-resistant depression: 1996–2013. Psychiatr Serv 65(8):977–987, 2014 24789696

Muzaffar S: "To treat or not to treat." Kerrie Wooltorton, lessons to learn. Emerg Med J 28(9):741–744, 2011 20923817

New Jersey Medical Aid in Dying for the Terminally Ill Act, N.J. Rev. Stat. § 26:16–3 (2019)

New Mexico End-of-Life Options Act, N.M. Stat § 24–7C-6 (2021)

Nicolini ME, Kim SYH, Churchill ME, et al: Should euthanasia and assisted suicide for psychiatric disorders be permitted? A systematic review of reasons. Psychol Med 50(8):1241–1256, 2020 32482180

Nowland R, Steeg S, Quinlivan LM, et al: Management of patients with an advance decision and suicidal behaviour: a systematic review. BMJ Open 9(3):e023978, 2019 30872542

Olick RS: Defining features of advance directives in law and clinical practice. Chest 141(1):232–238, 2012 22215831

Oregon Death With Dignity Act, OR Rev. Stat. § 127.880 (2023)

Owen GS, Martin W, Gergel T: Misevaluating the future: affective disorder and decision-making capacity for treatment: a temporal understanding. Psychopathology 51(6):371–379, 2018 30485862

Schuklenk U, van de Vathorst S: Treatment-resistant major depressive disorder and assisted dying. J Med Ethics 41(8):577–583, 2015 25935906

Sinyor M, Schaffer A: The lack of adequate scientific evidence regarding physician-assisted death for people with psychiatric disorders is a danger to patients. Can J Psychiatry 65(9):607–609, 2020 32452224

Sontheimer D: Suicide by advance directive? J Med Ethics 34(9):e4, 2008 18757623

Sullivan MD, Youngner SJ: Depression, competence, and the right to refuse lifesaving medical treatment. Am J Psychiatry 151(7):971–978, 1994 8010382

Vandenberghe J: Physician-assisted suicide and psychiatric illness. N Engl J Med 378(10):885–887, 2018 29514019

van Veen SMP, Ruissen AM, Widdershoven GAM: Irremediable psychiatric suffering in the context of physician-assisted death: a scoping review of arguments. Can J Psychiatry 65(9):593–603, 2020 32427501

van Veen S, Widdershoven G, Beekman A, et al: Physician assisted death for psychiatric suffering: experiences in the Netherlands. Front Psychiatry 13:895387, 2022 35795029

Vermont Patient Choice at End of Life, VT. Stat. Ann. 18 § 5281–93 (2023)

Volpe RL, Levi BH: Case study: exploring the limits of autonomy (commentary). Hastings Cent Rep 42(3):16–17, 2012 22670293

Washington Death With Dignity Act, Wash. Rev. Code § 70.245 (2023)

19

Structural and Implicit Bias in Violence Risk Assessments

Shoba Sreenivasan, Ph.D.

Melinda DiCiro, Psy.D., ABPP

James Rokop, Ph.D.

Linda E. Weinberger, Ph.D.

Violence risk assessment by forensic psychiatrists and psychologists has a significant role across various aspects of the criminal justice system: pre-adjudication assessments for viability of management in the community such as diversion and bail eligibility; sentencing; custody assessments for civil commitment; conditional release from state hospitals; risk management; prerelease planning; and postrelease rehabilitation. Such risk assessments affect broad competing interests: public safety, the protection of an individual's civil liberties, and the harm caused through undeserved incarceration and overly restrictive treatments. Actuarial risk tools use statistical algorithms to provide probabilistic estimates of future criminal recidivism; the risk markers are static (such as number of prior criminal offenses). Structured professional judgments (SPJs), unlike actuarial measures, do not assign a numeric value or probabilistic estimates of future risk but contain select risk factors identified in the literature as predictive of violent recidivism. SPJs include dynamic risk factors (such as participation in treatment) and protective risk factors (such as financial stability and social support) that may moderate risk (Singh et al. 2011). In both methods, criminal history carries significant weight. There has been growing concern regarding systemic bias in the criminal justice system against those from nondominant groups (Harcourt 2015; Vincent and Viljoen 2020) and whether as a consequence that violence risk may be overestimated (Trestman 2018). These concerns are relevant to forensic evaluators and decision-makers, particularly if the methodology used is biased against and inflates risk for subgroups. Understanding the impact of systemic bias, both implicit and explicit, is crucial for forensic psychiatrists and psychologists who conduct violence risk assessment and is essential for engaging in ethical forensic practice. In this chapter, we review the potential for violence risk assessments to be biased by criminal justice practices, discuss ethical obligations related to bias, and examine potential methods to mitigate bias.

Sources of Implicit Bias in Violence Risk Assessment

Implicit and other forms of bias are by their nature mostly hidden from awareness, are prone to error, and favor perception of danger from those outside one's own group (Jhangiani and Tarry 2014; Scherr and Dror 2021). Implicit bias can influence the level of risk assigned to the individual assessment. Biasing factors can unfairly impact risk assessments for people in certain racial and cultural groups, with mental health disorders, of lower socioeconomic status, and who are perceived as less likable and less attractive. Triers of fact and other decision-makers relying on these evaluations may not be aware of bias in assessments and may be subject to their own biases (Abrams et al. 2012). Thus, the potential for unwarranted detention or restriction is high. Given the potential for serious repercussions stemming from these evaluations' findings, variables that can impact opinion-making must be thoroughly considered. Forensic practitioners should strive to take conscious, intentional steps to avoid bias. They should strive to understand and account for structural and other systematic biases that affect violence risk factors; recognize and correctly manage the strengths and limitations of risk assessment methods; adhere to their ethical obligations to conduct fair, culturally sensitive assessments; and be aware of and effectively mitigate their own vulnerability to implicit biases. As experts, they are also obligated to alert decision-makers to potentially biasing factors and to educate them about empirically established relationships and their meanings.

Potentially biasing factors are often embedded in risk assessment instruments. Bias may not be obviously apparent, as it can be due to seemingly objective, statistically identified risk factors, such as criminal history. Criminal history is a dominant factor embedded in established risk assessment methods (Helmus et al. 2012; Singh et al. 2011) and may be especially subject to bias. Arrest and incarceration databases continue to demonstrate that Black males tend to be arrested and incarcerated at disproportionately higher rates than White males across all ages. Other empirically recognized risk factors that may disproportionately or unfairly and inaccurately elevate violence risk in evaluations of people in nondominant groups are substance use, antisocial associates, treatment compliance, parole and probation compliance, employment, and education. Substance use is more likely to be detected and formally documented in groups more subject to arrest, monitoring, and incarceration.

Additionally, particular substances predominantly used in certain groups may have greater rates of criminal justice intervention. To illustrate, in the 1990s, users of crack, who were more likely to be Black, were more subject to sanctions than were users of powder cocaine, who were more likely to be White. This bias was also evident in which substances were targeted and who was prosecuted in the War on Drugs (Fellner 2000). Trestman (2018) pointed to the Substance Abuse and Mental Health Services Administration (2014) and other sources showing that although Black and White individuals are equally likely to use drugs, Black people are more likely to be arrested for drug crimes (at a rate more than five times higher than other racial groups), including marijuana possession. Black youths are more likely to be arrested for drug use and sales, despite being less likely to be involved in these activities (Kakade et al. 2012). Monitoring, management, and treatment requirements may be especially burdensome for those of lower socioeconomic status. They may not have transportation to appointments, access to electricity to charge a GPS device, or the resources to live away from verboten locations or people. Members of some cultural groups are distrustful of mental health treatment, and some cultural groups ostracize or threaten people who participate in mental health treatment. Treatment noncompliance thus may have a different meaning for members of these groups. Moreover, economic conditions may have a disparate effect on members of certain racial and cultural groups, affecting employment and educational opportunities. To illustrate, Blacks and Hispanics suffered disproportionately higher levels of eviction, job loss, and unemployment during the COVID-19 pandemic of 2020 (Abedi et al. 2021). Economic factors also affect the ability to engage effective legal representation.

Racial Disparities in the Criminal Justice System

Perhaps the most salient and potent form of bias is the uneven way the American judicial system has treated minoritized racial and cultural groups. Bagaric et al. (2018) noted that the American criminal justice system held more than 2.2 million people in custody. Placing this finding in context, the authors concluded that the United States had approximately 4% of the world's population, but 21% of the world's prisoners. The U.S. Census Bureau (2019) estimated that Black people represented approximately 13%–14% of the U.S. population in 2019 but approximately 29% of those in legal custody—that is, 1,096 Black prisoners per 100,000 Black residents compared with 214 White prisoners per 100,000 White residents (Carson 2020b). For American Indian and Alaska Native (AIAN) group members, the rates of incarceration are second only to those of Blacks (Minton 2017; Perry et al. 2020). Therefore, in any violence risk scheme, the more such criminal history is weighted (e.g., criminal history increases the score, and higher scores mean higher risk), the more likely it is that the person is an individual of color.

Criminal justice involvement can unfairly impact risk assessment in a variety of ways. Structural disparities are wide and well documented, and these cause members of many nondominant groups to be unfairly categorized. Police misconduct (including falsification of evidence and coerced confessions) and bias in witness observation can lead to unwarranted arrests, convictions, and incarcerations. Violence risk assessment methods emphasize aspects of criminal justice involvement as key indicators of risk (Bonta and Andrews 2017). A person's involvement in the justice system alone can bias both evaluators and decision-makers, who themselves ordinarily have not experienced such involvement and the attendant injustices. Thus they may be prone to uncharitable perceptions, as a manifestation of the fundamental attribution error. A brief review of data showing racial and other disparities in criminal justice involvement and outcomes shows why the use of criminal history as a heavily weighted predictive factor can create an especially pernicious source of bias in violence risk assessments. Many nondominant groups are disproportionately represented in the American criminal justice system. Trestman (2018) described "cumulative disadvantage" to highlight how each element and stage of the justice system unfairly impacts nondominant groups, especially Black Americans. He cited studies showing that these groups are more subject to profiling, and therefore more likely to be arrested; once arrested, they are more likely to be incarcerated. They are also more likely to be arrested for substance use.

Bureau of Justice Statistics (BJS) data illustrate these disparities and highlight their potential impact. The data focus on adult male offenders, as do most violence risk assessment schemes. (Where data are available for adult female offenders, it is so specified.) In 2018 (Carson 2020a), Black males ages 18–19 were 12.7 times more likely to be imprisoned than White males in the same age bracket. In fact, across all age bands, from 18 to 65 and older, Black individuals had higher rates of imprisonment than White individuals. Black females were also more likely to be imprisoned across all age brackets compared with White females, with the greatest disparity in the 18- to 19-year-old bracket (more than 3.5 times as likely). Hispanic males ages 18–19 were 3.3 times more likely than White males in the same age bracket to be imprisoned. Despite a decline in the rates for all groups in the 10-year period of 2008–2018 (Zhen et al. 2020), jail incarceration rates remain higher for most non-White groups. By year-end 2018, White people were jailed at a rate of 187 per 100,000; Black people at a rate of 592 per 100,000; and AIAN people at a rate of 401 per 100,000. Hispanic people had a rate of jail incarceration of 182 per 100,000 Hispanic U.S. residents, similar to that of White people.

Recent data from BJS regarding correctional populations indicate that although a large number of people (6.4 million) were held in custody or under the supervision of parole or probation in 2018, the period marked a 19-year low in the correctional population (Maruschak and Minton 2020). Racial disparities are narrowing but nonetheless remain. Recent BJS data indicate that the imprisonment rate of Black U.S. residents in 2018 was the lowest since 1989: 1,134 per 100,000 (Carson 2020a). In addition, the number of Black prisoners sentenced to terms of more than 1 year decreased by 2.2% from 2017 to 2018. For White prisoners, the decline was 1.4%, and for Hispanic prisoners, 1.9%. For the 10-year period from year-end 2008 to year-end 2018, the imprisonment rate declined 15.2% for White adults (from 316 to 268 per 100,000) and 31.7% for Black adults (from 2,196 to 1,501 per 100,000). These declines were also noted among jail incarcerations (Zhen et al. 2020). For Black residents, the rate fell to less than 600 per 100,000 for the first time since 1990. For the 10-year period from 2008 to 2018, the Black jail population dropped by 21% and the Hispanic jail population dropped by 15%.

Despite these reduced rates and a narrowing gap in racial disparities, prison and jail incarceration rates remain higher for minoritized groups than for Whites. The imprisonment rate of Black males is 5.8 times that of White males; for Black females, the rate is 1.8 times that of White females (Carson 2020b). Those who have been incarcerated are more likely to be incarcerated again for offenses in the future. This is especially relevant for violence risk assessment, as prior sanctions and re-incarceration after sanction play prominent roles in evaluations. Racial disparities in incarceration rates can translate into a Black offender receiving higher risk scores than a White offender. Further, members of nondominant ethnic groups are more likely than White people to serve time for a violent crime. The BJS surveys for year-end 2018 found that among those sentenced to state prison, more Black (60%) and Hispanic (61%) people were serving terms for violent crimes in comparison to White people (48%) (Carson 2020a), despite similar rates of violent arrest (Beck 2021). Such data are not meant to be interpreted as nondominant groups being more violent than Whites; rather, this statistic reflects an imbalance in arrests, prosecutions, and convictions.

Vulnerability of Criminal History as Proxy for Race

Risk assessment tools offer empirical methods to address violence risk potential. Some researchers have suggested that if the instruments work equally well across racial groups in their prediction of violence—sometimes with recidivism rates as proxies for violence—then such tools may be less vulnerable to the criticism of racial bias (Skeem and Lowenkamp 2016). Actuarial instruments assign a numeric value to risk factors and provide probabilistic estimates of risk level using statistical algorithms (Singh et al. 2011). Actuarial instruments have the advantages of brevity, easily quantifiable and scorable items, and quantification of risk based on empirically derived risk factors. Their use of such factors and a theoretical basis may help reduce evaluator biases related to irrelevant offender characteristics (Neal and Grisso 2014).

Actuarial methods estimate the likelihood of criminal recidivism (violence, sexual violence), derived from nomothetical (group-based) risk factors. Prior arrests and convictions have been statistically associated with future violence risk and therefore play a prominent role in risk assessment schemes (Helmus et al. 2012). However, disparities by race in who is arrested and prosecuted may affect the utility of criminal history as a violence risk factor. Some argue that items such as criminal history (arrests, convictions, prior incarcerations) actually function as a proxy for race (Harcourt 2015) and serve to aggravate rather than mitigate racial disparities within the criminal justice system. Harcourt (2015, p. 240) asserted that criminal history is highly weighted in federal sentencing guidelines and is increasingly used as a proxy for future dangerousness:

> [R]eliance on criminal history [for sentencing and violence risk assessment] has proven to be devastating to African American communities and can only continue to have disproportionate impacts in the future.... In the end, the use of risk instruments focused on prior criminal history is toxic.

When a group is more likely to be perceived as dangerous, be arrested, be coerced into a confession, have ineffective counsel, and be convicted of violent crimes, then the use of actuarial instruments that heavily weight criminal history has the potential to be inherently unfair.

Nevertheless, some dispute that criminal history is a proxy for race. Skeem and Lowenkamp (2016) studied the relationship between race and risk assessment in 34,794 federal offenders on supervision, using the Post-Conviction Risk Assessment (PCRA) instrument and its ability to predict future arrest. PCRA predicted arrests equally well for Black and White offenders. Black offenders on average had higher scores than White offenders, however, and the racial difference was attributed to criminal history. The authors suggested that rather than criminal history functioning as a proxy for race, camouflaging discrimination, such history functions as a "mediator." Nonetheless, they acknowledged the potential for bias and recommended the development of risk instruments based on a broad range of factors that correlate less with race than criminal history. Of relevance is the conclusion by Vincent and Viljoen (2020, p. 6) that actuarial risk instruments, by the very nature of their construction (such as statistical modeling), are more likely to classify Black individuals in North America as higher risks than Whites:

Due to simple mathematics, we must expect that if Black defendants have a higher rate of official recidivism than White defendants, and an algorithm is highly predictive of or well calibrated to those outcomes, the algorithm will classify a greater proportion of Black defendants as high risk.

Moreover, they pointed out that a greater proportion of Black defendants will be (mis)classified as high risk, even though they ultimately do not recidivate. Vincent and Viljoen (2020, p. 6) noted the inherent unfairness, stating:

In short, we are confounding the question of who is likely to engage in illegal and potentially harmful conduct with who is likely to get apprehended, and we are shining a light on the long-standing problem of systemic injustices.

Methods to Mitigate Racial and Cultural Biases

Risk assessment instruments are alluring, given their apparent objectivity and their data- and algorithm-driven ability to provide information regarding future recidivism. However, they are susceptible to professional and ethical issues. Nilsson and colleagues (2009, p. 404) wrote:

Central to forensic psychiatry is the balance between conflicting individual interests, professional values, the public interest of safety, and important social values, such as justice.

Guidance for ethical risk assessment practice can be found in professional standards and in specialty guidelines for forensic psychiatrists (American Academy of Psychiatry and the Law 2005) and forensic psychologists (American Psychological Association 2013). They address considerations for mitigating racial, cultural, and other biases. The specialty guidelines for both professional groups agree in their core concerns about bias: external influences and awareness (and articulation in the assessment) of the limitations related to the risk methods used and the expert opinions formed (Weinberger and Sreenivasan 2018).

There are several ethical issues that the forensic psychiatrist and psychologist should consider. According to the Ethics Guidelines for the Practice of Forensic Psychiatry (American Academy of Psychiatry and the Law 2005), forensic psychiatrists should strive for objectivity, honesty, justice, and social responsibility. In Specialty Guidelines for Forensic Psychology, the American Psychological Association (2013, p. 10) noted that forensic practitioners need to consider issues that may impact a person's involvement in the legal system, including "factors associated with...race, ethnicity, culture, national origin,...language, socioeconomic status, or other relevant individual and cultural differences." In fulfilling their roles as consultants and experts, forensic psychiatrists and psychologists should not only acknowledge the risk instrument's limitations but also educate attorneys, judges, and juries about the difficulties in making risk assessment judgments. Clearly, risk assessment tools that use items that may be weak under a thorough analysis can lead to faulty interpretation and, more importantly, a potentially harmful outcome to the evaluee, society, or both. In light of this, great caution should be adopted when conducting risk assessment. The following methods reflect the need for professionals to be cognizant of the potential for bias, know its sources, and aspire to mitigate it. They are by no means a panacea, nor do they obviate the need for the forensic evaluator to be aware of personal reactions to the individual undergoing the assessment and the accusations against them, and whether any preformed biases about the evaluee exist.

Develop Structural Competency

Structural competency reflects proficiency in identifying how upstream social determinants impact the definition of a health issue, attitude, or problem (Metzl and Hansen 2014). With respect to violence risk assessments, forensic evaluators should be aware of how structural (or systemic) racial inequities may be embedded in violence risk assessment instruments. Moving away from a sole or heavy reliance on score-based classifications is also likely to reduce racial biases related to criminal history. If an arrest carries as much weight as a conviction regarding risk, then the factor is inherently biased based simply on the legal threshold necessary for an arrest (probable cause) versus a conviction (beyond a reasonable doubt). Some individuals may be more likely than others to be arrested based primarily on their racial or ethnic identity. Bearing this in mind, evaluations by risk assessment instruments that use arrest history as a risk factor have an ethical obligation to acknowledge this information and account for the tool's limitations in the findings and interpretation (American Psychological Association 2013, 2017). Extending this idea further is a possible interpretation that some risk assessment tools may not have established reliability and validity for use with members of certain groups. SPJ instruments classify violence risk as do actuarial instruments (Neal and Brodsky 2016; Singh et al. 2011) and can mitigate the biasing effects of unstructured clinical judgment (Neal and Grisso 2014), as well as reduce the reliance on criminal history that may inflate risk scores (Vincent and Viljoen 2020). The selection of the SPJ tool to be used should be based on not only the inclusion of relevant violence risk factors (such as the HCR-20V3 assessment tool; Douglas et al. 2013, 2014) but also allowance for the integration of culturally contextualized individual assessments (Shepherd and Willis-Esqueda 2017). Such an approach can reduce racial biases that may be more prominent within nomothetical risk schemes. SPJs can also be individualized by developing specific population-based risk templates with group-relevant risk markers.

Be Aware of How Risk Factors Are Identified

The use of risk assessment instruments is pervasive. Forensic psychiatrists and psychologists working in this area should have a thorough understanding of these tools, whether they use them or not. Before applying a risk assessment instrument, it is important to understand how that instrument was constructed, the statistical modeling method used, on what groups the norms were based, and how risk categories (e.g., low, medium, and high) were operationalized. It is also critical to know how the risk factors identified for inclusion were selected and weighted (e.g., criminal histories and prior sanctions). Statistical terms such as "moderate accuracy" may imply a higher level of certainty than is the case, and they should be explained in the report. Too often, particularly with actuarial risk assessments, risk percentages and risk labels may provide a false sense of certainty as to the quantification of risk (Sreenivasan et al. 2010) to both the evaluator and the trier of fact. Some researchers have noted the paucity of racial and ethnic minoritized groups in adult violence risk instruments, possibly lowering the predictive accuracy of such instruments in non-White samples (Shepherd and Willis-Esqueda 2017).

Normative data within actuarial instruments, even when they include minoritized groups, may not correct for cultural and structural biases such as governmental policies that led to loss of language and culture and generational disintegration of family and led to unstable psychosocial histories. Such data have built-in biases when factors such as employment history are protective or unstable childhood is a risk factor (Shepherd and Willis-Esqueda 2017). Although SPJs can individualize assessment, biases may still exist, including those related to the inclusion of historical risk factors derived largely from the majority culture or exclusion of culturally relevant protective factors (e.g., having elder mentors and cultural support, as found in AIAN groups). Notably, it has been reported that risk assessment instruments have differential predictive validity based on race. In a systematic review and meta-analysis of nine commonly used risk instruments (Historical Clinical Risk Management-20 [HCR-20], Level of Service Inventory-Revised [LSI-R], Psychopathy Checklist-Revised [PCL-R], Spousal Assault Risk Assessment [SARA], Structured Assessment of Violence Risk in Youth [SAVRY], Sex Offender Risk Appraisal Guide [SORAG], Static-99, Sexual Violence Risk 20 [SVR-20], and Violence Risk Appraisal Guide [VRAG]), the highest predictive validity was found for White individuals who were older (Singh et al. 2011). Singh et al. advised evaluators to use caution when using risk assessment tools in groups that are not similar to the validation sample.

Consider Juvenile History Appropriately

Juvenile history plays a prominent role in adult violence risk. Disparity in policing and sanctions across racial groups characterize the juvenile justice system in a manner similar to that in the adult system. Risk classifications impact whether the juvenile offender experiences treatment-based rehabilitative efforts or punitive criminal juvenile justice sanctions (Campbell and Miller 2018), as well as their ability to successfully reintegrate into society. Most juvenile risk assessment measures have been developed on White, mostly male groups and have potentially lowered applicability to females and nondominant groups. At minimum, at the structural level, juvenile tools should be validated on the targeted jurisdiction population and address potential racial bias in items, cutoff scores, and measurements of risk. A study on a group of youths who committed offenses of moderate severity found that they were more likely to receive harsher punishment depending on aspects of their physical appearance (Chen et al. 2021). Forensic evaluators should be aware of the tendency to rapidly form impressions based on physical appearance and take steps to mitigate bias by engaging in "blind" reviews of case files before seeing identifying information about the offender. On the individual evaluator level, evaluators 1) should be aware of potential areas of bias in specific risk instrument factors and domains such as juvenile justice history, which might encompass age at first arrest and prior incarceration; and 2) should consider a youth's self-reported criminal history as a source of information that can bypass the bias of justice system responses to offending (St. John et al. 2020).

Use Culturally Informed Practices

Rogers (2000) characterized as "lopsided" evaluations that emphasize aggravating static factors (such as criminal history) to the exclusion or minimization of other case-based elements. Relatedly, risk assessments that consider only the viewpoint of the majority culture—as is the case with most current standard methods—may be lopsided. Integrating culturally informed practices remains a gap in violence risk assessment (Shepherd and Willis-Esqueda 2017). Alternatively, instruments and evaluators themselves may ignore culturally relevant interventions and practices or not view them legitimate, even when a person is participating and benefiting from them (Gone and Calf Looking 2011). Evaluators should take care to consider cultural influences regarding the presence or absence of risk and protective factors. Shepherd and Willis-Esqueda (2017) solicited responses from legal and health care professionals who worked with at-risk youth who self-identified as American Indian/First Nations. The 28 participants thematically reviewed the SAVRY items. Four recurrent themes emerged: negative labeling; cultural decontextualization (e.g., questions did not consider why there may have been a failure to comply with the intervention or whether individuals were compliant with cultural versus court-ordered treatment); absence of cultural manifestations of behavior (e.g., lack of awareness that Aboriginal/Indigenous youth tend to be quiet or shy, which may be misinterpreted as poor coping ability); and absence of cultural norms and practices (e.g., lack of integration of traditional teaching, nuclear families that are mistakenly labeled "extended families" by non-Natives, differences between Native and non-Native child-rearing practices, lack of consideration of tribal ceremonies as prosocial involvement). The responses to individual SAVRY items illuminate the contextual aspects of violence risk assessment items.

Conclusion

Forensic specialists are not immune to biases, either implicit or explicit. Awareness of biases can be enhanced through periodic case discussions with other professionals and development of cultural competence and awareness through education and training (Neal and Brodsky 2016). The ethics codes for both psychiatrists and psychologists emphasize that one should engage only in practices in which one has competence (special training, knowledge, skill, and experience). In this respect, the many limitations and strengths of the predominant forms of risk assessment must be considered and articulated by the expert. Such transparency not only projects objectivity but also supports ethical behavior. Notably, this professional obligation is critical when the issues at hand carry significant consequences for both the examinee and the public, as in violence risk assessments.

References

Abedi V, Olulana O, Avula V, et al: Racial, economic, and health inequality and COVID-19 infection in the United States. J Racial Ethn Health Disparities 8(3):732–742, 2021 32875535

Abrams D, Bertrand M, Mullaninathan S: Do judges vary in their treatment of race? J Legal Stud 41:347–383, 2012

American Academy of Psychiatry and the Law: Ethics Guidelines for the Practice of Forensic Psychiatry. Adopted May 2005. Bloomfield, CT, American Academy of Psychiatry and the Law, 2005. Available at: https://www.aapl.org/ethics-guidelines. Accessed October 1, 2020.

American Psychological Association: Specialty guidelines for forensic psychology. Am Psychol 68(1):7–19, 2013 23025747

American Psychological Association: Ethical Principles of Psychologists and Code of Conduct. Washington, DC, American Psychological Association, 2017

Bagaric M, Wolf B, Rininger W: Mitigating America's mass incarceration crisis without compromising community protection: expanding the role of rehabilitation in sentencing. Lewis Clark Law Rev 22(1):1–60, 2018

Beck AJ: Race and Ethnicity of Violent Crime Offenders and Arrestees, 2018. U.S. Department of Justice, Office of Justice Programs, Bureau of Justice Statistics, NCJ 255969, January 2021. Available from: https://bjs.ojp.gov/content/pub/pdf/revcoa18.pdf. Accessed August 14, 2021.

Bonta J, Andrews D: The Psychology of Criminal Conduct, 6th Edition. New York, Routledge, 2017

Campbell CA, Miller W: A Review of the Validity of Juvenile Risk Assessment Across Race/Ethnicity. Oxford Research Encyclopedia of Criminology and Criminal Justice, February 26, 2018. Available at: https://oxfordre.com/criminology/display/10.1093/acrefore

/9780190264079.001.0001/acrefore-9780190264079-e-345. Accessed July 18, 2024.

Carson EA: Prisoners in 2018. Washington, DC, Office of Justice Programs, U.S. Department of Justice, NCJ 253516, April 2020a. Available at: https://bjs.ojp.gov/redirect-legacy/content/pub/pdf/p18.pdf. Accessed July 18, 2024.

Carson EA: Prisoners in 2019. Washington, DC, Office of Justice Programs, U.S. Department of Justice, NCJ 255115, October 2020b. Available at: https://bjs.ojp.gov/redirect-legacy/content/pub/pdf/p19.pdf. Accessed July 18, 2024.

Chen J, Fine AD, Norman J, et al: Out of the picture: Latinx and White male youths' facial features predict their juvenile justice system processing outcomes. Crime Delinq 67(6–7):787–807, 2021

Douglas KS, Hart SD, Webster CD, et al: HCR-20V3 Assessing Risk for Violence (User Guide). Burnaby, BC, Canada, Mental Health, Law, and Policy Institute, Simon Fraser University, 2013

Douglas KS, Hart SD, Webster CD, et al: Historical-Clinical-Risk Management-20, version 3 (HCR-20V3): development and overview. Int J Forensic Ment Health 13:93–108, 2014

Fellner J: Punishment and Prejudice: Racial Disparities in the War on Drugs. U.S. Department of Justice, Office of Justice Programs, Bureau of Justice Statistics, NCJ 183785, May 2000. Available at: https://www.ojp.gov/ncjrs/virtual-library/abstracts/punishment-and-prejudice-racial-disparities-war-drugs. Accessed April 10, 2021.

Gone JP, Calf Looking PE: American Indian culture as substance abuse treatment: pursuing evidence for a local intervention. J Psychoactive Drugs 43(4):291–296, 2011 22400459

Harcourt B: Risk as a proxy for race: the dangers of risk assessment. Federal Sentencing Reporter 27:237–243, 2015

Helmus L, Thornton D, Hanson RK, et al: Improving the predictive accuracy of Static-99 and Static-2002 with older sex offenders: revised age weights. Sex Abuse 24(1):64–101, 2012 21844404

Jhangiani R, Tarry H: Principles of Social Psychology, 1st International HP5 Edition. Victoria, BC, Canada, BCcampus, 2014. Available at: https://opentextbc.ca/socialpsychology/. Accessed April 10, 2021.

Kakade M, Duarte CS, Liu X, et al: Adolescent substance use and other illegal behaviors and racial disparities in criminal justice system involvement: findings from a US national survey. Am J Public Health 102(7):1307–1310, 2012 22594721

Maruschak LM, Minton TD: Correctional populations in the United States, 2017–2018. Office of Justice Programs, U.S. Department of Justice, NCJ 252157, August 2020. Available at: https://bjs.ojp.gov/library/publications/correctional-populations-united-states-2017-2018. Accessed April 10, 2021.

Metzl JM, Hansen H: Structural competency: theorizing a new medical engagement with stigma and inequality. Soc Sci Med 103:126–133, 2014 24507917

Minton TD: American Indian and Alaska Natives in Local Jails, 1999–2014. U.S. Department of Justice, NCJ 250262, September 2017. Available at: https://bjs.ojp.gov/library/publications/american-indian-and-alaska -natives-local-jails-1999-2014. Accessed April 10, 2021.

Neal TMS, Brodsky SL: Forensic psychologists' perceptions of bias and potential correction strategies in forensic mental health evaluations. Psychol Public Policy Law 22:58–76, 2016

Neal TMS, Grisso T: The cognitive underpinnings of bias in forensic mental health evaluations. Psychol Public Policy Law 20(2):200–211, 2014

Nilsson T, Munthe C, Gustavson C, et al: The precarious practice of forensic psychiatric risk assessments. Int J Law Psychiatry 32(6):400–407, 2009 19800123

Perry SW, Durose M, Antenangeli L: Tribal Crime Data-Collection Activities, 2020. U.S. Department of Justice, NCJ 254789, July 2020. Available at: https://www.bjs.ojp.gov/content/pub/pdf/tcdca20.pdf. Accessed April 10, 2021.

Rogers R: The uncritical acceptance of risk assessment in forensic practice. Law Hum Behav 24(5):595–605, 2000 11026213

Scherr K, Dror IE: Ingroup biases of forensic experts: perceptions of wrongful convictions versus exonerations. Psychol Crime Law 27:89–104, 2021

Shepherd SM, Willis-Esqueda C: Indigenous perspectives on violence risk assessment: a thematic analysis. Punishm Soc 20:599–627, 2017

Singh JP, Grann M, Fazel S: A comparative study of violence risk assessment tools: a systematic review and metaregression analysis of 68 studies involving 25,980 participants. Clin Psychol Rev 31(3):499–513, 2011 21255891

Skeem J, Lowenkamp CT: Risk, race, and recidivism: predictive bias and disparate impact. Criminology 54:680–712, 2016

Sreenivasan S, Weinberger LE, Frances A, et al: Alice in actuarial-land: through the looking glass of changing Static-99 norms. J Am Acad Psychiatry Law 38(3):400–406, 2010 20852227

St. John V, Murphy K, Liberman A: Recommendations for addressing racial bias in risk and needs assessment in the juvenile justice system. Child Trends, February 2020. Available at: https://cms.childtrends.org/wp -content/uploads/2020/01/Duke-Risk-Assessment-FAQ_ChildTrends _Jan2020-1.pdf. Accessed April 13, 2021.

Substance Abuse and Mental Health Services Administration: Results from the 2013 National Survey on Drug Use and Health: Summary of National Findings (NSDUH Series H-48, HHS Publ No SMA-14–4863). Rockville, MD, Substance Abuse and Mental Health Services Administration, 2014. Available at: https://www.samhsa.gov/data/sites/default/files/NSD

UHresultsPDFWHTML2013/Web/NSDUHresults2013.pdf. Accessed July 18, 2024.

Trestman RL: Is justice really blind? J Am Acad Psychiatry Law 46(4):416–418, 2018 30593470

U.S. Census Bureau, Population Division: 2019. Available at: https://www .census.gov/programs-surveys/acs/news/updates/2019.html. Accessed April 10, 2021.

Vincent CM, Viljoen JL: Racial algorithms or systemic problems? Risk assessments and racial disparities. Crim Justice Behav 47:1576–1584, 2020

Weinberger LE, Sreenivasan S: Addressing ethical dilemmas in violence risk assessment from a forensic psychologist's perspective, in Ethics Dilemmas in Forensic Psychiatry and Psychology Practice. Edited by Griffith E. New York, Columbia University Press, 2018, pp 284–303

Zhen Z, Minton TD, Miller S: Jail Inmates in 2018. U.S. Department of Justice, Office of Justice Programs, Bureau of Justice Statistics, NCJ 253044, March 2020. Available at: https://bjs.ojp.gov/content/pub/pdf/ji18.pdf. Accessed April 10, 2021.

20

Structural Racism and Ethics

Cheryl D. Wills, M.D.

> "I will willingly refrain from doing any injury or wrong from false-hood ... whatever may be the rank of those who it may be my duty to cure."
>
> —Classic Hippocratic Oath

Medical ethics are the foundation of precision health care delivery. The Hippocratic tradition admonishes physicians to avoid harm when practicing. The four-principles model of biomedical ethics (Beauchamp and Childress 2001)—respect for autonomy, beneficence, nonmaleficence, and justice—is the cornerstone of ethical medical practice (Shea 2020). Upholding these standards is particularly important in psychiatry because mental disorders and pharmacotherapy can result in changes that compromise a person's perceptions and stream of thought. These changes can impede the individual's capacity to provide a coherent history or give informed consent for psychiatric care.

The forensic psychiatrist strives to appreciate the evaluee's narrative—including experiences involving culture, trauma, and racism—that informs the diagnostic process and expert opinion. Vitiation of this endeavor by partiality-based misinformation and stereotypes can abase people's autonomy and quality of life. This chapter examines how being cognizant of the effects of structural racism can be conducive to ethical forensic psychiatric practice.

The American Academy of Psychiatry and the Law (2005) and the Canadian Academy of Psychiatry and the Law (2018), the largest forensic psychiatry professional organizations in North America, offer ethics guidance for forensic psychiatric practice. Both stress the importance of the forensic psychiatrist being fair and rendering dispassionate opinions. The practitioner must be mindful that trauma, including events involving racism, can affect the narrative of an evaluee. Disparities in race-based mortality rates during the 2020–2022 COVID-19 pandemic and events such as the deaths of unarmed Black people, including George Floyd, by U.S. law enforcement officers have magnified the importance of considering the impact of race-based experiences in psychiatric assessments.

Definitions

Race is a social construct or interpretation based on one's physical characteristics. *Racism* is a system that uses race to assign merit and opportunities and undermines progress of the nondominant group. *Discrimination* is an action based on *prejudice*, which is a belief frequently based on unfair assumptions about race, nationality, class, ability, gender, sexual orientation, age, etc. *Intersectionality* refers to the complex cumulative, and at times synergistic, ramifications that various forms of discrimination have on an individual.

In 1970, U.S. psychiatrist Chester M. Pierce coined the term *microaggression*, to describe subtle comments or behaviors, intentional or otherwise, that denigrate a member of a marginalized group (Pierce 1974). Although Pierce's definition referred to the disparaging of Black people by Whites after the civil rights movement, the term, which was added to the Merriam-Webster Dictionary (2022) in 2017, has expanded to include the derogation of members of other minority and marginalized groups. Repeated exposure to microaggressions can erode the coping skills of the denigrated individual and can increase the risk for suicide spectrum behavior, as a manifestation of depression, in Black youth, Black adults, and others (Goodwill et al. 2021; O'Keefe et al. 2015). *Microinequity* refers to the experience of being undervalued, marginalized, overlooked, and devalued because of one's status as a minority (Silver et al. 2018).

Structural racism or *systemic racism* is an amalgamation of public and institutional policies, practices, and protocols, along with social forces and beliefs, that intentionally restrict privileges and opportunities based on race. Individuals can indirectly engage in structural racism by knowingly enforcing racist policies. Racism systematically impedes progress and affects the quality of life, morbidity, and mortality of non-dominant groups.

Race-based discriminatory policies and practices have long affected where individuals are born, live, work, are educated, access health care, shop, worship, socialize, and age. These social determinants of health (SDOH) are responsible for up to 80% of outcomes in physical and mental health (Hood et al. 2016).

Racism in Organized Medicine

In 2020, amid the pandemic and civil unrest, the American Medical Association reiterated that race is a social construct and that "racism is a threat to public health" (American Medical Association 2020b). The organization admonished clinicians and researchers to "focus on genetics and biology, the *experience of racism* and social determinants of health"—and not race—"when describing risk factors for disease" (emphasis added) (American Medical Association 2020a). The forensic psychiatrist can accomplish this by modifying the traditional psychiatric interview that includes inquiries about the SDOH in developmental, educational, and social histories. A receptive exploration of the examinee's culture, experiences with racism, and history of personal, vicarious, and transgenerational trauma can add depth to the evaluee's narrative and decrease evaluator bias.

DSM-5-TR (American Psychiatric Association 2022), which advises psychiatrists to consider the evaluee's ethnic and cultural circumstances in every psychiatric assessment, includes a semistructured Cultural Formulation Interview (CFI). The CFI is designed to glean information about the evaluee's identity, emotions, behaviors, health, sense of identity, and perspective on health, including mental health. The text contains commentary on how racism and discrimination can influence psychiatric assessment and diagnosis (American Psychiatric Association 2022).

Individuality and Bias

The forensic psychiatrist's work product should be devoid of evaluator bias, such as stereotypes and clichés. There are two types of bias, explicit and implicit. Explicit bias consists of acknowledged beliefs, based on assumptions, that select against a person, item, or group (e.g., Sam dislikes white sneakers because they are hard to keep clean). Implicit bias involves beliefs, ideas, and perspectives imprinted by one's past experiences. The person may not immediately be aware of the bias but can use it to provoke or discriminate against others. For example, Jane constantly insists on treating everyone fairly, but she always assigns individuals wearing red shirts to stand at the end of the line, even when they present VIP passes.

Bias in Patient Care

Bias informs the quality of health care service delivery and the patient's experience. This may be attributed, at least in part, to the bias that accompanies individuals who enter the health profession. Dyrbye et al. (2019) studied 3,400 White medical residents and showed that resident burnout was directly related to their explicit bias against Black patients. The residents' implicit bias against Black patients was not affected by the residents' perceived level of stress. This association affects the quality of the patient experience for Black people.

Bias in Psychiatry

Racial bias in psychiatric care is a major concern. Schwartz and Blankenship (2014) determined that in a 24-year period, Black people were three to four times more likely, and Latinx/Hispanic people three times more likely, to be diagnosed with schizophrenia than White patients. The pattern has been observed in adolescents as well; White teens with clinical presentations similar to those of Black teens diagnosed with schizophrenia are more likely to be given a diagnosis of mood disorder (Kilgus et al. 1995). The bias persists even when the evaluator conducts a semistructured interview to ascertain the diagnosis (Olbert et al. 2018).

Black people are more likely to be prescribed antipsychotic medications at higher dosages, thereby increasing the risk for adverse side effects and related disability. They also disproportionately receive first-generation antipsychotics and long-acting injectable medications (Herbeck et al. 2004; Kuno and Rothbard 2002). Metzl (2010) showed that the authors of schizophrenia research articles that included the races of patients were more likely to use adjectives like "violent," "hostile," "aggressive," and "paranoid" to describe behavior.

But diagnostic partiality goes beyond schizophrenia. Black patients are disproportionately diagnosed with personality and substance use disorders and are less likely to be prescribed the latest treatment modalities for substance use and other mental disorders, even when they are discharged from inpatient psychiatric units (Thompson et al. 2003). Additionally, Black patients are disproportionately restrained in emergency departments (Schnitzer et al. 2020) and on inpatient psychiatric units (Smith et al. 2022).

Lithium therapy, which psychiatrists have used to treat bipolar disorder for more than 60 years, can potentiate renal failure (Aiff et al. 2014). The diagnosis was determined by race-based computations of estimated glomerular filtration rate (eGFR). The metric, which is not evidence-based, resulted in Black people being initially diagnosed at a more advanced stage of the disease. This increased their morbidity and mortality and reduced their eligibility for renal transplantation because they were less healthy when they applied (Morris and Mohan 2020).

In July 2022, the Organ Procurement and Transplantation Network (OPTN) mandated using race-neutral calculations to estimate glomerular filtration rate in all transplant candidates (Mohottige et al. 2023). Also, in December 2022, OPTN required every transplant center to use race-neutral calculations to ascertain renal functioning in all Black transplant candidates (Mohottige et al. 2023). Those whose applications were delayed owing to race-based eGFR had their transplant eligibility backdated. By May 2024, more than 14,700 Black renal transplant candidates had received 1–3 years' wait-time credit (Organ Procurement and Transplantation Network 2024). This affirms that equitable assessment of renal function can improve health outcomes for Black patients.

Solutions

The forensic psychiatrist uses their unique skill set while striving to practice ethically. They are mindful of personal biases while endeavoring to appreciate how cultural experiences, including systemic inequities, inform the experiences of colleagues, subordinates, and examinees. This set of conditions adds complexity to a challenging assessment process.

Failure to consider, when relevant, the impact of structural racism on the evaluee's mental health introduces bias into the examination. Addressing minute details of the evaluee's personal history, however, may detract the expert from proffering a focused opinion about the forensic question. These competing interests can be more effectively balanced by becoming familiar with the CFI and considering three principles: structural competence, cultural competence, and structural humility.

Structural Competence

Structural competence (Metzl and Hansen 2014) involves acknowledging that many adverse health outcomes, such as disparities in renal failure prognoses, are not due to biology or genetics. Instead, the long-term effects of structural bias in policies and protocols, which are mediated by SDOH and the experience of racism, include health disparities in targeted groups. For example, zoning laws and infrastructure can affect health outcomes by restricting access to quality housing, education, groceries, exercise, transportation, employment opportunities, green spaces, and health care services.

Cultural Competence

Cultural competence involves being sensitive to the complexities of the examinee's ideology, biases, and life experiences—including those involving health care and lifestyle management—beyond the scope of evidence-based medicine. The forensic psychiatrist should endeavor to learn about other cultures, values, and norms while noting that the quality of research publications and other resources can vary widely. Cultural competence has been criticized for being an academic, determinate process (Trinh et al. 2020) that risks introducing bias into evaluations by reinforcing stereotypes instead of focusing on psychosocial and cultural inquiries (Whitley 2007). Cultural knowledge can be thoughtfully implemented by the forensic psychiatrist who is endeavoring to be culturally humble.

Cultural Humility

Cultural humility is a dynamic mindset based on core psychotherapy principles: critical self-reflection, nonjudgment, curiosity, and openness (Comas-Díaz et al. 2019). These skills are conducive to facilitating communication with the evaluee and illuminating evaluator bias. For example, Dr. Blue, who has experienced discrimination, can use critical self-reflection and seek consultation from others before deciding to evaluate the defendant in a hate crime case. If she accepts the case, being curious and nonjudgmental will be conducive to learning about the evaluee's cultural beliefs, past experiences, and perhaps, motives for engaging in the alleged offense.

Conclusion

The forensic psychiatrist should be cognizant of how bias, including structural racism, can affect every evaluee's presentation and history. The CFI and other resources facilitate ascertaining this information in the psychiatric interview. These data impact diagnoses, opinions, and recommendations and can greatly affect the autonomy and quality of life of others. Medicine is in the introductory stages of realizing the damage that structural racism has on health care. The profession has a long way to go.

References

Aiff H, Attman PO, Aurell M, et al: End-stage renal disease associated with prophylactic lithium treatment. Eur Neuropsychopharmacol 24(4):540–544, 2014 24503277

American Academy of Psychiatry and the Law: Ethics Guidelines for the Practice of Forensic Psychiatry. Adopted May 2005. Bloomfield, CT, American Academy of Psychiatry and the Law, 2005. Available at: https://www.aapl.org/ethics-guidelines. Accessed October 1, 2020.

American Medical Association: New AMA Policies Recognize Race as a Social, Not Biological, Construct. November 16, 2020a. Available at https://www.ama-assn.org/press-center/press-releases/new-ama-policies-recognize-race-social-not-biological-construct. Accessed January 30, 2022.

American Medical Association: New AMA Policy Recognizes Racism as a Public Health Threat. November 16, 2020b. Available at https://www.ama-assn.org/press-center/press-releases/new-ama-policy-recognizes-racism-public-health-threat. Accessed January 30, 2022.

American Psychiatric Association: Diagnostic and Statistical Manual of Mental Disorders, 5th Edition, Text Revision. Washington, DC, American Psychiatric Association, 2022

Beauchamp TL, Childress JF: Principles of Biomedical Ethics, 5th Edition. New York, Oxford University Press, 2001

Canadian Academy of Psychiatry and the Law: Ethical Guidelines for Canadian Forensic Psychiatrists. Ottawa, ON, Canadian Academy of Psychiatry and the Law, 2018. Available at: https://capl-acpd.org/wp-content/uploads/2019/06/CAPL-Ethics-FIN-Rev2019-EN.pdf. Accessed January 30, 2022.

Comas-Díaz L, Hall GN, Neville HA: Racial trauma: theory, research, and healing: introduction to the special issue. Am Psychol 74(1):1–5, 2019 30652895

Dyrbye L, Herrin J, West CP, et al: Association of racial bias with burnout among resident physicians. JAMA Netw Open 2(7):e197457, 2019 31348503

Goodwill JR, Taylor RJ, Watkins DC: Everyday discrimination, depressive symptoms, and suicide ideation among African American men. Arch Suicide Res 25(1):74–93, 2021 31597538

Herbeck DM, West JC, Ruditis I, et al: Variations in use of second-generation antipsychotic medication by race among adult psychiatric patients. Psychiatr Serv 55(6):677–684, 2004 15175466

Hood CM, Gennuso KP, Swain GR, et al: County health rankings: relationships between determinant factors and health outcomes. Am J Prev Med 50(2):129–135, 2016 26526164

Kilgus MD, Pumariega AJ, Cuffe SP: Influence of race on diagnosis in adolescent psychiatric inpatients. J Am Acad Child Adolesc Psychiatry 34(1):67–72, 1995 7860460

Kuno E, Rothbard AB: Racial disparities in antipsychotic prescription patterns for patients with schizophrenia. Am J Psychiatry 159(4):567–572, 2002 11925294

Merriam-Webster Dictionary: Microaggression. Available at: https://www.merriam-webster.com/dictionary/microaggression. Accessed January 30, 2022.

Metzl JM: The Protest Psychosis: How Schizophrenia Became a Black Disease. Boston, MA, Beacon Press, 2010

Metzl JM, Hansen H: Structural competency: theorizing a new medical engagement with stigma and inequality. Soc Sci Med 103:126–133, 2014 24507917

Mohottige D, Purnell TS, Boulware LE: Redressing the harms of race-based kidney function estimation. JAMA 329(11):881–882, 2023

Morris H, Mohan S: Using race in the estimation of glomerular filtration rates: time for a reversal? Curr Opin Nephrol Hypertens 29(2):227–231, 2020 31895163

O'Keefe VM, Wingate LR, Cole AB, et al: Seemingly harmless racial communications are not so harmless: racial microaggressions lead to suicidal ideation by way of depression symptoms. Suicide Life Threat Behav 45(5):567–576, 2015 25556819

Olbert CM, Nagendra A, Buck B: Meta-analysis of Black vs. White racial disparity in schizophrenia diagnosis in the United States: do structured assessments attenuate racial disparities? J Abnorm Psychol 127(1):104–115, 2018 29094963

Organ Procurement and Transplantation Network (OPTN): Over 14,700 waiting time modifications completed for Black kidney patients one year after policy. OPTN, 2024. Available at: https://optn.transplant.hrsa.gov/news/over-14-700-waiting-time-modifications-completed-for-black-kidney-patients-one-year-after-policy-implementation. Accessed October 22, 2024.

Pierce CM: Psychiatric problems of the Black minority, in American Handbook of Psychiatry. Edited by Arieti S. New York, Basic Books, 1974, pp 512–523

Schnitzer K, Merideth F, Macias-Konstantopoulos W, et al: Disparities in care: the role of race on the utilization of physical restraints in the emergency setting. Acad Emerg Med 27(10):943–950, 2020 32691509

Schwartz RC, Blankenship DM: Racial disparities in psychotic disorder diagnosis: a review of empirical literature. World J Psychiatry 4(4):133–140, 2014 25540728

Shea M: Forty years of the four principles: enduring themes from Beauchamp and Childress. J Med Philos 45:387–395, 2020

Silver JK, Rowe M, Sinha MS, et al: Micro-inequities in medicine. PM R 10(10):1106–1114, 2018 30366648

Smith CM, Turner NA, Thielman NM, et al: Association of Black race with physical and chemical restraint use among patients undergoing emergency psychiatric evaluation. Psychiar Serv 73(7):730–736, 2022 34932385

Thompson EE, Neighbors HW, Munday C, et al: Length of stay, referral to aftercare, and rehospitalization among psychiatric inpatients. Psychiatr Serv 54(9):1271–1276, 2003 12954945

Trinh NH, Tuchman S, Chen J, et al: Cultural humility and the practice of consultation-liaison psychiatry. Psychosomatics 61(4):313–320, 2020 32299622

Whitley R: Cultural competence, evidence-based medicine, and evidence-based practices. Psychiatr Serv 58(12):1588–1590, 2007 18048561

21

Priority-Setting in the COVID Pandemic

Perspectives From Sweden

Lars Sandman, Ph.D.

Manne Sjöstrand, M.D., Ph.D.

Svante Nyberg, M.D., Ph.D.

Christoffer Rahm, M.D., Ph.D.

Niklas Juth, Ph.D.

In a budget-constrained health care system, priority-setting is always on the agenda, aiming to strike a reasonable balance between efficiency and equity. The publicly financed health care system of Sweden is no exception. Sweden is one of the top spenders on health care in Europe in terms of percentage of gross domestic product, but there are signs of a gap between available resources and needs because of a combination of demographic changes, technological development, and increasing public expectations. At the same time, the Swedish health care system generally has good health outcomes from an international perspective, with a high level of population health.

In this chapter, we discuss ethical challenges of prioritization during the COVID pandemic in Sweden. We describe the Swedish framework for priority-setting and how it was adapted and interpreted during the pandemic, with particular focus on intensive care and vaccine distribution. In this context, we also discuss the question of whether it is justifiable to prioritize health care staff. Last, we discuss priority-setting in psychiatric care, using experiences from one of the largest psychiatric services in Sweden, Psychiatry South Stockholm. Countries have handled these ethics priorities in various ways; this chapter aims to illustrate the rationale for the priorities in Sweden, which we hope may be of interest to others.

A general rationale is that priority-setting should be transparent and guided by explicit ethical principles. To handle health care priority-setting, the Swedish parliament in 1995 adopted a framework (Socialdepartementet 1995), often referred to as the *ethics platform for priority-setting*, that is based on three ethical principles:

1. The *human dignity principle,* a basic formal equality principle, explicitly claims that aspects such as social standing and situation, economic situation, chronological age, and previous lifestyle should not be taken into account. (It does allow considerations related to biological age and future lifestyle if such factors affect treatment outcome.)
2. The *needs-solidarity principle* claims that the greater the health care need, the greater the claim to health care resources—under the condition that these resources can bring benefit to the patient. Explicitly, the needs of vulnerable patients must be observed.
3. The *cost-effectiveness principle* claims that health care interventions should have a reasonable balance between cost and effect in terms of improved health and increased quality of life.

The three principles are codified into the general health care law and have a rank order, implying that the human dignity principle must be fulfilled first (i.e., no unjustified discrimination). Patient need is given higher weight than cost-effectiveness, implying that a higher threshold for cost-effectiveness is acceptable for more severe conditions.

Swedish health care is organized into 21 self-governing regions, with taxation rights and the right to organize and distribute health care according to regional political decisions, within the requirements of the national health care legislation. Hence, the exact interpretation and implementation of the stated principles might differ between regions.

This potential difference (and in some cases observed difference) in what is available for citizens has led to a number of national initiatives to harmonize priorities across regions when it comes to new pharmaceuticals or medical technologies.

COVID-19: Priority-Setting in the Intensive Care Setting

When the COVID pandemic hit Sweden in March 2020, it was expected that need for intensive care would outweigh available resources. The National Board of Health and Welfare therefore issued priority guidelines for intensive care, that is, applying the Swedish law and prioritization guidelines to a situation of acute rationing. Two issues raised in particular prompted discussion: how to take into consideration patients' life expectancy (and therefore indirectly age), and whether health care staff should get priority. The ban against taking chronological age into account while allowing consideration of biological age, in combination with 20 years of priority practice in which treatments resulting in longer survival had been prioritized (ceteris paribus), led to three priority levels (Table 21.1) (Socialstyrelsen 2020a).

In the intensive care profession, the guidelines were largely accepted as reasonable in the circumstances, but they also received criticism. Later public investigations criticized how elderly patients were prioritized for health care and how some operationalizations of the guidelines used chronological age limits as proxies, without criticizing the guidelines per se (IVO 2020).

In April 2020, the National Board of Health and Welfare published priority guidelines for routine care. These provided a rank order for rationing in health care while, at the same time, emphasizing the patient's right to be diagnosed and have access to palliative interventions and care if active treatment is rationed (Socialstyrelsen 2020b). This general rank order was then translated into concrete guidance in different parts of the health care system.

Prioritizing Health Care Personnel

The issue of prioritizing health care personnel (HCP) received attention early in the pandemic. The intensive care guidelines decided against prioritizing HCP, but the question has been continuously discussed, and as detailed later in this chapter, HCP were eventually prioritized

Table 21.1 Priority-setting in intensive care

Priority level	Condition
1	Patients with severe illness or injury, expected survival >12 months, and an indication for intensive care and who do not have impaired chances of survival if treated. *To the extent that prioritization must be made between patients at priority level 1, priority is based on biological age in terms of life expectancy.*
2	Patients who meet any of the following criteria (or a combination of several criteria): a. One or more serious systemic diseases with marked functional limitation. b. Expected survival 6–12 months, based on underlying disease.
3	Patients with an overall expected low probability of survival initially and for whom intensive care is normally used only to enable a reassessment and consultation with relatives.

for vaccination. The arguments for prioritizing HCP boil down to three kinds of considerations: instrumental considerations of usefulness or utility, considerations of need or equity, and considerations of reciprocity. The first kind of consideration is of a consequentialist kind; the last two are based on ethical considerations of justice.

Considerations of Usefulness

The most common version of utility-based arguments in the debate has undoubtedly been the following: HCP are a limited resource and are essential to reduce the overall health impact of the pandemic. If HCP are prioritized in health care, they are more likely to stay at work or return to work faster. Prioritizing HCP will, therefore, lead to a net gain of health and saved life years. Thus HCP should be prioritized in health care.

There are at least four problems with the argument. First, it is not established to what extent the empirical presupposition of the argument is correct (that prioritizing HCP leads to a net benefit in terms of health or saved life years). Some data suggest that HCP is one of the occupational categories with the highest rates of COVID-19 infection, perhaps even the highest of all (Nguyen et al. 2020). Even though HCP are better trained and equipped to protect themselves than most or all other occupational categories, they are also more exposed than others. However, this is not sufficient to conclude that not prioritizing HCP leads to worse outcomes than if they were prioritized.

Second, even if it is true that prioritizing HCP would lead to better overall health and more life years saved, it does not settle to what extent HCP should be prioritized compared with other occupational groups and other grounds of prioritization. According to the argument of usefulness, it seems that HCP should be prioritized to the extent that they benefit others (in terms of health or life years). But other occupational groups may also contribute to health and saved life years, such as workers who are essential to maintaining critical services and infrastructure. A few examples are safety personnel ensuring that distances are kept, police enforcing pandemic rules, and public officials formulating and communicating pandemic rules. Some of these may be thought to be more replaceable than HCP, but such a conclusion is far from obvious. In the end, if we want to avoid COVID-19 exceptionalism, then when we refer to usefulness, anyone who is more useful to others should have higher priority. This is not only difficult to determine in practice but also morally questionable. Moreover, being useful to others is arguably not the only factor that should determine priority-setting; it should be balanced with other factors, such as need and effect of treatment for the patient in question. Guidelines settling how this weighing should be done have not yet seen the light of day.

Third, it is unclear what HCP should be prioritized—a common suggestion is those who are directly involved in treating patients with COVID-19. This is not as clear-cut as it may look: almost all HCP may encounter patients with COVID-19, with different degrees of probability. But even if we set aside this practical difficulty, the suggestion is still not aligned with the rationale. The rationale is that HCP should be prioritized because they are useful. If so, it should not matter whether they deal with COVID-19 patients or not. Again, the general usefulness argument is not grounds for COVID-19 exceptionalism. If we invite this line of reasoning, then we would have to rank all HCP (and others) according to usefulness (in terms of health and saved life years).

Last, even if the difficult issues of how we should prioritize with reference to usefulness could be settled satisfactorily, there is still the moral problem: should how useful you are really be allowed to determine how you are prioritized? Of course, one could argue that social usefulness, in the end, is morally more important than other considerations. But this would contradict the most fundamental principle in the Swedish priority platform—the principle of human dignity—and Swedish health care law (Socialdepartementet 1995). From a perspective of need, it is obvious that being unable to be productive or useful to others should not be a reason to lessen a person's priority. Indeed, those who lack the ability to be productive or useful are often the ones most in need of health care.

Considerations of Need

When it comes to prioritizing in Swedish health care, the principle of need is, in practice, the most important. The principle of human dignity is fundamentally a ban against unjust discrimination, which rules out certain grounds for prioritization. The principle of need, on the other hand, says something substantial about how to prioritize. The magnitude of need, in turn, is to be determined by the severity of the condition and, at least to some extent, the effect of the treatment (Gustavsson 2017).

In consideration of preventive measures, such as vaccines, severity is translated into risk. The concept of risk is composed of two elements: (size of) probability and (size of) negative outcomes. Although there are no grounds for claiming that HCP would get more severely ill than the average citizen if infected with COVID-19, there are grounds for claiming that HCP have a higher probability of contracting COVID-19. Hence, there is a needs-based claim to prioritize HCP, at least to some extent, when it comes to vaccination.

What the principle of need, as formulated in the ethical platform, does not reveal is how the probability factor and the negative-effect factor should be weighed against each other. Older citizens have a lower probability of being infected by COVID-19, but if they are infected, they are much more likely to suffer seriously and die prematurely. Thus, compared with HCP, older people would score higher on the severity factor and lower on the probability factor. The most straightforward interpretation of the recommendations of the Public Health Agency of Sweden (2021) is that severity is assigned greater weight than probability. This interpretation has not been explicit, however, and it is not a direct implication of the ethics platform. How to weigh probability against severity is one of the many issues that need to be addressed in the future.

Considerations of Reciprocity

The idea of reciprocity has intuitive appeal: HCP take risks to reduce risk and harm to others. They are assigned by society to do this; therefore, they have a special claim to be protected against these very risks. There at least three kinds of ethical justice–based reasons to accept considerations of reciprocity: 1) the contractualist idea that society or the state asks HCP to take risks (e.g., of being infected) and that a fair service in return is that society provide extra protection for these very risks (Walker 2010); 2) the desert-based backward-looking idea that HCP should get something in return for the sacrifices made in the line of duty (Persad et al. 2009); and 3) the similar idea of compensation for taking on higher risks. Regardless of what the basis is, the conclusion is that HCP have special claims to priority.

If one refers to reciprocity, one must also settle how strong the claim is. The most radical proposition would be that HCP should always have the highest priority. But that seems difficult to defend, especially in the intensive care setting. It is counterintuitive that considerations of patients' occupations should always trump obviously relevant considerations such as need and effect of treatment. The weakest suggestion would be to say that considerations of reciprocity are a mere tiebreaker when other considerations are equal, making the suggestion practically irrelevant. As with utility, considerations of reciprocity would contravene the Swedish priority platform and health care legislation.

Vaccine Distribution

At the end of 2020, the Public Health Agency of Sweden issued priority guidelines for vaccine distribution. As of May 2021, four phases of priority were set (Public Health Agency of Sweden 2021):

Phase 1

- People in nursing homes for the elderly or receiving home social care according to Swedish social services legislation
- Staff in elderly care, health care, and other professions working closely with the cohort above
- Close family contacts—that is, adults living with people receiving home social care

Phase 2

- People older than 65 years, starting with the oldest
- People who have undergone bone marrow or organ transplant and their domestic contacts
- People who need dialysis and their domestic contacts
- People older than 18 years who receive assistance compensation according to the Swedish social insurance act—starting with the oldest
- Staff in health care and social care working closely with the cohorts above

Phase 3

- People ages 60–64 with a disease or condition that implies increased risk of serious illness in COVID-19 (see list that follows)
- People ages 60–64 not in the cohort above
- People ages 18–59 with a disease or condition that implies increased risk of serious illness in COVID-19 (see list below)
- People with a condition implying that they have difficulty following advice to contain the spread of the pandemic (those ages 18–59 with cognitive or psychiatric disabilities; socially vulnerable populations)

Diseases or conditions with an increased risk of developing serious illness in COVID-19

- Chronic cardiovascular disease, including stroke and hypertension
- Chronic obstructive pulmonary disease; severe or unstable asthma

- Other conditions that result in reduced pulmonary function or that may affect respiratory function in other ways (e.g., severe obesity or neuromuscular disease)
- Chronic liver or kidney failure
- Diabetes type 1 or 2
- Conditions featuring a severely impaired immune system
- Down syndrome

Phase 4

- People older than 18 years who were not prioritized in the previous phases

The Public Health Agency did not present any detailed rationale for these priorities. To a large extent, they seem to be in line with the platform for priority-setting, prioritizing the patients at risk of being worse off if they contract COVID-19. At the same time, the focus on nursing homes and people in need of home care lacks a clear medical rationale per se and seems to serve only as a proxy for vulnerability and old age. Based on the priority platform, it could be argued that other patient groups should also be part of Phase 1. Critics of the plan for vaccine distribution have suggested that there are political considerations behind this priority, given the high level of deaths from COVID-19 within Swedish nursing homes and the consequent criticism of the Swedish government and authorities (Sjögren and Milstaed 2021).

A somewhat more controversial standpoint, given the ethics platform, is to allow staff and those residing with prioritized persons to be vaccinated at an early stage. The human dignity principle does not allow considerations of social situation, function, or standing. However, there are several reasonable ethical rationales for this deviation from the platform. First, for vulnerable patients in need of daily care, social isolation becomes more difficult. In addition, it is not far-fetched to believe that the high rate of deaths at Swedish nursing homes was driven by patients being exposed to staff contacts. A more general argument is that healthy and functioning staff are necessary to attend to people's health care needs. According to the ethics platform, it might be argued that tending to the needs of severely ill people (regardless of the reason) should get a higher priority, thus limiting which staff should get priority. This argument might be supported by both utilitarian ethics and the theories of John Rawls (Tännsjö 2019). The Rawlsian basis implies that we accept unequal treatment (in this case prioritizing health care staff) to benefit the worst off (patients at risk of severe

illness as a result of COVID-19). Within Sweden, to prevent staff shortages, many regions chose to broaden the scope of priority to include
staff involved in acute and intensive care, or health care more generally.

An important issue, in the context of this chapter, is whether patients
with psychiatric diagnoses should be given priority. In the guidelines,
patients with psychiatric conditions were mentioned only as a population potentially unable to follow recommendations. However, studies
have shown that psychiatric disorders may be a risk factor for severe
COVID-19 (Nemani et al. 2021), and patient interest groups have argued
that those with severe psychiatric disorders should also be prioritized
for vaccination (RSMH 2021). In April 2021, the Swedish National Board
of Health and Welfare included schizophrenia and bipolar disorder in
their updated guidelines of conditions with an increased risk of severe
COVID-19 (Socialstyrelsen 2021).

There is a related reason to prioritize vaccination of psychiatric
staff. Severely ill patients with acute psychosis or mania may not be
able to follow guidelines of social distancing, handwashing, or mask
wearing and may be at elevated risk of exposing others to the disease.

Prioritizations in Psychiatric Care: Psychiatry South Stockholm

The new priority guidelines were intended for intensive care, but other
areas of health care, including psychiatry, faced similar questions of rationing. We now turn to one of the largest psychiatric services in Sweden,
Psychiatry South Stockholm (PSS). PSS is a public psychiatric service for
inpatient and outpatient psychiatric care in southern Stockholm with 12
inpatient wards, 224 hospital beds, and 11 specialized outpatient units.

It was expected early that health care resources would have to be
redistributed to care for patients with COVID-19. It was decided that
psychiatry should support the geriatric clinics, which needed more
resources because of the pandemic. However, it was also expected that
staff would be infected themselves, resulting in reduced personnel
and, consequently, reduced capacity. Moreover, there was a risk that
COVID-19 would spread at psychiatric wards, necessitating realloca-
tion of resources to contain outbreaks, such as reducing the number
of patients or closing affected wards. Hence, PSS decided to adjust the
priority guidelines of psychiatric care as shown in Table 21.2.

As a general rule, patients in group 2 or 3 who were caregivers of
minors would be moved up one priority level.

Table 21.2 Priority guidelines revised for COVID-19

Priority at Psychiatry South Stockholm	Patients with
1. Indispensible need for care; acute and life-threatening conditions	Imminent risk of suicide Imminent risk of harm to others Very severe eating disorders (in cooperation with somatic care) Acute psychotic or manic conditions Catatonic conditions
2. Other serious conditions	Severe depression Severe eating disorders or self-destructive behavior Severe anxiety conditions Psychotic or bipolar conditions
3. Other patients not included in 1 or 2	

The main guiding principle was to prioritize according to need. From the perspective of the priority platform, however, at least two questions are potentially controversial. First, is it justified to prioritize patients based on their risk of harming others? In one interpretation of the Swedish priority platform, it is the patients' own need for care and not societal interests that should be considered. For patients with psychiatric disorders, however, risk of harm to others is an indication of the severity of the patient's psychiatric condition—and may be a reason for involuntary commitment according to the Swedish Mental Health Act (1991). Moreover, risk of harm to others is a valid consideration for prioritizing measures in other areas of health care, particularly in the context of infectious diseases. Arguably, an overarching reason for prioritizing treatment and prevention of COVID-19 is to prevent harm to individuals and society at large.

Second, is it right to prioritize caregivers of minors? This prioritization was based on a children's rights perspective. The rationale is not that caregivers are more deserving of care than others but that the interests of the minors they care for are given particular weight. If the consideration is valid in psychiatry, however, it seems equally valid in general health care. This is not directly recognized in the priority platform.

Based on the prioritization plan, a number of strategies were formed to prepare and handle the COVID pandemic at PSS:

- HCP strategy: staff members who self-identified as belonging to an at-risk group for severe COVID-19 were asked to report it to their supervisor and were offered alternative task assignments. No medical certificate was required.
- One 16-bed psychiatric ward including staff was reassigned to geriatric care in collaboration with a neighboring geriatric hospital.
- Cohort care plan: one specific psychiatric ward was designated to handle COVID-19–positive patients.
- Pharmacologic treatment recommendations were made for psychiatric patients comorbid with COVID-19.
- Implementation of telepsychiatry: the option of video-based consultations was introduced for both inpatients and outpatients and rapidly became widely used.
- Procedures were made for seclusion of COVID-19 patients at inpatient wards according to the Swedish Communicable Diseases Act (2004) in collaboration with infection control physicians at Region Stockholm.

A few preliminary conclusions may be drawn:

- The HCP strategy did not lead to a shortage of staff in critical clinical care. Only a few staff members reported being in an at-risk group, and the vast majority continued to work with patients while wearing protective equipment.
- The number of HCP staff members absent on sick leave was much higher than the previous year. The increased cost for temporary staff was specifically recorded and reimbursed by dedicated state funds.
- All through the pandemic, beds were available. In fact, the number of available beds increased during both the first and second waves of COVID-19 (March and October 2020), but less so during the third wave (March 2021).
- The cohort care plan in PSS did not have to be implemented. Figure 21.1 shows the total number of COVID-19–positive patients admitted to public psychiatric hospitals in the larger Stockholm area, including general psychiatry, forensic psychiatry, and child and adolescent psychiatry, with about 1,000 beds

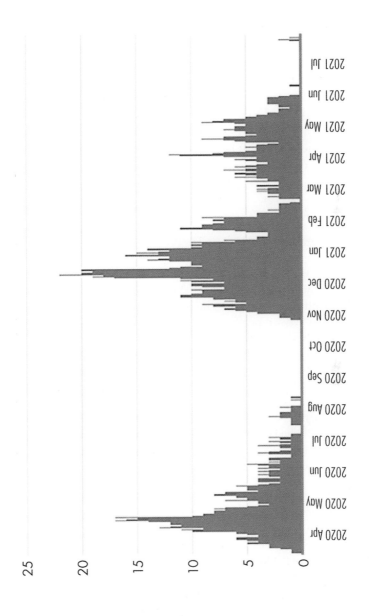

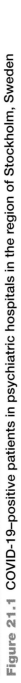

Figure 21.1 COVID-19-positive patients in psychiatric hospitals in the region of Stockholm, Sweden

in total. There was one peak during the first wave with about 15 patients and one during second wave with about 20 patients, the majority due to two outbreaks at forensic psychiatric units.

Ultimately, limited resources did not turn out to be a clinical problem for psychiatric care. A more urgent analysis is whether prioritized patient groups have refrained from seeking care. It is possible that patients did not seek care out of concerns about contracting COVID-19 or because they did not want to burden the health care system. Future prioritization plans need to prepare psychiatric services not only situations of health care rationing but also for the opposite scenario, when beds are available and there is a risk that prioritized patient groups refrain from seeking care.

References

Gustavsson E: Characterising Needs in Health Care Priority Setting. Linköping, Sweden, Linköping University, 2017

IVO: IVO Deepens the Examination of Care and Treatment in Special Housing For the Elderly [in Swedish]. IVO News, July 7, 2020. Available at: https://www.ivo.se/aktuellt/nyheter/2020/ivo-fordjupar-granskningen-av-vard-och-behandling-pa-sarskilda-boenden-for-aldre. Accessed October 30, 2024.

Nemani K, Li C, Olfson M, et al: Association of psychiatric disorders with mortality among patients with COVID-19. JAMA Psychiatry 78(4):380–386, 2021 33502436

Nguyen LH, Drew DA, Graham MS, et al: Risk of COVID-19 among front-line health-care workers and the general community: a prospective cohort study. Lancet Public Health 5(9):e475–e483, 2020 32745512

Persad G, Wertheimer A, Emanuel EJ: Principles for allocation of scarce medical interventions. Lancet 373(9661):423–431, 2009 19186274

Folkhälsomyndigheten [The Public Health Agency of Sweden]: National Plan for COVID-19 Vaccination. Interim Report by the Public Health Agency on Government Assignment S2020/04550/FS, February 4, 2021 [in Swedish]. Solna, Sweden, Folkhälsomyndigheten, 2021

RSMH: Prioritize People With Serious Mental Illness for Vaccination Against COVID-19 [in Swedish]. RSMH, March 3, 2021. Available at: https://rsmh.se/wp-content/uploads/2021/03/Skrivelse-om-prioritering-av-covid-19-vaccin-till-personer-med-allvarlig-psykisk-sjukdom.pdf. Accessed October 30, 2024.

Sjögren A, Milstaed S: Despite the Criticism, Tthe Public Health Agency Does Not Change Its Course Regarding Vaccination Strategy [in Swedish].

Aftonbladet, Sweden, January 2, 2021. Available at: https://www
.aftonbladet.se/nyheter/a/bnX7xB/trots-kritiken-fhm-andrar-sig-inte-om
-vaccinationsstrategin. Accessed October 30, 2024.

Socialdepartementet [The Ministry of Health and Social Affairs]: The
Difficult Choice of Healthcare [in Swedish]. Stockholm, Sweden,
Socialdepartementet, 1995

Socialstyrelsen: National principles for prioritization in intensive care
under extraordinary circumstances [in Swedish]. Stockholm, Sweden,
Socialstyrelsen, 2020a

Socialstyrelsen: National principles for proritization of routine care
during the COVID-19 pandemic [in Swedish]. Stockholm, Sweden,
Socialstyrelsen, 2020b

Socialstyrelsen [The National Board of Health and Welfare]: Final Report
on the Government Assignment Regarding the Risk of Severe
Disease Progression in COVID-19 [in Swedish]. Stockholm, Sweden,
Socialstyrelsen, 2021.

Swedish Communicable Diseases Act, Smittskyddslag, SFS 2004:168

Swedish Mental Health Act, Lag om psykiatrisk tvångsvård, SFS 1991:1128

Tännsjö T: Setting Health-Care Priorities: What Ethical Theories Tell Us. New
York, Oxford University Press, 2019

Walker T: Who do we treat first when resources are scarce? J Appl Philos
27(2):200–211, 2010

Index

AAPL *see* American Academy of
Psychiatry and the Law
AAPL Annual Meeting, 3
AAPL Ethics Guidelines, 2–3, 10–11,
18, 28, 54, 69, 83, 111, 120, 123, 129,
132, 135–136, 149, 295
honesty and objectivity, 157
AAPL Presidential Address, 12
in 1997, 11
in 2014, 12
in 2017, 11
ABA *see* American Bar Association
Abortion, 249
adolescent decision-making, 262
breast cancer, 256
capacity for informed consent, 263
conscientious objection to, 254
counseling requirement for, 251
decisional capacity, 249
differences in state laws, 250, 264
financial barriers to, 251
guardianship, 260
illness exacerbations, 251
impact on mental health, 252
increased risk of fertility, 256
judicial bypass by minors, 261–263
mental disorders and incapacity,
257
mental or physical health, 250
minors and parental consent, 260
right to privacy, 250
serious mental illness, 250
ultrasounds before, 256
Abortion informed-consent law, 255
autonomy and privacy, 257
provisions of, 256
state-produced materials, 255
Adshead, Gwen, 40, 42
Advance directives, 270
decision-making capacity, 271
durability and consistency, 274

evaluation after suicide attempt, 274
intent, 273
intent and causation, 273
Kerrie Wooltorton case, 271,
274–276
legal foundations of, 271
present vs. future self, 274
suicidal behavior, 272
suicide attempt, 271–272
treatment preferences, 270
Wooltorton case, 271
Advocacy in forensic psychiatry, 147
advocacy from within, 148
advocacy from without, 151
death penalty, 148
insanity cases, 151
selective participation, 147–148
Algorithms in the courtroom, 99
artificial neural networks, 99
electronic medical record (EMR),
99
human biases, 101
violence risk assessment, 100
violent behavior prediction, 99
AMA Ethics Opinion, 161
AMA Institute of Ethics, 60
American Academy of Forensic
Sciences (AAFS), 16, 18
American Academy of Psychiatry
and the Law, 37
American Academy of Psychiatry
and the Law (AAPL), 1, 10, 12, 18,
23, 37, 51, 53, 55, 59, 82, 111, 120,
161, 304
Committee on Ethics, 2
Peer Review of Psychiatric
Testimony committee, 75
American Bar Association (ABA),
121–122
American Board of Forensic
Psychiatry, 1

American Board of Medical
    Specialties (ABMS), 1
American College of Obstetricians
    and Gynecologists (ACOG), 254
American criminal justice system,
    290–291
    correctional populations and race,
        291
    incarceration and racial
        disparities, 292
    individuals of color, 290
    racial profiling, 291
    violence risk assessment, 290
American Educational Research
    Association, 107
American Legal Institute (ALI), 151
American Medical Association
    (AMA), 129, 155
American Psychiatric Association,
    18, 83
American Psychological Association,
    18, 119
American Psychological
    Association's Ethical Principles
    of Psychologists and Code of
    Conduct, 174
    confidentiality and legal
        constraints, 174
Americans with Disabilities Act, 186
AOT *see* Assisted outpatient
    treatment
APA Council on Psychiatry and Law,
    176
Appelbaum, Paul S., 9, 16, 27
    forensic roles, 9
    interests of justice, 37
    overidentification of psychiatrists, 9
    principle of respect, 10
    principlism approach, 16
    truth-telling, 10
Artificial intelligence (AI), 89, 98
Assembly Bill (AB) 2888, 208
Assisted outpatient treatment (AOT),
    183
    autonomy, 186
    autonomy and coercive
        infringement, 184
    benefits of, 185, 187, 189, 192–193
    commitment orders and racial
        bias, 192
    contentious aspects of, 195
    cost-effectiveness of, 190
    cost of, 189

enhancing individual's autonomy,
    191
ethical considerations, 184, 191
groups and competing interests,
    184
length of time for treatment, 186
mental health funding, 190
outpatient mental health
    treatment, 184
protection of civil rights, 195
racial bias and social control, 192
reports of coercion, 188
schizophrenia and psychotic
    disorders, 188
self-determination of treatment, 186
service costs for SMI, 190
socioeconomic bias and structural
    racism, 196
states with statutory authorization
    for, 189
systemic discrimination, 193
trade-offs, 188
violence and racial bias, 192
Autonomy, 16, 20, 27, 95, 207, 222, 233,
    253–254, 303
    defined, 275

Barefoot v. Estelle, 83, 159
Bazelon, David, 151
Behavioral Science of Firearms
    (Pirelli et al.), 212
Bellotti v. Baird, 260
Beneficence, 16, 20, 27, 171, 194, 219,
    222–225, 254, 303
    described, 275
Biomedical ethics principles, 20, 90,
    171, 218, 223, 225, 275, 303
    beneficence, 132
    justice, 275–276
    nonmaleficence, 132, 275
British Mental Capacity Act of 2005,
    275
Brooks, Peter, 34, 41
Buchanan, Alec, 59

Canadian Academy of Psychiatry
    and the Law, 304
Candilis and Martinez, 16
Candilis, Paul J., 39, 124
Canterbury v. Spence, 245
Carlsen v. Koivumaki, 173
Casuistry, 20
Charon, Rita, 35

Code of Federal Regulations, 202
    commitment to a mental
        institution, 202
    possessing firearms and mental
        illness, 202
Colbach, Edward, 147
Community settings, 225
    beneficence and nonmaleficence,
        226
    ethical challenges, 226
    ethical dilemmas and additional
        services, 228
    implicit rationing, 226
    limits on length of stay, 227
    resource limitations, 227
Competence-to-be-executed case, 161
Competency restoration, 222
Competency to stand trial (CST-CR),
    222
    assessment, 223
    correctional and community
        settings, 224
    CST evaluation, 222
    ethical challenges, 223
    treatment modalities, 223
Competency-to-stand-trial
    evaluation, 69
Confidentiality, 234
    autonomy and privacy, 235
    discretionary exceptions, 236
    duty to protect, 236
    duty to warn, 236
    governmental incursion, 240, 242
    HIPAA regulations, 235
    medical gag rule, 246
    overdose crisis, 239
    prescription monitoring, 239
    protect third parties, 237
    role of governmental regulation,
        239
    testimonial privilege, 238
COVID-19 pandemic, 225
    decision-making processes, 225
    state hospital settings, 225
Cultural Formulation Interview
    (CFI), 305, 307
    cultural competence, 307–308
    cultural humility, 308
    structural competence, 307–308
    structural humility, 307

Darby, William Connor, 22, 121
Daubert case, 82

Decision-making capacity (DMC), 271
    depression, 282
    state statutes, 277
Deep learning, 97
    artificial neural networks, 98
    error rates, 98
    explained, 98
Dialectical principlism, 15, 23
    application of, 27
    conflicting ethics considerations,
        23
    dialectics, 27
    ethics considerations, 24
    ethics duties and principles, 16
    examples of, 27
    principlism, 24
    proximal vs distal duties, 24
    special situations, 15
    violating fundamental ethics
        values, 18
Diamond, Bernard, 1, 22, 56, 74, 123
    diminished capacity, 56
Distal duties, 16–17
    conflicts, 28
    examples of, 26, 28
    significance of risks, 175
District of Columbia v. Heller, 201
*Dobbs v. Jackson Women's Mental
    Health Organization*, 250
DSM-5, 74
Durham v. United States, 151
Duty to protect, 169–170, 175, 178
    suicide attempt, 178
    suicide or violence, 179
Duty to warn, 165, 168–170, 175–176
    California Civil Code Section
        43.92, 176
    immunity from liability, 176
    liability to patient and potential
        victim, 177
    predicting violence, 168
    protective privilege vs. public
        peril, 168, 170

EAS *see* Euthanasia and assisted
    suicide
EPPCC *see* Ethical Principles of
    Psychologists and Code of
    Conduct
Estelle v. Smith, 83, 158
Ethical challenges of testimony, 81
    capital cases, 160
    confirmation bias, 85

Ethical challenges of testimony
    (*continued*)
  honesty and objectivity, 87
  jurisdiction-specific evidentiary
      rules, 82
  objectivity, 150
  reasonable medical certainty, 82
Ethical dilemmas, 52
  competency assessment, 52
  distorting of data, 84
  honesty and objectivity, 86
  legal-moral challenge, 53
*Ethical Principles of Psychologists and
    Code of Conduct (EPPCC)*, 107,
    114–115
  releasing test data, 115
  test scoring and interpretation, 108
  use of assessments in, 107
Ethical report writing, 67
  data collection, 70
  ethical evaluation, 68
  ethical questions and
      transparency, 70
  ethical values, 68
  ethics of forensic psychiatry, 67
  feedback from attorney, 74
  forensic psychiatric evaluation, 68
  honesty, 68
  honesty and objectivity, 72
  inconsistencies in, 71
  informed consent, 68
  objectivity, 68
  transparency and thoroughness, 74
Ethics in Forensic Psychiatry: A
    Cultural Response to Stone and
    Appelbaum (Griffith), 11
Ethics of caring, 19
  professionalism in, 61
Ethics theories and forensic work, 19
Euthanasia and assisted suicide
    (EAS), 276, 281
  American Psychiatric Association
      on, 278
  capacity assessment, 282
  decision-making capacity, 281–282
  ethical permissibility, 280
  false positives, 280
  physician-patient relationship, 282
  terminal physical conditions, 276

Feigning psychosis/malingering, 5
Firearms and Clinical Practice
    (Pirelli and DeMarco), 212

Floyd, George, 304
Foot, Philippa, 148
Ford v. Wainwright, 160
Forensic assessments, 4
  capacity or competency, 4
  criminal-responsibility, 5
  cultural context, 6
  empathy, 39
  exaggeration of findings, 8
  honest forensic testimony, 7
  Miranda rights, 5
  social motive, 6
Forensic consultant role, 128
  deposition and trial tasks, 128
  dubious or limited evidence, 131
  and ethical issues, 132
  ethical principles for, 129
Forensic evaluation process, 67
  areas of inequity, 76
  forensic psychiatric evaluations,
      68
  narrative approach, 76
  obtaining consent, 69
  structural inequities, 76
Forensic evaluator role, 122, 124
  challenges to the credibility, 126
  ethical issues, 125
  fiduciary responsibility, 123
  responsibilities of, 124
  retention of medical values, 124
  therapeutic bias, 123
Forensic mental health, 54, 119
  diagnosis, 203
  ethical considerations in, 120
  firearm possession, 203
Forensic practice, 17
  adversarial legal system, 56
  assessment of suicide or violence,
      99
  bias and unfairness, 58
  defined, 61
  empathy and compassion, 71
  ethical dilemmas, 52
  ethics dilemmas, 18
  formation of professional identity,
      62
  goals and purposes, 54
  Hippocratic ethics, 23
  implicit bias assessment tools, 70
  multiplicity of roles, 122
  objectivity and detachment, 56
  presence, 71
  principles of, 27

qualities/attributes in, 53
respect for persons, 56
robust professionalism, 61
role-based justifications, 57
social goods, 54
truth-telling, 56
understanding of the role, 121
Forensic professional ethics, 21
robust professionalism, 22
Forensic professionalism, 60
cultural formulation, 59
moral dilemmas and obligations,
61
robust professionalism, 60
Forensic psychiatric ethics, 11
culture-free, 11
narrative, 33
political dimension of, 34
Forensic psychiatric evaluation, 156
aggravating/mitigating factors,
159
capital cases and conviction, 157
death penalty, 157
death row inmates, 162
defendant's mental status, 158
ethical challenges, 156
incompetence after conviction,
160
insanity defense and death
sentence, 158
penalty phase, 159
pretrial phase, 157
Forensic psychiatry, 1, 17
application of psychiatric
knowledge, 134
apprenticeship model, 1
artificial intelligence algorithms,
97
aspirational professional qualities,
62
compassion, 39
cultural formulation, 38
deception of the evaluee, 10
defined, 120
determinism versus free will, 7
ethical boundary, 3, 7
evaluation and testimony, 53
evolution and modernization of,
40
fellowship training programs, 1
fiduciary duties, 234
forensic assessment, 82
goals and purposes of, 53

identification of forensic role,
120–121
identity and purpose, 51
legal value system, 2
legitimacy, 4, 7
moral questions, 5
narrative and ethics in, 37
opining on legal issues, 150
primary societal value, 17
principle of legal dominance, 55
prostitution of the profession, 8,
10
psychoanalysis, 144
psycholegal cases, 4
rehabilitation vs. punishment, 144
robust professionalism, 52
search for truth, 43
treatment vs. legal settings, 234
Forensic psychiatry ethics, 37, 120,
147
advocacy, 149
dual roles, 52
human dignity, 44
legal questions, 52
narrative understanding, 73
principles of, 75
Forensic psychology, 51
Forensic report, 40
disagreements, 83
forensic case conference, 75
forensic empathy, 72
formulation and conclusion of, 73
giving voice, 72
narrative section of, 72
parts of, 45
performative techniques, 46
quality of, 75
Forensic role, 2
after death penalty conviction, 160
confirmation bias, 11
ethical problems, 18
expert evaluator and clinician, 57
honest opinion, 2
honesty and objectivity, 11
mixed model, 21
skillful vs. unethical evaluation, 8
societal value, 27
Forensic roles and primary duty/
obligation, 138
Forensic scientific expert role, 125,
130
advocacy-based testimony, 126
case-blind didactic expert, 125

Forensic scientific expert role
   (*continued*)
   impartiality, 125
   issues, 128
   objectivity and credibility of
      testimony, 130
Frye case, 82

Gigante, Vincent, 84
Gilligan, Carol, 19
Gold, Robert, 166
Gould, Jonathan, 129
Governmental institutions, 221
   ethical challenges of working at,
      221
Governmental systems, 218
   budget limitations, 219
   competing priorities of actors, 220
   differences among actors, 218
   ethical/personal dilemmas
      stemming from, 219
   use of resources, 219
Griffith, Ezra, 6, 11, 16, 57, 124
   inequities in justice system, 59
   narrative approach, 16
Griffith, Véronique, 36
Grigson, James, 83
Guardianship, 258
   best interests standard, 259
   defined, 258
   incapacity to consent to abortion,
      259
   substituted judgment, 259
Gun Violence and Mental Illness
   (Gold and Simon), 212
Gun Violence Restraining Order
   (GVRO) law, 208–210
   firearm rights termination, 209
   states with, 209
Gutheil, Thomas, 52, 170
Guttmacher, Manfred, 150
   dual concerns, 151

Hargrave v. Vermont, 186
Hastings Center, 60
HCP *see* Prioritizing health care
   personnel
Health care practice, 60
   common goals for, 60
   social goods, 60
Health Insurance Portability and
   Accountability Act (HIPAA) of
   1996, 235

Heller decision, 202
   possession of firearms and mental
      illness, 202
HIPAA *see* Health Insurance
   Portability and Accountability
   Act (HIPAA) of 1996
Hired gun, 81
   problem, 82–84, 86
Hired-gun problem, 10, 56

Illinois Judicial Bypass Coordination
   Project, 262
Informed consent, 100, 234, 242, 253
   abortion, 254
   autonomy, 100
   basic components of, 253
   controversial limits to, 244
   decisional capacity, 257
   emergency situations, 244
   engagement in the consent
      process, 243
   exceptions to, 244
   integrity/autonomy, 243
   medical decision-making
      capacity, 253
   nocebo effect, 245
   patient/subject choice, 243
   patient values/preferences, 254
   requirements by states, 253
   substitute decisionmaking, 244
   therapeutic privilege, 245
   therapeutic waiver of consent, 244
   Tuskegee syphilis experiments,
      242
Insanity acquittees, 224
   conditional release, 224
   length of psychiatric
      hospitalization, 225
   modalities of treatment, 224
   safety of the community, 224
Insanity defense cases, 5
   not guilty by reason of insanity, 6
Involuntary psychiatric treatment,
   167, 228
   unintended financial burdens, 228
Iphigenia in Forest Hills (Malcolm),
   34

Jaffee v. Redmond, 172
*Journal of the American Academy of
   Psychiatry and the Law, The*, 57, 86
Jurek v. Texas, 159
Justice, 20, 171, 223, 303

Kleinman, Arthur, 36
Kohlberg, Lawrence, 19
 developmental principlist model,
  19
 moral development, 20

Lanterman-Petris-Short Act, 167, 169
*Lefebvre v. N. Broward Hospital
 District*, 259
Lockett v. Ohio 1978, 159

Machine learning, 97
Malcolm, Janet, 34
Maleficence, 221
Mandatory disclosures, 237
 mental disorders and
  discrimination, 237
 public health purpose, 237
Martinez, Rene J., 39
Mayberg, Helen, 91
Medical ethical principles, 184
Mehl-Madrona, Lewis, 33
Mental health, 204
 access to firearms and risk of
  suicide, 207
 assaultive patients and arresting,
  229
 capacity assessments, 272
 criminal justice system, 228
 ethical concerns about firearms,
  207
 ethical questions about
  involuntarily admission, 205
 firearm laws, 207
 firearm prohibition, 204
 firearm-related ethical issues, 206
 firearm rights, 205, 212
 involuntary commitment and
  firearm rights, 206
 involuntary detention, 204
 violation of autonomy and firearm
  rights, 207
Method for distinguishing roles and
 contracts, 127
Minnesota Multiphasic Personality
 Inventory (MMPI), 106
Mol, Annemarie, 35
Morality test, 5

Narrative approach to ethics, 34
Narrative medicine, 36
Narrative model, 22
 conflicting duty considerations, 22

cultural considerations, 22
 empathy and compassion, 44
 perspectival narrative, 42, 46
 psychoanalysis, 45
 racism and injustice, 44
Narrative psychiatry, 36
 cross-examination tests, 41
 immigrant-refugee credibility, 41
 irresponsible authorship, 43
 narrative glue, 42
National Association of State Mental
 Health Program Directors, 225
National Council on Measurement in
 Education, 107
National Instant Criminal
 Background System, 237
Neuroimaging in the courtroom, 89
 acquired antisocial behavior, 94
 causal inferences, 92
 constitutional rights, 95
 Daubert, 93
 DTI fiber-tracking maps, 96
 fMRI for lie detection, 96
 Frye v. U.S., 93
 group-to-individual (G2i)
  inference, 93
 interpretation of neuroimages, 96
 issues with, 93
 lesion network mapping, 94
 lie detection, 95
 major functions of, 91–92
 neuroimaging evidence, 90
 neuroimaging evidence and
  judicial decisions, 96
 neuroimaging techniques, 91
 reverse inference, 92
 single-subject abnormality, 93
Neuroscience in the courtroom, 89
 DNA evidence, 91
 ethical use of neuroscience, 91
 impaired behavioral capacities, 92
 judicial decisions, 91
 lack of replication, 93
 limitations of, 93
 neuroscience evidence, 90
 normative data set selection, 113
 trier of fact, 97
*Nguyen v. Massachusetts Institute of
 Technology*, 178
Nonmaleficence, 16, 20, 27, 171, 195,
 207, 219, 222–225, 254, 303
 described, 275
Norko, Michael, 11, 16, 43, 59

Norko, Michael (*continued*)
    compassion, 59
    compassion model, 16
Normative ethics, 19
    consequentialism, 19
    deontological ethics, 19
    virtue ethics, 19

OPTN *see* Organ Procurement and
        Transplantation Network
Organ Procurement and
        Transplantation Network
        (OPTN), 307
Oxford Community Treatment Order
        Evaluation Trial, 186

Panetti v. Quarterman, 160
PDMPs *see* Prescription Drug
        Monitoring Programs
Personality Assessment Inventory
        (PAI), 106
Physician-assisted death (PAD), 270,
        276
    legalization of, 277
    mental illness, 283
    nonterminal conditions, 282
    parity, 278
    permissibility of, 278
    resistance to treatment, 279
    terminal disease, 277
Pierce, Chester M., 304
Planned Parenthood v. Casey, 255
Poddar, Prosenjit, 166–169
Policy roles and ethical issues, 137
Pollack, Seymour, 2, 56, 74, 123
Porter v. McCollum, 159
Post-Conviction Risk Assessment
        (PCRA), 293
Prescription Drug Monitoring
        Programs (PDMPs), 240–241
    curb on overprescription, 241
    opioid prescriptions, 240
    triplicate prescription program, 240
Principles of Medical Ethics (AMA),
        132–133, 135
    legislative advocacy, 136
    policy role, 135
    promoting legislative changes,
        136
    serving society, 135
*Principles of Medical Ethics With
        Annotations Especially Applicable
        to Psychiatry (APA)*, 110, 175

confidentiality, 175
Principlism, 20
Principlism approach, 9
Prioritizing health care personnel
        (HCP), 315, 319
    argument of net gain, 317
    argument of usefulness, 317
    considerations of reciprocity, 319
    human dignity principle, 321
    moral problem with, 318
    principle of need, 318
    probability and negative-effect
        factors, 319
    vaccine distribution phases in
        COVID pandemic, 320–321
Priority guidelines revised for
        COVID-19, 323
    caregivers of minors, 323
    prioritization plans for psychiatric
        services, 326
    risk of harming others, 323
Priority-setting in COVID pandemic,
        313
    ethical challenges of, 314
    intensive care, 315
    in intensive care, 316
    prioritizing health care personnel,
        315
    psychiatric care, 322
    psychiatric disorders, 322
Professional organizations, 220
    advocacy, 221
    ethical difficulties, 221
    policy statements and ethical
        issues, 221
Proximal duties, 16–17
    defined, 16, 26
Psychiatric disorder, 4
    criminal responsibility, 7
Psychiatric experts, 143
    advocacy and partiality, 146
    bias, 145
    cross-examination, 146
    impartiality, 144, 147
    impartiality and objectivity, 149
    insanity defense, 151
    professional bias, 147
    rules of evidence, 145
    subjectivity, 145
Psychiatric practice, 155
    capital punishment, 155
    death penalty, 156
    paranoid schizophrenia, 166

Psychiatric treatment role, 132
  confidentiality, 133
  fiduciary responsibility, 134
  honesty and respect, 133
  informed consent, 133
  testimonies, 134
Psychological testing, 105
  cultural appropriateness, 111
  integrity and security of, 114
  interpretation of, 113
  neuropsychology testing, 106
  objective psychodiagnostic tests,
    106
  obtaining informed consent, 112
  optimal test conditions, 112
  psychodiagnostic testing, 106
  referral, 110
  reliability and validity of, 114
  tests for forensic issues, 106
  validity scales, 114

Rappeport, Jonas, 2, 73
Rawls, John, 17
  reflective equilibrium, 20, 23
  reflective equilibrium method, 17
Reasonable degree of medical
    certainty (RMC), 73
Relief from disabilities (RFD), 204,
    211
  ethical principles in, 211
  RFD evaluation, 212
  RFD petition, 210
  RFD procedures, 210
  RFD process, 210
  risk assessment, 211
Reporting laws, 234
Reporting past crimes, 239
RFD *see* Relief from disabilities
RMC *see* Reasonable degree of
    medical certainty
Roe v. Wade, 250, 252, 263
Rorschach Inkblot, 106
Rosen case, 177
  duty of care, 177
  unintended consequence of, 179

Sadoff, Robert, 86
*Salgo v. Leland Stanford Junior
    University Board of Trustees*, 243
SAVRY *see* Structured Assessment of
    Violence Risk in Youth
Second Amendment to the US
    Constitution, 201

right to possess firearms, 201
Secure Ammunition and Firearms
    Enforcement Act (SAFE Act), 209
Serious mental illness (SMI), 183
Singleton v. Norris, 161
SMI *see* Serious mental illness
Specialty Guidelines for Forensic
    Psychologists (APA), 54, 120, 295
Specialty Guidelines for Forensic
    Psychology (SGFP), 108, 114
  assessment, 108
    forensic contexts, 108
    procedures, 108
    results, 109
    forensic contexts, 108
    procedures, 108
    results, 109
  compliance with court orders, 114
*Standards for Educational and
    Psychological Testing*, 107
State-of-mind evaluation, 69
Stone, Alan, 3–4, 7, 9, 37
  Black army sergeant case, 4
  Dr. Leo case, 58
  obust professionalism, 59
Structural competency, 295
Structural racism, 303
  antipsychotic medication
    prescriptions, 306
  bias, 305
    explicit and implicit, 305
    in psychiatric care, 306
  defined, 304
  discrimination, 304
  impact of race-based
    discriminatory policies, 305
  intersectionality, 304
  lithium therapy, 307
  microaggression, 304
  microinequity define, 304
  in patient care, 306
  prejudice defined, 304
  race-based glomerular filtration
    rates, 307
  race defined, 304
  racism defined, 304
  social determinants of health, 305
Structured Assessment of Violence
    Risk in Youth (SAVRY), 298
Structured professional judgments
    (SPJs), 287, 296–297
Substance Abuse and Mental Health
    Services Administration, 289

Swedish ethics platform for priority-
    setting, 314
  cost-effectiveness, 314
  ethical principles of, 314
  human dignity, 314
  needs-solidarity, 314

Tarasoff duty, 27, 52, 176, 179–180
  duties to avoid liability, 174
  duties to potential victims, 172
  duties to society, 173
  duties to the patient, 171
  ethical principles, 171
  increase in violence, 172
  legal consequences, 180
  patient confidentiality and public
      safety, 180
  public safety vs. individual
      privacy, 174
  third-party safety, 171
  unintended consequences of, 172
Tarasoff I, 168
  amicus brief, 168
  confidentiality, 168
Tarasoff II, 169
  confidentiality vs. privilege, 170
  effectiveness of psychiatry, 170
Tarasoff v. Regents of the University of
    California, 165, 179
Thematic Apperception Test (TAT),
    106
A Theory of Ethics for Forensic
    Psychiatry (Weinstock), 9
TRD see Treatment-resistant
    depression
Treatment in forensic settings and
    ethical issues, 135
Treatment refusals, 275
  life-sustaining treatment, 276
  severe mental illness, 276
  suicide attempts, 275
Treatment-resistant depression
    (TRD), 279
  subjectivity, 280

treatment resistance, 280
Turner v. Rivera, 176

U.S. Public Health Service and the
    Centers for Disease Control, 242
U.S. v. Gigante, 84–85

Vacco v. Quill, 273
Violence Risk Appraisal Guide
    (VRAG), 99
Violence risk assessment, 287
  actuarial risk tools, 287, 293
  biasing factors, 289
  Black vs. White individuals, 291
  Black youths, 289
  commonly used risk instruments,
      297
  criminal recidivism, 293–294
  culturally informed practices, 298
  dynamic risk factors, 288
  implicit bias, 288
  juvenile history, 297
  juvenile history bias mitigation,
      297
  limitations of instruments, 295
  mental health treatment and
      culture, 289
  mitigating bias, 294
  operationalization of risk
      categories, 296
  reliability and validity of
      instruments, 296
  risk factors, 289
  systemic bias, 288, 296–297
  use of criminal history in, 291, 293

Washington v. Harper, 161
Weinstein, Henry, 3
Weinstock, Robert, 3, 9, 21, 121, 147
  response to ethical boundary
      questions, 9
Whalen v. Roe, 241
Wiggins v. Smith, 159